Critical Appraisal of Epidemiological Studies and Clinical Trials

FOURTH EDITION

Mark Elwood

Professor of Cancer Epidemiology
University of Auckland, New Zealand

OXFORD
UNIVERSITY PRESS

OXFORD
UNIVERSITY PRESS

Great Clarendon Street, Oxford, OX2 6DP,
United Kingdom

Oxford University Press is a department of the University of Oxford.
It furthers the University's objective of excellence in research, scholarship,
and education by publishing worldwide. Oxford is a registered trade mark of
Oxford University Press in the UK and in certain other countries

Third Edition published in 2007
Fourth Edition published in 2017

Impression: 1

Published in the United States of America by Oxford University Press
198 Madison Avenue, New York, NY 10016, United States of America

British Library Cataloguing in Publication Data
Data available

Library of Congress Control Number: 2016943648

ISBN 978–0–19–968289–8

Printed and bound by
CPI Group (UK) Ltd, Croydon, CR0 4YY

To Candace,
Jeremy and Briana,
Jasper, Chiara, Holly, and Ariana

Preface and acknowledgements

This book is a revised and expanded successor to *Causal Relationships in Medicine: A Practical System for Critical Appraisal*, published by Oxford University Press in 1988, and *Critical Appraisal of Epidemiological Studies and Clinical Trials*, Second Edition, 1998, and Third edition, 2007. In 1988, the book broke new ground in bridging the gap between epidemiological and clinical reasoning by applying a consistent system of critical appraisal to questions of aetiology, clinical therapy, and health care management. Now, systematic methods of critical appraisal are accepted as central to rational health care, whether applied to individuals or communities. Critical appraisal is the central core of evidence-based health care.

The book is designed to encourage readers to apply their existing skills and knowledge within a framework of critical appraisal that can be applied to any type of study assessing the relationship between what is experienced and what eventuates. The essential issue in questions of the aetiology of disease, the effectiveness of clinical management, and the efficacy of health services is often whether a cause and effect relationship holds between the intervention or exposure and the relevant outcome. The method presented is applicable to a wide range of health care issues, to both medical and non-medical disciplines, and to many areas outside health care.

The new edition is revised throughout. The core text is the first ten chapters. These are followed by six examples of the application of critical appraisal to a particular study. Appendix 2 summarizes statistical methods and useful statistical tables. The approach to statistics is to treat the assessment of chance variation as one aspect of critical appraisal, and to review statistical methods specifically in Chapter 8. The rest of the text can be read with only simple arithmetic; the essential logic of the critical appraisal approach does not require any mathematical expertise.

The extensive list of acknowledgments to colleagues, students, and other friends given in the three earlier editions applies also to this volume. Again I thank my family for their support and patience.

I am grateful to the publishers of *The Lancet*, *The New England Journal of Medicine*, and the *Journal of the National Cancer Institute*, and to the first authors, for permission to reproduce parts of the papers shown in Chapters 12–17.

Contents

Chapter 1

Introduction

There is occasions and causes, why and wherefore in all things.

—William Shakespeare: *Henry V*, v; 1599

The structure of this book

This book presents a system of critical appraisal to help the reader evaluate studies in the health and medical fields, and also to carry out their own studies more effectively. The method emphasizes the central importance of cause and effect relationships. Over several years, many doctors, nurses, health educators, health managers, and students, as well as epidemiologists and researchers, have found it interesting and useful. The great strength of the method is that it is applicable to a wide range of issues, both to intervention trials and observational studies.

The scheme is shown in Figure 1.1. We start with a discussion of the concept of causation (Chapter 2), and then discuss the types of study design which can be used to demonstrate causation (Chapter 3) and the ways in which their key results can be expressed precisely and simply (Chapter 4). We then consider how the subjects in a study should be chosen (Chapter 5). Chapters 2–5 cover the essentials of study design, and we give examples of each of the major study designs to illustrate the concepts and some practical aspects.

We then move to the central issue of the interpretation of the results of any one study. We consider in turn each of the three non-causal explanations that have to be considered before a judgement of a causal explanation can be made. These are observation bias (Chapter 6), confounding (Chapter 7), and chance variation (Chapter 8).

In Chapter 9, we move from one study to many, reviewing the methods of systematic review and meta-analysis, the process of combining data from many studies.

We then consider features which positively support causation and how the results from one study or set of studies can be generalized more widely (Chapter 10). Putting these steps together leads to an overall method of critical appraisal, based on the evaluation of causal relationships, which can be applied to important issues within the reader's own field of interest. This section concludes by reviewing the applications of critical appraisal to evidence-based medicine, knowledge-based health care, and health practice and policy.

Chapters 12–17 give six examples of the application of the scheme to studies of different designs and topics: a randomized trial of medical treatment, a randomized trial of

ASSESSMENT OF CAUSATION

Figure 1.1 The assessment of causation. The overall strategy presented in the book for assessing the evidence for and against causality in a particular issue. Numbers indicate the relevant chapter.

a preventive measure, a prospective and a retrospective cohort study, a small matched case–control study, and a large case–control study. Sections of the original papers are reproduced in these chapters, although the reader will obtain the best value from them by first reading the whole of the original paper before working through the appraisal given in each chapter.

Most of this book can be understood without complex mathematics. Statistical issues are dealt with in Chapter 8 and in part of Chapter 9. The statistical methods of most value are summarized for reference in Appendix 2. Statistical questions form only one aspect of the evaluation of evidence. Readers who wish to ignore the mathematical parts of this book should feel free to do so.

Chapter 2

The importance of causal relationships in medicine and health care

Intellectual progress is by no one trait so adequately characterized as by the development of the idea of causation.

—Herbert Spencer: *The Data of Ethics*, IV; 1879

Introduction

The study of causal relationships is essential to medicine and health care (Figure 2.1). In treating a patient, the decision to offer a treatment is based on the assumption that that treatment will *cause* an improvement in the patient's condition. The study of the causes and prevention of a disease involves determining which factors *cause* the disease to occur. In health service management, the decision to provide a certain type of service or facility assumes that it will *cause* an improvement in the health of the individuals or the community that it serves. On my desk today there are new studies on whether the prenatal environment leads to diabetes; assessments of new treatments for heart disease, malaria, and bladder cancer; and a discussion on whether clinical leadership improves the performance of health services. These articles essentially ask questions of causality. Does a specific treatment cause an improvement in the patient's condition? Do particular factors cause diseases to occur? Do different systems of health management cause improvements for the users of the service? Most critical issues in health care and most controversial issues depend on the assessment of whether a cause and effect relationship exists.

In this book, we will explore the methods available to us to test whether relationships are in fact causal, and therefore to decide whether the assumptions behind decisions relating to therapy, aetiology, and health service management are true or false.

This *critical appraisal* process is central to the related topics of *meta-analysis* and *evidence-based medicine*. The evaluation of what is done and what is not done in health care, in terms of its basis in scientific evidence, depends on correct judgements being made about causal relationships.

We will concentrate on the critical appraisal of epidemiological studies and clinical trials. We will present a practical system for critical appraisal, which can be applied to any of the main types of study that assess relationships between an *intervention* or

RELEVANCE OF CAUSATION

Figure 2.1 The relevance of causal relationships in health care. Decisions on therapy, aetiology, or health service provision all make assumptions of cause and effect relationships.

exposure and an *outcome*. The central issue is whether any association seen between the intervention or exposure and the outcome indicates a cause and effect relationship; if so, appropriate action can follow. If a cause and effect relationship does not exist, the association must be due to other mechanisms; this conclusion has different practical consequences.

Definition of causation, and types of causation

To discuss causal relationships, we must have a definition of causation, and this definition will determine how causation can be demonstrated or disproved. The concept of causation often brings to mind only the extreme and limiting situation, which is the situation where a certain event *always and invariably* follows another event. This is a familiar notion because it is regularly observed in the physical sciences. For example, Boyle's law states that at a given temperature, the volume of a fixed mass of a gas is inversely proportional to its pressure. Thus a change in pressure results invariably and automatically in a corresponding change in volume (Figure 2.2). The effect is instantaneous, can be replicated easily, and can be expressed as a simple mathematical relationship. Therefore, there is little difficulty in accepting the notion that a change in pressure *causes* a change in volume. Similarly, there is little difficulty in the concept that applying heat to a metal bar *causes* it to expand; again there is an invariable and almost immediate relationship between the 'outcome', that is, the change of length of the bar, and the 'exposure', that is, the heat applied to the bar.

SIMPLE CAUSATION

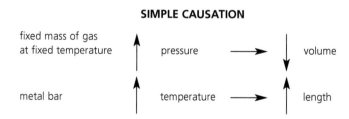

Figure 2.2 Simple causal relationships. Causal relationships in the physical sciences are often simple, as in Boyle's law relating pressure and volume of a gas, or the effect of heat on a metal bar. The causal agent is sufficient, the time relationship is short, and replication is easy.

This type of causation has a number of special properties. The chief among them is that the causal agent is *sufficient*; in other words, the operation of the one defined causal agent invariably produces the outcome. Secondly, the time relationship between the action of the causal agent and the effect produced is very short. Thirdly, because the situation can be modelled in an experiment, it can be replicated with ease under controlled conditions.

Situations that are relevant to human health and disease are rarely as simple. In human health and disease not all causal agents are sufficient. For example, the disease tuberculosis is caused by infection of the human body by the tubercle bacillus (Figure 2.3). However, infection by the tubercle bacillus does not invariably lead to clinical tuberculosis. Only a small proportion of those who are infected by the bacillus develop clinical disease, and a number of other factors influence whether the disease develops, such as poor nutrition (Figure 2.4). Thus a combination of tubercle bacillus infection and poor nutrition, with perhaps other factors, is required for clinical disease. We must consider both the tubercle bacillus and poor nutrition as causal factors; indeed, improved nutrition was the main cause of the reduction in tuberculosis in the first half of the twentieth century.

The tubercle bacillus in this situation is a 'necessary' cause of the disease. We can now define two categories of causal factors. A *sufficient* causal factor, acting on its own, will always produce the outcome. A *necessary* causal factor is one without which the outcome cannot occur; it has acted in all instances of the outcome (Box 2.1). In the Boyle's law situation, a change in pressure was both necessary and sufficient for

CAUSATION IN HEALTH (1)

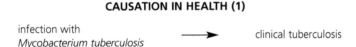

infection with
Mycobacterium tuberculosis
⟶
clinical tuberculosis

Figure 2.3 Simple causal relationship? An apparently simple causal relationship in medicine. But while the causal agent is necessary, it is not sufficient and the time relationship is uncertain.

CAUSATION IN HEALTH (2)

infection with *Mycobacterium tuberculosis*

poor nutrition

age

genetic factors?

environmental conditions

clinical tuberculosis

Figure 2.4 Simple causal relationship? A somewhat more complete diagram of the causes of clinical tuberculosis.

Box 2.1 The different types of causal relationships. The last category is by far the most important

Types of causal Relationships

Necessary: the outcome occurs only if the causal factor has operated.

Sufficient: the operation of the causal factor always results in the outcome.

Both: the causal factor and the outcome have a fixed relationship; neither occurs without the other.

Neither: the operation of the causal factor increases the frequency of the outcome, but the outcome does not always result, and the outcome can occur without the operation of the causal factor.

---

a change in volume, given that the other circumstances were fixed. In the metal bar example, heat was a sufficient but not a necessary cause; there are other ways of lengthening a metal bar.

Most situations in health and disease do not fulfil the criteria for either necessary or sufficient causation. If an otherwise healthy man is admitted to hospital with multiple fractures, having been hit by a bus just outside the hospital, we would conclude that there was a causal relationship between being hit by the bus and having multiple fractures. But the relationship implies neither that the cause is sufficient nor that it is necessary. Not all people hit by buses have multiple fractures. Not all patients with multiple fractures have been hit by buses.

A frequent error of logic is to define causation in a way that describes only the limiting case of the necessary and sufficient cause. Thus the fact that Uncle Joe is alive and well at age 95, having smoked 20 cigarettes a day since age 10, does not show that smoking is not harmful; it shows only that smoking is not a sufficient cause of death or disability before age 95. This one observation can disprove a hypothesis of sufficient causation. But to assume, on this evidence, that no type of causation exists between smoking and disease is like concluding that the existence of elderly veterans of a war means that war does not kill people.

We must use a concept of causation that is relevant to health issues, and define a causal association in a way that is applicable to real situations. The definition of cause we will use is: *a factor is a cause of an event if its operation increases the frequency of the event* (Box 2.2).

Box 2.2 The general definition of cause. Necessary and sufficient causation are merely extremes within this definition

Definition of cause

Cause: a factor is a cause of an event if its operation increases the frequency of the event.

The opposite of a causal factor is, of course, a preventive factor, whose operation decreases the frequency of the outcome event. The concept of causality, and the evidence required to assess it, applies equally to preventive issues.

Returning to the man with multiple fractures, what led us to the conclusion that these were caused by having been hit by a bus? The main evidence is the immediate time relationship. Consider another situation. A woman has persistent headaches and gives a history of a head injury some months previously. Can we assume a causal relationship in this case? We cannot easily make such a judgement, because the time relation is not so clear and so many other events may have occurred. Suppose, however, we study a number of patients who have persistent headaches, and we find that most of them give a history of a head injury. We should then be justified in suspecting that the apparent connection between the two events indicates a cause and effect relationship. However, we need to be cautious about our method of recording a history of previous injury. Some people who have had an injury may not be able to remember it, and similarly, many of the injuries reported might be expected as part of normal life. To go much further we need to ask whether the *frequency* with which such events have been experienced by subjects with persistent headaches is different from 'what we would expect'. To know 'what we would expect', we need to determine, by comparable methods, the frequency of such injuries in similar people who do not have persistent headaches.

So, where the time relation is not clear, and the concepts of necessary and sufficient cause do not hold, we need a *quantitative* assessment of the relationship, based on observations not on one individual but on a number of individuals. Hence the definition of causation is quantitative.

A direct test of causation: the randomized trial

A direct test of the quantitative definition of causation is given if we have two groups of individuals, who are very similar in all relevant characteristics, and apply to one group the putative causative factor. 'Relevant' characteristics are those factors, other than the one under study, which affect the frequency of the outcome event. If a causal relationship exists, the frequency of the defined outcome will be higher in the group exposed to the causal factor. A study design that uses this approach is the *randomized trial*, that is, the assignment of the treatment for each subject is made by a random or chance procedure (Figure 2.5).

DIRECT TEST OF CAUSATION

Figure 2.5 One way to test causation. When applied to therapy for patients, this is the randomized clinical trial. It is also the basic controlled experiment of biology and other sciences.

Randomized trials were used first in agricultural science, where, for example, fertilizers were applied to plots of soil and identical untreated plots were used for comparison; subsequently, crop yields were measured. The causal relationship between fertilizer application and crop yield was seen in the difference in crop yield between treated and untreated plots. The application of this technique to medicine dates from the late 1940s; a trial of therapy for tuberculosis (Figure 2.6) is often regarded as the first such study [1], although some other early clinical trials will be mentioned in Chapter 3. The method has been used most extensively in trials of methods of treatment, where the methods compared are generally similar, for example, the choice between giving one drug and giving a different drug. The ways in which randomization contributes to the study design will be discussed in later chapters; at present it is useful to note the two main features. Because the groups receiving each of the treatments being compared are selected by a chance assignment, they are likely to be similar to each other in regard to any factors (other than the treatment) which influence the outcome; therefore, differences in the outcome can be attributed to the treatment. Because the different groups are being treated and assessed at the same time, it is possible to design the study so that neither the subjects nor the investigators are aware of which treatment has been given, and this *double-blind* method will allow the observations of outcome to be made in the same way for all subjects. Since that first trial, many thousands of randomized trials have been carried out.

As an aside, the tuberculosis trial arose because there was only a small amount of streptomycin in the United Kingdom immediately after the Second World War, and most of it was used for patients with advanced tuberculosis, for which the benefits were clear even without a trial, as in the absence of treatment nearly all patients would

AN EARLY RANDOMIZED TRIAL

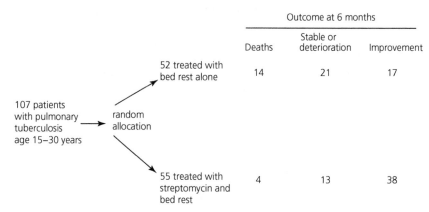

Figure 2.6 A trial of chemotherapy for advanced pulmonary tuberculosis, which was organized by the British Medical Research Council and which began in 1946. Often regarded as the first randomized clinical trial.

Source: data from Medical Research Council, 'Streptomycin treatment of pulmonary tuberculosis,' *British Medical Journal*, Volume 2, Issue 4582, pp. 769–782, © 1948. [1].

die [2]. The distinguishing mark of this trial was its use of true randomization, using random sampling numbers and sealed envelopes. The trial involved six centres, and subsequently a combined analysis of this and later trials was published, which is one of the first meta-analyses (meta-analysis will be covered in Chapter 9). There was no informed consent procedure as it was felt that if more therapy were available it would be used as the treatment of choice without specific consent, and that the consent situation for trials should not differ from routine practice.

There is no argument with the statement that the 'double-blind, randomized, prospective trial' is the ideal way to test a causal relationship applying to human subjects. However, the procedure is not simple to carry out, not so much for scientific reasons as for practical and ethical ones. For example, to compare two types of treatment whose aim is to reduce the mortality from a chronic disease such as cancer, a large number of patients who all have a similar type of disease will have to be randomized, receive treatment, and be followed up for many years. Such a trial is obviously an expensive undertaking and will require many logistical problems to be overcome. Its results apply to the therapies used during the trial, which may be made obsolete by new therapies by the time the results of the trial are available. The absolute limitation of the prospective, randomized trial is that it can be used only to assess interventions that are likely to be beneficial. It is clearly unethical to randomize individuals to receive a potentially harmful exposure, such as being exposed to smoking, industrial pollutants, or other toxins. Even when the comparisons are to be made between exposures that we would hope are beneficial, for example, different treatments, there may well be sufficient disparity of professional opinion that many individual physicians may not judge it ethical to enter patients under their care into randomized trials.

One response to this situation is to define causation as that which can be demonstrated in a randomized trial, and to discount all other situations. This is an unrealistic stance. On this definition, we could not assume a causal relationship between the multiple fractures and the bus accident. This viewpoint that a particular scientific method determines the definition of causation is the root of the commonly made assertion that epidemiological or observational studies can show 'only associations'. This is not true. In the mid 1970s, several case–control studies (an epidemiological study design which will be explained in Chapter 3) suggested that women using hormonal therapy for menopausal symptoms had a substantially increased risk of cancer of the uterus. As hormonal therapy had been used for many years, the issue was very controversial and many experts strongly criticized these studies. Some of the criticism was that these were not double-blind, randomized, prospective trials. In a letter in response to a *Lancet* editorial which took this approach, it was pointed out that to ignore evidence other than that derived from randomized trials 'is to dismiss most of our working understanding of biology, including, for example, our presumptions about the cause of that other common intrauterine tumour, pregnancy' [3].

The argument presented in this book is that the decision as to whether a certain relationship is causal must in all cases be a balanced professional judgement. We will argue that even prospective, randomized trials do not 'prove' causation, because even these trials do not give certainty; there are many practical and methodological limitations of their results. It will be argued that causation can be adequately demonstrated by other scientific methods, and that the acceptance of causation on the basis of results of such methods is essential to health care practice and planning. Only a small fraction of therapeutic decisions in health care can be supported by the results of randomized trials. Very few managerial or policy decisions can be so supported. Few conclusions as to the causes and natural history of disease can be supported by such evidence. For most of our knowledge of human health in terms of therapy, aetiology, and health care planning, we must use observational studies because of the ethical and logistical impossibility of mounting randomized trials in more than a tiny proportion of circumstances. Therefore we must be skilful in assessing such evidence and judging whether it supports a causal relationship.

Methods of counting events: prevalence and incidence

We have seen that causation needs to be defined in terms of probabilities, and so we need to use quantitative methods. This section reviews the terminology used in counting events in epidemiology, which may well be familiar ground to many readers.

The simplest measure of frequency is *prevalence*: the frequency of a characteristic, or the proportion of a group which has the characteristic, at one point in time. It is a simple proportion, has no units, and is measured at one point in time. In Table 2.1, there is a population of 100 000 in a community and a survey shows that at one point in time there are 800 cases of a disease present: the prevalence rate (or ratio) is 800 per

Table 2.1 The relationship between incidence, prevalence, and duration of disease, assuming a steady state and a substantial population size.

	Time point	Time period
	31 Dec 2001	1 Jan 2001–31 Dec 2002 (2 years)
Population (average or at one time point)	100 000	100 000
Number of cases at one time point	800 = prevalence Prevalence rate = 800 per 100 000	
Number of new cases diagnosed over a time period		400 = incidence Incidence rate = 200/100 000 per year
Number of deaths over a time period		40 = mortality Mortality rate = 20/100 000 per year
Average duration of disease		$P = I \times D$ so $D = P/I = 800/200$ = 4 years

100 000. The following are real examples of prevalence rates. In a survey of 1547 people aged over 65 years in London, 563 (36 per cent) had cataract in one or both eyes; the prevalence rose from 16 per cent in men aged 65–69 to 76 per cent in women aged 85–100 [4]. This is a prevalence measure as it applies to the frequency of a condition at one point in time.

Similarly, we could say that 23 per cent of students in a university are smokers, 25 per cent are obese, and 8 per cent have red hair. In a series of autopsies, pathologists might find that the prevalence of arteriosclerosis was 60 per cent (this in particular seems to be very frequently mislabelled as incidence in pathology texts and conversation). A slightly more difficult one is that the frequency of Down syndrome in live births is about 1.5 per 1000; this is a prevalence rate, as it is the proportion of term births which show the syndrome, and may be referred to specifically as a 'prevalence rate at birth'.

An *incidence rate* is the frequency of incidents, events such as deaths or new diagnoses of disease, over a defined time period; it has units of time^{-1}. For example, an annual mortality rate is the number of deaths occurring in 1 year divided by the population at risk. The annual incidence of a disease is the number of new cases occurring in a year, while the prevalence at a particular date is the number of cases existing at that date. Incidence rates are numbers of cases divided by the population size. In Table 2.1, 400 new cases of the disease are diagnosed over 2 years, and so the incidence rate is 200 per 100 000 per year. In Australia in 2012, there were 120 710 people diagnosed with cancer, in a mid-year population of 22 728 254, giving an average incidence rate for the year of 531.1 per 100 000 per year. In a study of workers at an atomic weapons establishment, 22 552 workers were identified and the average follow-up was 18.6 years, so that the total person-years of follow-up was 22 552 × 18.6 = 419 467 person-years. There were 3115 deaths during this period, giving an average death rate over the whole time period of 7.43 deaths per 1000 person-years [5]. Therefore measurement of the incidence rate requires counting events over a period of time. The term is frequently misused in place of prevalence.

In all these examples of incidence rate, the number of events (incidents) is precisely recorded, but the denominator is an approximation, representing the average or typical number of individuals at risk, or number of person-time units at risk in a whole study. This is routinely done in analysis of vital statistics and other large bodies of data. Obviously, this type of approximation is not good enough in small sets of data. More precise analysis involves life-table methods, in which the number of individuals actually at risk at any point in time is calculated precisely, and incidence rate is based on these calculations. These methods are described in Chapter 8.

The *population at risk* is the appropriate denominator for many rates, although in practice the total population is often used. The population at risk may be defined quite precisely in detailed studies. For example, although men can get breast cancer, in general, breast cancer rates are related to the female population, and in more detailed studies the population at risk of newly incident breast cancer may be defined more accurately by excluding women who have already developed the disease. In studying an infectious disease, the population at risk may exclude immunized subjects; in a food poisoning outbreak, the population at risk from each type of food can be defined as those who consumed that food.

Cumulative incidence is the proportion of a group of subjects who experience an event from the start to the end of a specified time period, that is, the cumulative frequency of the event. Being a measure based on incidents, it requires counting events over a period of time, but as it relates to one point in time, it is a simple proportion with no units. In a study of retinopathy (damage to the retina of the eye) in subjects with diabetes, the cumulative incidence by 1 year in 3743 subjects with no retinopathy at the baseline survey and an average age of 63 was 5.3 per cent, rising to 38.1 per cent by 5 years [6]. The outcome from major chronic diseases in patients is often expressed as a fatality rate up to a certain point in time; for example, the cumulative incidence of death for patients diagnosed with breast cancer in Norway between 1968 and 1975 reached 40 per cent at the end of 5 years after diagnosis, and, correspondingly, the survival at that point (the 5-year survival rate) was 60 per cent. In a major study of treatment of myocardial infarction, the outcome measured was cumulative mortality over 35 days since the infarction, which was about 7 per cent; that is, by the end of 35 days, 7 per cent of the original group had died and 93 per cent were still alive [7].

If an infectious disease, or a single-source epidemic such as food poisoning, passes through a community, at the end of the epidemic we can calculate the proportion of all people who were infected as a cumulative incidence rate over the whole time period; we might find that 20 per cent of the population was affected. This is the cumulative incidence, and is also referred to as the *attack rate*. This rate is often calculated in terms of the population at risk; for example, the attack rate of measles may be calculated specifically for those who are susceptible, excluding others who are not because of immunization.

Relationship between prevalence and incidence

Where a disease is in a stable situation in a large population (a situation of 'dynamic equilibrium'), the number of people who have a disease at one point in time (the prevalence) will depend on the incidence rate (the rate at which people develop the disease) multiplied by the average duration of the disease, ending in recovery or death. In fact, prevalence rate (P) equals average incidence rate (I) multiplied by average duration (D), or $P = I \times D$. Thus, if there are 200 new cases of disease each year in a community, as shown in Table 2.1, and the disease lasts 4 years on average, the prevalence at one point in time will be 800 cases. The steady-state assumption also means that, to keep the prevalence constant, 200 cases each year must finish; as 40 deaths each year are shown in Table 2.1, this implies that 40 of the 200 cases (20 per cent) are fatal, and the other people affected are either cured or die from other causes.

Self-test questions

Answers in Appendix 1, p.395.

Q2.1 Give a definition of a cause or causal factor.

Q2.2 What type of causation is shown in each of the following?

(a) A person falls 50 feet off a roof onto concrete and sustains a fractured leg.

(b) Exposure to the poliomyelitis virus and clinical polio.

(c) A man smokes heavily from age 14 and develops lung cancer at age 52.

(d) The association of extra chromosome 21 material with Down syndrome.

(e) A change in health service purchasing policy and a reduction in health care costs.

Q2.3 What rate and what units are given by:

(a) Out of 40 children in a class, 8 wear glasses.

(b) In a community of 50 000 people, there have been 100 road accidents in the last 2 years.

(c) Of 100 patients who have a certain surgical operation, 14 die in hospital.

(d) In an autopsy series, microscopic evidence of breast malignancy is found in 10 of 40 examinations.

Q2.4 Of 1000 obese subjects, 160 already have hypertension. Over 3 years, 120 more are diagnosed with hypertension.

(a) What is the initial, and the final, prevalence of hypertension?

(b) What is the cumulative incidence over 3 years in the population at risk?

(c) What is the average annual incidence rate?

Q2.5 Consider the following data on HIV seroconversion (from negative to positive) in a high-risk group of 1000 subjects. Assume that HIV positivity is permanent, and there are no entries to or losses from the group of subjects. On 1 January 2001 there are 180 positives, on 1 January 2002 there are 200 positives, and on 1 January 2003 there are 250 positives. Calculate:

(a) the population at risk on 1 January 2001

(b) the prevalence rate on 1 January 2002

(c) the cumulative incidence over 2 years from 1 January 2001

(d) the incidence rate in 2002.

References

1. **Medical Research Council**. Streptomycin treatment of pulmonary tuberculosis. *BMJ* 1948; **ii**:769–782.

2. **Yoshioka A**. Use of randomisation in the Medical Research Council's clinical trial of streptomycin in pulmonary tuberculosis in the 1940s. *BMJ* 1998; **317**:1220–1223.

3. **Mack TM, Pike MC**. Hormone replacement therapy and endometrial carcinoma. *Lancet* 1977; **i** (8026):1358.

4. **Reidy A, Minassian DC, Joseph J, Joseph J, Farrow S, Wu J, et al**. Prevalence of serious eye disease and visual impairment in a north London population: population based, cross sectional study. *BMJ* 1998; **316**:1643–1646.

5. **Beral V, Fraser P, Carpenter L, Booth M, Brown A, Rose G**. Mortality of employees of the Atomic Weapons Establishment, 1951–1982. *BMJ* 1988; **297**:757–770.

6. **Younis N, Broadbent DM, Vora JP, Harding SP**. Incidence of sight-threatening retinopathy in patients with type 2 diabetes in the Liverpool Diabetic Eye Study: a cohort study. *Lancet* 2003; **361**:195–200.

7. **ISIS-4 (Fourth International Study of Infarct Survival Collaborative Group)**. ISIS-4: a randomised factorial trial assessing early oral captopril, oral mononitrate, and intravenous magnesium sulphate in 58 050 patients with suspected acute myocardial infarction. *Lancet* 1995; **345**:669–685.

Chapter 3

Study designs which can demonstrate and test causation

All true and fruitful natural philosophy hath a double scale or ladder, ascendant and descendent, ascending from experiments to the inventions of causes, and descending from causes to the invention new experiments.

—Francis Bacon: *The Advancement of Learning*, II; 1605

Introduction

Clinical and epidemiological studies of causation are defined by two features: how the study subjects are selected, and the time dimensions of the study.

Part 1. Types of study

The relationship of study design to the definition of causation

The definition of a causal factor given in Chapter 2 was, '*a factor whose operation increases the frequency of an event*'. This implies that (1) people who are exposed to the causal agent will have a higher frequency of the outcome, and also (2) individuals with the outcome will have a greater frequency of past exposure to the causal agent.

Thus there are two general types of comparative study. To test statement (1), we compare a group of people exposed to the putative causative factor with a group not exposed, a *cohort* study. To test statement (2), we compare a group of people who have already experienced the outcome with a group of people without the outcome, a *case–control* study.

These studies are set up to test causal hypotheses. For the extreme hypotheses, that the causal agent is either necessary or sufficient, or both, a study may not be needed. One definitive instance of mesothelioma (a type of cancer) occurring without any exposure to asbestos shows that asbestos is not a *necessary* causal factor for mesothelioma. A single demonstration of a normal baby born to a mother who had taken thalidomide (a drug) shows that thalidomide is not a *sufficient* cause of birth defects.

Although true in logic, a single demonstration would not be enough, as the reliability of the observations would be questioned. So it is easy to disprove necessary or sufficient causation; but it is impossible to confirm it; it is only possible to conclude on the basis of all reliably ascertained situations that the cause appears to be necessary or sufficient. The usual question is to assess causation that is neither necessary nor sufficient. This causation gives a quantitative relationship between the causative factor and the outcome, and therefore the evidence for it must be expressed in quantitative terms.

A classification of comparative studies: classification by the groups of people compared

Cohort and intervention studies

In *cohort* and *intervention* studies, groups of individuals are defined in terms of their exposure to the putative causative factor. The outcome in the 'exposed' group is compared to the outcome in the 'unexposed' group (Figure 3.1). To find out if oral contraceptives cause, or protect against, heart disease, we could identify a group of women starting to use oral contraceptives, and a group of non-users, and follow them over

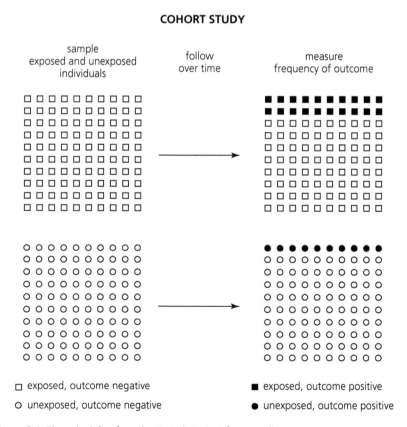

COHORT STUDY

sample exposed and unexposed individuals

follow over time

measure frequency of outcome

□ exposed, outcome negative

○ unexposed, outcome negative

■ exposed, outcome positive

● unexposed, outcome positive

Figure 3.1 The principle of a cohort study to test for causality.

Table 3.1 Cohort results

	Outcome		Total subjects
	Yes	No	
Exposed group	20	80	100
Unexposed group	10	90	100

time to record the frequency of heart disease in each group. This is a cohort study (as it compares 'exposed' and 'unexposed' groups, or 'cohorts').

Groups of individuals are chosen, 'exposed' and 'unexposed' to the putative causal factor. The frequency of the outcome is measured in each group (see Table 3.1 for the results).

This is an *observational* study—the researchers observe the natural events, they do not influence which women use oral contraceptives. In *intervention* studies, the investigators control the assignment of individuals to the intervention, so intervention studies are a special type of prospective cohort study.

Thus, in the example given in Chapter 2, the outcome in a group of tuberculosis patients treated with an antibiotic was compared to the outcome in a group treated without the drug.

The term 'cohort' merely means a group of people with some characteristic; for example, a 'birth cohort' is a group of people born in the same year or time period. Some studies merely describe the experience of one such group. Thus to measure the incidence of eye disease (retinopathy) in subjects with diabetes, 3700 patients with diabetes in England who had no retinopathy at the start of the study were followed over 5 years and the new cases of retinopathy recorded [1].

Case–control studies

In *case–control* studies, groups of individuals are defined in terms of whether they have or have not already experienced the outcome under consideration, and the exposure is then measured (Figure 3.2). For example, children with asthma (the 'cases') might be compared to unaffected children of the same age (the 'controls') in terms of aspects of their home environment.

Example

One of the earliest case–control studies of non-infectious disease was done in London in 1930, comparing patients with various types of cancer to subjects of the same age and sex without cancer, selected by the doctors of the cancer patients [2]. Many factors, such as keeping a dog or cat, having constipation, and pipe smoking were assessed, but the conclusion emphasized by the authors was that the cancer patients ate vegetables less frequently than did the controls, suggesting a protective effect. This association was statistically significant, and the authors concluded that it 'seemed to be inexplicable from random causes' and suggested that further comparative studies, or

CASE–CONTROL STUDY

Figure 3.2 The principle of a case–control design.

an intervention study, could be undertaken to clarify it further. There is now substantial evidence that the intake of fresh vegetables and fruit is protective against several types of cancer.

A group of individuals who have experienced the outcome under assessment, and a group who have not, are assessed and the frequency of exposure measured in each group (see Table 3.2).

Surveys

Surveys are carried out on subjects chosen as all members or a representative sample of a population, but the sampling is not based on any defined exposure or outcome. Thus a national census, studies of all hospital admissions, or reviews of all patients in a practice or all members of a school or work force are surveys. As will be seen, different types of comparison may then be made within the surveyed group.

Table 3.2 Case–control results

	Cases	Controls
	Outcome positive	**Outcome negative**
Exposed	20	12
Unexposed	30	38
Total subjects	50	50

Classification by time relationships

Prospective studies

The studies are also defined in terms of their relationship to time (Figure 3.3). A study in which subjects are entered and some data are collected at this entry time, and then the subjects are followed and further events recorded as they happen, is a *prospective* study. The study suggested earlier, to identify a group of women starting to use oral contraceptives, and a group of non-users, and follow them over time to record the frequency of heart disease in each group, is prospective; examples of such studies will be given in Chapter 5.

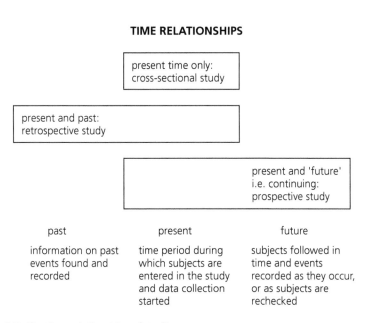

Figure 3.3 The time relationships of studies.

Retrospective studies

A *retrospective* study includes observations relating to the time of study entry and previous time. Case–control studies are always retrospective, because the outcome has already happened. To study the relationship between heart disease and oral contraceptive use, we could select a group of women with heart disease (cases) and a group of generally similar women without heart disease (controls), and assess for each person their use of oral contraceptives prior to the diagnosis of heart disease. If oral contraceptive use increases the risk of heart disease, the frequency of past use will be higher in the cases than in the controls.

Retrospective cohort studies

A cohort study can be retrospective, in that cohorts can be defined and information collected which applies to past time. We could identify from medical records a group of women who 10 years ago were using oral contraceptives, and a group of women who were not. We could then go to these women, or use subsequent medical records, to review their subsequent history from that time point to the present in terms of developing heart disease. This is a *retrospective cohort study*. It is retrospective because it deals with current and past events (and so may be done fairly quickly), but it is a cohort study as the comparison made is between women who used oral contraceptives and those who did not.

Example

In 1983, the UK Ministry of Defence commissioned a study of the health of servicemen exposed to nuclear bomb tests between 1952 and 1958 in Australia and the South Pacific. In this retrospective cohort study, some 21 000 men who participated in the tests were identified and their mortality and cancer incidence from 1952 up to 1998 were compared to a comparison group of other servicemen who served in tropical and subtropical areas but were not involved in the tests. The results showed no clear increase in mortality or in any type of cancer, but there was some evidence suggesting a raised risk of some types of leukaemia [3,4]. Although the data are based on up to 45 years' follow-up, the study was done relatively quickly as it was retrospective. A major limitation is that information on other relevant exposures, including radiation exposure other than from these tests, was not available, although the choice of controls makes it likely that factors like smoking, for example, would be similar in the two groups. Also, by relying on the Ministry of Defence records to identify both exposed and unexposed groups, an estimated 15 per cent of exposed men were not identified and it has been claimed that that omission could bias the results [5].

Cross-sectional studies

The simplest, but weakest, type of study is one where all the information is related to one point in time and is collected at that time. Thus to assess the association between eye colour and hair colour, we could survey a group of subjects, and assess eye and (natural) hair colour. This is a *cross-sectional* study, as the data collected relate to a cross-section in time. Where both the putative causal factor and the outcome state are stable, this study design may be adequate. More commonly, the exposure or outcome changes over time, and so this design is weak. For example, to assess an association between oral contraceptive use and high blood pressure in women, a cross-sectional study comparing current oral contraceptive use with current blood pressure is a very poor method. The results will be misleading, for example, if women who develop high blood pressure stop taking oral contraceptives, or if hypertension develops only after several years of oral contraceptive use.

Example

To assess the relationship between housing conditions and current health, a questionnaire was sent to a 10 per cent sample of residents in one area of England [6]. Nine per cent of the respondents reported that their housing was damp, and amongst these, 49 per cent reported longstanding illness, compared to 37 per cent of those in dry housing. The researchers also assessed social class, employment, and various other measures. They were aware of the limitations of the cross-sectional design, and so in their discussion they consider the possibilities that the damp housing caused the ill health, but also that people with longstanding illnesses might have more difficulty maintaining their homes, and that people who are ill may gravitate to poorer housing.

More complex designs

The selection of subjects, and the exposure–outcome association being assessed, defines the study. If the groups compared are defined by their exposure, it is a cohort study; if the groups are defined by their outcome, it is a case–control study. This principle is useful when more complex designs are considered.

Case–control study 'nested' within a cohort

In a cohort study, a large number of subjects may be enrolled while only a few suffer the outcome of interest. It may be useful to compare these subjects specifically with a sample of those without the outcome: this gives a case–control study within a cohort.

Example

In a large prospective study in Japan, over 65 000 subjects were surveyed and serum samples collected and stored in 1988 to 1990. In 2002, an analysis was done comparing the 169 subjects who had subsequently developed colorectal cancer with 481 controls from the same cohort, using the data and samples collected earlier, and showed associations between serum fatty acid levels and cancer risk [7]. The study required analysis of a few hundred serum samples, rather than many thousands. As the case–control study is 'nested' within the larger prospective cohort study, this can be referred to as a 'nested' case–control study.

Cohort and case–control analyses within a cross-sectional survey

Most analyses of a cross-sectional survey will examine the frequency of characteristics and associations between them in the whole sampled group. In addition to such 'survey' analysis, exposure- or outcome-based comparisons can be made. In the survey data, subgroups with different exposures can be compared, giving a cohort design, and subgroups with different outcomes can be compared, giving case–control comparisons. Extensions to the study could add data for future outcomes in the cohort design, or for past exposures in the case–control design.

Summary: types of study design

As an example, the different types of study are illustrated by work on a vitamin, folic acid, and a type of birth defect, neural tube defects, over some 20 years [8]. Descriptive epidemiological and clinical studies showed features suggesting a nutritional aetiology (such as a higher frequency in births to less affluent mothers, and time and geographical associations). Then a *case–control* study comparing mothers of affected babies with comparison mothers suggested lower levels of folic acid in the 'case' mothers [9]. Then, in a *prospective cohort* study, researchers measured blood levels of folic acid in about 1000 women in early pregnancy and showed that the frequency of these defects was higher in births to women with low folic acid levels [10]. Subsequently, in a *non-randomized intervention* study, women offered dietary folic acid dietary supplements were compared to others not given supplements: the frequency of the defects in births was reduced in those receiving supplementation, but the result was not easy to interpret as there were other differences between the two groups [11]. Finally, a *randomized intervention* study was done, in which women were randomly assigned to receive either supplements with folic acid, or others without folic acid: this also showed a large reduction in the frequency of subsequent birth defects, which is a definitive result as no other factor differed between the groups of women being compared [12]. This led to public health programmes in many countries to add folic acid to foodstuffs; so, returning to descriptive studies, such studies showed reductions in the frequency of these defects after supplementation [13].

By defining both the sampling system and the time relationships, studies can be categorized in a way that is useful in their interpretation (Table 3.3). The main study designs have different applications, and answer different questions; the best design will depend on the question to be answered, and will be influenced by practical and resource restraints. The main designs have different strengths and weaknesses, so in assessing a study it is important to identify the design used, and then to keep these likely strengths and weaknesses in mind when appraising it. The method of analysis depends on the sampling system used (cohort or case–control) rather than on the time relationships, so understanding the study design shows the correct method of analysis.

Incorrect terminology for study design can be confusing. For example, one study in a major journal was called a 'retrospective case–control study' in the title, but an 'historical cohort study' in the abstract [14]. The confusion is often because 'case–control' is sometimes used for any study that has cases and controls, which of course can be almost any design. In this study, a series of patients with cancer was used to provide two cohorts: relatives of these patients (their 'exposure' was their family history of this cancer), and relatives of the spouses of the original case patients (the unexposed group). The outcome was the occurrence of cancer in these two cohorts, so this is a cohort study. In another example, the incidence of malaria was monitored in villages in Ethiopia close to small dams recently constructed to assist irrigation and found to be seven

Table 3.3 The different types of study design.

Sampling system	Time relationship	Type of analysis
COHORT: Select on exposure	Prospective, retrospective, or cross-sectional	Cohort
INTERVENTION: Assign exposure	Prospective	Cohort
CASE–CONTROL: Select on outcome	Retrospective or cross-sectional	Case–control
SURVEY: Total or sample of a defined population	Cross-sectional or retrospective	Survey, plus cohort or case–control analyses comparing subgroups

times higher than in comparison villages not near dams [15]. This is also a prospective cohort study, yet the accompanying editorial comments on the 'weakness of the case–control design'.

Part 2. The strengths, weaknesses, and applications of the main study designs, and examples

Intervention trials

Objectives

An intervention trial measures the effect of the intervention on certain predetermined outcomes. It is a direct test of the causal hypothesis that the intervention, being a change in the exposure factor, produces a change in the outcome. Key features of intervention studies are shown in Table 3.4.

Unlike observational studies, the investigators control the intervention, giving it to selected subjects, with their consent: so trials are limited, in humans, to assessing interventions that are expected to be beneficial. Interventional trials can be randomized; for the assessment of treatment, the randomized clinical trial (RCT) is accepted as the optimal method. They are increasingly being applied to preventive programmes and to management questions as well. Non-randomized interventional studies will be discussed later.

Randomized interventional studies (randomized trials)

Design

Ideally, the subjects receiving the intervention should be similar to those in the comparison group, both in regard to any other care they receive and in regard to other characteristics that might influence the outcome being assessed. This is best achieved

Table 3.4 Key properties of intervention studies

Design	Intervention trials
Question asked	What is the effect of this intervention?
Applicability	Controlled interventions of likely benefit
	Primary methods of studying new therapies
Major strengths	Allows randomization
	—best way to control confounding
	Allows double-blind assessment—best way to control bias
Major weaknesses	Ethical limitations
	Organizational problems
	Timescale

by using *randomization*; that is, by selecting people who are eligible for either the intervention under test or the comparison procedure, and then selecting by a random process those who will receive the test intervention. Usually, consent is obtained before randomization, so that each subject needs to give consent to all the possible interventions offered, and to the randomization process. In large trials with an option of normal care, it may be appropriate to seek consent only from those offered the new intervention, after randomization.

Ethical issues

Randomized clinical trials are appropriate when a new therapy looks as if it may give better results than an established therapy. A trial will be unethical if the new therapy has very little chance of being better, or if the new therapy is clearly much better, making it the treatment of choice. So there can be much disagreement over the necessity for a clinical trial; for example, there was a large debate about the need for, and the ethics of, the randomized trial of folate supplementation described earlier. The usual ethical basis of involvement of randomized trials is the uncertainty principle, or clinical equipoise. To invite a patient to give consent to enter a randomized trial comparing a new and an established treatment, the trial investigators and the clinicians responsible for that patient's care are assuming that first, it is unknown which of the trial treatments would be best for that particular patient, and second, that there is no medical or non-medical reason why any of treatments would be inappropriate for that patient. Of course, these are complex issues; for example, the balance of responsibility between the research investigators and the individual clinician can be debated [16].

Historical examples

As described in Chapter 2, one of the first randomized clinical trials was of streptomycin treatment for tuberculosis in 1946–48. It was a small, quick trial (107 patients, and the main result in 6 months), which was possible because the effect size was large: a decrease in death rate from 27 per cent to 7 per cent (Figure 2.6). The *British Medical Journal* devoted its 31 October 1998 issue to the fiftieth anniversary of this trial [17], including a reprint of the original report and several interesting papers on both past trials and issues for the future [18,19].

Randomization, as a statistical method, was developed and used first in agricultural research by R.A. Fisher and others [20]. Prior to the 1940s, some comparative trials used alternating treatments by order of entry or by day of admission, such as Fibiger's trial of serum treatment of diphtheria in Denmark in 1896–97 [21], and several British studies in the 1930s. A large British trial in 1944 to assess the antibiotic patulin as a cure for the common cold used an alternate allocation system with two active and two placebo preparations [22]; the results showed no benefit. From 1939, in Massachusetts, USA, in a remarkable trial of a social programme to reduce delinquency, some 500 boys aged 5 to 13 were assigned 'by the toss of a coin' to a therapy programme or to a non-intervention control group, presumably without informed consent. A report after 30 years' follow-up [23] shows worse outcomes in the intervention group in several respects. Lind's work on scurvy in 1747 used simple allocation between patients, as described in Chapter 5, and similar studies were proposed but not carried out by van Helmont in 1662.

Advantages

The randomized intervention study has advantages that are shared by no other type of study. So whenever a major question arises, consideration must be given to whether a randomized intervention trial can be mounted. Often the possibility is too readily dismissed. Ineffective interventions may continue to be used, or effective interventions not widely adopted, because of the inconclusive results from less rigorous study designs. This applies not only to aspects of therapy, but also to questions of prevention, public education, and the provision of services. There is a strong case for using randomized intervention studies more in other social areas, such as education, management, and law [24].

The prime advantage is that randomization is usually the best method of obtaining two or more groups of subjects whose outcome rates, in the absence of any treatment effect, are likely to be the same. This serves to minimize the effect of other factors on the outcome (confounding, discussed in Chapter 7), and also fulfils some statistical criteria (see Chapter 8).

Blind assessment

A randomized design makes it easier to use techniques such as single- or double-blind methods to minimize bias in the recording of the outcome, as will be discussed in Chapter 6. Trials in which two or more drugs are compared, all being given in similar ways, allow very comparable protocols and make double-blind designs fairly easy, where neither the patient nor the clinicians looking after the patient are aware which of the randomized treatments were given. Where different types of care are being compared, this is more difficult. For example, until the 1970s it was generally assumed that even uncomplicated suspected myocardial infarction required hospital treatment. To test this was challenging [25]. In the trial, a skilled mobile team responded immediately when a primary care practitioner notified them of a patient with suspected myocardial infarction, and assessed the patient at home. Patients for whom the options of hospital and home care both appeared reasonable, and who consented to participate, were randomized between general practitioner care and immediate hospitalization. Contrary to most prior opinion, there was no difference in mortality.

Disadvantages

Aside from their fundamental limitation to interventions that are likely to be beneficial, the main disadvantages are their requirements in organization, time, cost, and resources, and in the ethical questions they raise. Clinical trials of therapy to assess modest, although important, improvements in treatment need large numbers of subjects, as will be discussed in Chapter 8. Such studies require a high degree of commitment and cooperation from health professionals and from their patients. For outcomes in chronic diseases, many years of follow-up may be required, so the therapy assessed is obsolescent by the time the results are available.

As a result, not all randomized trials are good studies, and their results may be wrong or irrelevant. A survey of 2000 randomized trials in the treatment of schizophrenia in 1998 reported that most were of less than 6 weeks' duration, included only a small number of patients, and were poor quality [26], and many reviews in other topics have given similar conclusions.

Large trials

While trials with short time frames and large anticipated effects can be quite small (like the streptomycin trial), to detect a modest, but important, improvement in outcome may require a very large trial. To assess the effects of three different medications in the treatment of suspected myocardial infarction, a trial involved some 58 000 patients in over 1000 hospitals in 32 countries, in a study that cost about £6 million sterling [27]. This study showed no benefit of one widely used treatment, and benefits of a new treatment, and thus changed international medical practice.

In the first trial of screening for breast cancer, some 62 000 women aged 40–64 in a health maintenance organization in New York were randomized into two equally sized groups: one group was offered the new screening intervention, mammography. The other group received their normal care. Informed consent was obtained after randomization only from the group who were offered the extra intervention of mammographic screening; some 65 per cent of those women accepted the offer. No extra intervention or consent procedure was used for the comparison group, who did not necessarily know about the trial. Long-term follow-up to assess particularly the occurrence and mortality from breast cancer was instituted and is continuing. After 10–14 years of follow-up, the death rate from breast cancer in the women randomized to being offered mammographic screening was 30 per cent less than that of the comparison group [28].

The National Cancer Institute in the United States is running a complex randomized trial to assess, in the same trial, screening techniques for prostate, lung, colorectal, and ovarian cancer, which together make up almost half of all cancers diagnosed (the PLCO trial). Over 150 000 volunteers are involved in the trial. Enrolment started in 1993 and was completed in 2001; subjects are followed for at least 13 years so follow-up is continuing. Updates are available at the trial website (http://prevention.cancer.gov/plco).

Standardized reporting

Standard formats for reporting of results of clinical trials have been developed, which ensure that all subjects assessed for eligibility are accounted for, whether excluded or randomized, such as the CONSORT recommended system [29]. These criteria and recommended formats are kept under review and are available from websites such as http://www.consort-statement.org/. See Chapter 5; the CONSORT standard reporting template for a randomized trial is shown in Figure 5.4.

Registration

Another emphasis has been on ensuring all trials that are performed are reported, so that all the results can be assessed, to avoid publication bias; this is discussed further in Chapter 9. Investigators are encouraged to register their trial and submit the protocol when the trial is designed. Many leading medical journals will now only publish the results of trials which have been registered in advance, and which are reported according to standard criteria.

Some specific designs

Crossover trials

Where a treatment is designed to give short-term benefit in the continuing disease, different treatments can be tested by giving them at different times to the same patients. In a randomized crossover trial, each patient is allocated each of the treatments, in random order. To ensure the effects of one treatment have completely disappeared before the other treatment is tried, a suitable 'washout period' may be set. There are several specific statistical issues, such as assessing if the time period or order of the treatments is important [30]. As an example, to assess a new drug compared with placebo in the prevention of migraine [31], participants who were regular migraine sufferers were observed during a 4-week run-in period during which they were given (unknown to them) the placebo drug, and then were randomized into two groups. Thirty patients received the active drug for 12 weeks, discontinued it for a 2-week washout period, and then were given the placebo for a second 12-week period. The other group of 30 had the placebo drug first, and the active drug later. The patients kept a daily diary of migraine attacks and other symptoms. The trial was double-blind. Based on hours and days with headache and days with migraine, the active drug was shown to be beneficial.

Individual patient (*n*-of-1) trials

The '*n*-of-1' study is a crossover design using randomization between different treatments, in one patient, and is applicable to longstanding diseases where the objective is to improve function or decrease symptoms or disability, rather than to cure the disease.

The objective is to assess the better intervention for this patient, rather than the one which is better on average; but a series of such studies can assess treatments more generally [32]. An example is a comparison of two different medications for osteoarthritis, assessing 2-week courses of each of the treatments, in randomized order [33]; other uses have been in hypertension and chronic respiratory disease.

Community-based randomized trials

It may be appropriate to randomize groups of people, such as families, school classes, medical practices, or whole communities, rather than randomize individuals. This can be referred to as 'cluster randomization'. To evaluate health promotion activities, comparisons between towns, workforces, or schools may be appropriate: for example, studies of the prevention of coronary heart disease have compared workforces receiving a complex intervention programme to those not receiving it. There are differences in the calculation of the necessary size of the study, and many other methodological issues, involved where communities rather than individuals are compared [34].

Examples of cluster randomized studies

In an intervention study in Ethiopia, households were randomized, and provided with either iron cooking pots or aluminium pots, and the change in haemoglobin level in one child per household assessed over 12 months; this showed that children in households supplied with iron pots had lower risks of anaemia and improved growth [35].

A trial of a new method for the diagnosis of skin lesions in primary care, with the objective of reducing unnecessary excisions, involved randomizing 223 general practices in Perth, Australia, equipping and training the 468 doctors in the intervention practices to use the new method, and comparing the ratios of benign to malignant lesions excised in the intervention and in the control practices over a year [36]. The design avoided the consent processes needed if patients were to be individually randomized, and was relevant as the new system would be implemented at a practice level; but the results showed no benefit of the new method.

Non-randomized intervention trials

Studies of treatments, historical controls

These are studies assessing an intervention, but without randomization, such as comparing outcomes between patients treated with a new method and previous patients ('*historical controls*'), or patients treated in different countries, cities, or hospitals. Lacking the strengths that randomization gives in avoiding biases, non-randomized intervention trials are more difficult to interpret and are best considered as observational cohort studies. For example, there are many factors that may influence why a particular patient is offered or accepts the new treatment. A slightly better comparison may be to compare all patients undergoing treatment in a particular facility after the new treatment is introduced with all patients seen at the facility before it was introduced, thus avoiding the problems of individual selection and acceptance of the new treatment. However, this still assumes that there have been no changes in the factors that influence patients to go to that particular facility (i.e. the referral patterns). Also, when a new intervention is introduced, the professionals who deliver it may well act differently to those who continue to use the conventional programmes. A new educational approach in schools, for example, is very likely to be first taken up and promoted by particularly interested teachers, and it may be the differences between these teachers and others which affect the educational outcome, rather than particular properties of the new programme.

So, for studies of treatment of patients, non-randomized studies are usually regarded as unsatisfactory, and are often ignored if some randomized studies are available. There are many examples of situations in which apparently similar groups of patients treated by apparently similar methods give considerably different outcomes, with no ready explanation. Several examples in surgery, such as gastric freezing, were documented in an influential book [37]. This treatment for peptic ulcer, using a gastric balloon with a coolant, was widely used in the United States in the 1960s with the idea that cooling reduces gastric acid secretion and the unsystematic comparison of results after the treatment with past experience. A randomized trial then showed no benefit, and indeed somewhat worse results, when the treatment was compared with a sham treatment [38]. However, non-randomized comparisons comprise most of the 'evidence' presented in support of alternative medicine treatments, dietary supplements, and so on, in the general media, as shown in Ben Goldacre's excellent books [39] and comments (http://www.badscience.net/).

Examples

Non-randomized studies are useful in situations where randomization would be very difficult or unacceptable, and have been important for large-scale interventions. For example, communities using fluoridated water were compared to generally similar communities continuing with unfluoridated supplies [40]. The Stanford Heart Disease Prevention Program compared intensive methods of health education in two communities, comparing them with rather similar communities that did not receive the intervention [41,42]. A more recent non-randomized study of cancer screening had very clear results. Neuroblastoma is a cancer affecting young children, which can be detected by a urine test, and screening has been advocated, especially in Japan. In Canada, a comparison was made between a cohort of births in Quebec, where a screening programme was set up, and a comparison cohort, unscreened, in Ontario. This showed that screening produced a great increase in the incidence rate of neuroblastoma, but the mortality rate was not reduced. The interpretation was that screening led to 'overdiagnosis', that is, the diagnosis of 'silent tumours': tumours diagnosed and treated as neuroblastoma, but which if left alone would not have produced any clinical problems [43]. Even without any randomized studies, these results prevented further programmes being set up, and led to the discontinuation of neuroblastoma screening in Japan.

In contrast, other non-randomized trials have given results that have been later confirmed by a randomized study. In a non-randomized study of the prevention of congenital defects by dietary supplementation, women who came for genetic counselling in good time for their next pregnancy were offered and accepted the dietary supplement. They were compared to women who did not get the supplement, in most cases because they did not seek professional help early enough in regard to their next pregnancy. The comparison, published in 1981, showed a considerable reduction in birth defects in women receiving the supplement, but this could obviously be influenced by a large number of factors which would be related to whether the woman sought professional help in time for her to be offered supplementation [11]. A further study, however, showed that in the area of England where this study was carried out, the recurrence rate of the defect in *all* births to at-risk women fell over time, at the same time as the proportion of all at-risk women receiving this dietary supplementation rose [44]. While still a non-randomized comparison, and open to the major problem that something else might be changing over time which affects the recurrence rate, this second comparison does avoid the individual selection effects which complicate the comparison between women being offered and not being offered the supplement. As noted earlier, these results were later confirmed by a randomized trial, which reported in 1991 [12]; but it is an interesting question whether more action should have been taken after the 1981 results, rather than waiting 10 years for the later results.

Observational cohort studies

Objectives

The other types of studies involve observation rather than intervention; that is, the researcher does not control the intervention, but merely observes its effects. A cohort study is designed to answer the question: 'What are the effects of this particular exposure?' The studies compare a group of people with the exposure to a group without the exposure, or with a different level of exposure. In a prospective cohort study, the exposure is defined and the subjects selected before the outcome events occur. This ensures that the time relationship between exposure and outcome is appropriate; the follow-up procedures allow direct measurement of the incidence rate of the outcome(s) in each of the groups being studied. Key features of cohort studies are shown in Table 3.5.

Table 3.5 Key properties of cohort studies

Design	Cohort studies
Question asked	What are the effects of this exposure?
Applicability	Any exposure for which adequate numbers of exposed subjects can be found and studied, and outcome can be assessed
	Primary method of studying unusual or new exposures
Major strengths	Allows multiple endpoints to be assessed
	Cause to effect time sequence clear
	All measures of risk can be assessed
	Exposure is assessed prior to outcome, avoiding bias
Major weaknesses	Usually requires large numbers
	Long timescale for some effect

Applications

Cohort studies are therefore the appropriate method to study the effects of a certain exposure. Thus, cohort studies were set up to follow survivors of the atomic bomb explosions in Japan in 1945 and those affected by the Chernobyl nuclear plant accident in 1986, assessing many end points, for example, total mortality and the incidence of leukaemia. The effects of many occupational hazards have been established by studying cohorts of exposed workers, comparing their subsequent mortality or morbidity either to defined comparison groups or to the general population, which can be regarded as unexposed to the particular chemical or process. Several studies before the Second World War showed lung scarring, and suggested a possible increase in lung cancer, in workers exposed to asbestos. Increases in several types of cancer were then shown in cohort studies, first in Britain and then in the United States [45]. These studies led to much stricter control of asbestos exposure in work places and in the general population, and also to legal actions that forced a major asbestos manufacturer into bankruptcy.

Time required

A major disadvantage of prospective cohort studies relates to the time required. If the outcome does not follow the exposure until after a long period, the study has to have many years of follow-up. A retrospective cohort design will overcome this problem, but is possible only if there are adequate records for the appropriate subjects and the time period.

Numbers needed

If the outcome does not occur frequently, the cohort study must involve large numbers of subjects to observe even a reasonable number of events, as discussed in Chapter 8. The effective size of a study depends primarily on the number of outcome events that are observed; in Chapter 4 we show a prospective study of 2332 pregnancies, but to assess the relevant outcome, the critical figure is the number of malformed births occurring to mothers exposed to a particular drug, which was only six.

Examples: general

Subjects may be chosen for cohort studies not because they are particularly unusual in terms of exposure, but because they can be kept under surveillance over a long period. A cohort study of the effects of smoking in British doctors started in the 1950s, selecting doctors not because their smoking habits were particularly unusual, but because they could be followed through annual registration procedures and their rate of cooperation was expected to be high [46,47]. Using similar logic, a cohort study of American nurses was started in the late 1970s as an opportunity to assess many major health issues in women [48,49].

A cohort can be set up by performing an initial survey of a sample of subjects or of a whole community, chosen not because of any unusual characteristic of exposure but because of availability and practical considerations. Such general population follow-up studies are analysed as cohort studies comparing subjects with different exposures from within the same initial group. An important example is the Framingham Heart

Study, started in the 1950s by asking for volunteers from the small town of Framingham, a short distance from Boston, Massachusetts, enrolling those who volunteered, and following them up over a long period of time [50,51].

Several cohort studies have started at birth or early childhood with active follow-up. A study based on a sample of 4454 people born during a single week, 3–9 March 1946, in England, Scotland, and Wales has followed them through childhood and adolescence into adulthood; active follow-up is continuing [52]. Cohort studies of people born in single week in 1958 and in 1970, and of 19 000 children born in 2000–01 in the UK are in progress (http://www.cls.ioe.ac.uk/). A study in New Zealand of a group of children identified at birth in 1972–73 in one town has continued by inviting participants to come for a 1- or 2-day assessment of psychological and physical characteristics about every 3 years, and is now being extended to assess the children born to the original cohort members (http://dunedinstudy.otago.ac.nz/studies/main-study/description) [53]. An ambitious proposal for a 'conception to death' cohort study is aimed at addressing prenatal influences and events [54].

Examples: large cohort studies

In several countries, large, long-term cohort studies have become important national projects [55]. The UK 'Biobank' study is a cohort study of over 500 000 volunteers aged 45–69 with emphasis on assessing biochemical and genetic parameters, using an initial questionnaire and blood sample with analyses based on different biological parameters being done later [56,57] (http://www.ukbiobank.ac.uk/). Follow-up is continuing using death and cancer incidence records and hospital admissions; linkages to primary care records and other databases are planned. Similar large cohort studies are in progress or underway in other countries, such as Canada (http://www.partnershipagainstcancer.ca/priorities/research/strategic-initiatives/canadian-partnership-for-tomorrow-project/).

The 'Million Women Study' was set up in the United Kingdom originally to study the relationship between hormone replacement therapy and breast cancer, but now includes diet, exercise, employment patterns, oral contraceptive use, childbirth and breastfeeding, and family history of illness, in relation to a wide range of cancers and to other conditions such as fractures, gallbladder problems, and cardiovascular disease. After pilot studies involving 6000 women, from 1997 to 2001, women coming for breast cancer screening in the United Kingdom were invited to join the study and to provide important baseline information. Follow-up was by linkage within the NHS central register to cancer registrations and deaths. Over 1.3 million women joined the study, with an average age of 56, and over 50 per cent had used hormone replacement therapy at some time. By June 2009, over 90 000 cancers and 35 000 breast cancers had been reported in these women. The study website provides current updates and lists of publications (http://www.millionwomenstudy.org/).

The Million Women Study emphasizes relatively simple data collection at one point in time and routine follow-up through data linkage to achieve a very high sample size. In contrast is the European Prospective Investigation into Cancer and nutrition (EPIC), which started in 1992 and includes over 500 000 participants in 10 European countries. The participants were asked to provide extensive data including food consumption questionnaires, lifestyle data, and blood samples, resulting in the collection of 9 million specimens, the largest repository of biological material in a study in the world [58]. Participants have been followed up regularly by multiple methods, and over 26 000 cancer cases have been reported. Many of the analyses will be in the form of nested case–control studies; a useful website gives current information at http:// epic.iarc.fr/.

Case–control studies

Objectives

The question asked in a case–control study is: 'What caused this event?' Case-control studies start after the outcome event, and can therefore assess multiple causes relating to this event. They are therefore the prime method to assess the causes of a new problem. For example, cancer of the vagina had been generally described as rare, and occurring in older women. Between 1966 and 1969 seven occurrences in women aged 15–22 were reported in Boston, Massachusetts [59]. To investigate possible causes, these cases, plus one further patient seen in another Boston hospital, were studied, and for each 'case', four control subjects were chosen, women born within 5 days and in the same hospital as the case women. Interviews were carried out in an identical fashion on all 40 subjects. These interviews explored a wide range of possible factors, and the greatest difference between the cases and controls was in the use of diethylstilboestrol (DES) by their mothers during the pregnancy, which was documented for seven of the eight cases, but for none of the 32 controls. This suggested that it was the key causal agent, a result confirmed by further studies.

Key features of case–control studies are shown in Table 3.6. The case–control study is a natural development from the case series. We start looking for possible causes by considering the characteristics of affected subjects, and we then have to assess how common those characteristics would be in an unaffected population.

Table 3.6 Key properties of case–control studies

Design	Case–control studies
Question asked	What were the causes of this event?
Applicability	Any event for which groups of cases and appropriate controls can be found, and exposure factors can be assessed retrospectively
	Primary method of studying unusual or new outcomes
Major strengths	Usually can be done with moderate numbers of subjects; feasible even on small numbers
	Retrospective method is rapid
	Multiple exposure factors can be assessed
Major weaknesses	Retrospective method limits exposure information, and is open to bias
	Adequate control group may be difficult to define or obtain

Advantages

The major *advantage* of case–control studies is that they are highly efficient in terms of the numbers of subjects required. Thus, in a study of the causes of breast cancer, in principle the amount of information given by studying 100 women who have developed breast cancer and 100 controls, is similar to that produced by asking the same questions of a group of some 50 000 middle-aged women and following them for a year, during which 100 of them might develop breast cancer.

Disadvantages

This advantage of numbers is because the outcome has already happened. However, that fact also results in the great *disadvantage* of case–control studies that all information on previous events has to be collected after the outcome has happened. This gives two major problems. Firstly, the relevant causal events may have happened a considerable time in the past, and therefore the information obtained is likely to be incomplete and inaccurate. The greater problem, however, is that the case subjects, who have suffered the outcome under investigation, may tend to give different responses than the control subjects, thus introducing a bias into the information obtained on previous exposures. These problems, and methods to overcome them, will be discussed further in Chapter 5.

The advantages in the numbers of subjects and the time required for a case–control study must be compared with the disadvantages of unreliability of exposure information and possible bias in the recall of events. Often these biases are severe enough to justify a more expensive and time-consuming cohort study. Case–control studies have been of immense importance in elucidating the causes of chronic diseases, such as cancer, and the first indications of causes have often come from such studies.

Example: smoking and lung cancer

Between 1922 and 1947, the number of deaths from lung cancer in England and Wales increased by 15 times. While some thought this might be an artefact of diagnosis or recording, investigations suggested that the increase was real, and the most favoured explanations were an effect of atmospheric pollution, or of smoking tobacco, and small studies were available on each. In 1947, the British Medical Research Council decided to carry out a more thorough investigation. To do this, patients with lung cancer and some other cancers in some 20 London hospitals were interviewed, along with control patients who had a range of diseases excluding cancer. The results showed that 647 out of 649 men with lung cancer were smokers (99.7 per cent), but 622 out of 649 (95.8 per cent) of the control patients were also smokers. The results by detailed smoking history are more useful, and showed that the risk of lung cancer increased strongly with the amount smoked. The original reports of this investigation [60,61] are well worth reading because of the detail given to the methodology and the consideration of biases and possible explanations of the results. For example, the issue of possible bias by the subject or by the interviewer is addressed by looking at the results from a number of patients who, at the time of interview, were thought to have lung cancer, but in whom the final diagnosis was something else. The smoking habits of these patients were clearly different from those of patients who actually had lung cancer, but were similar to the non-cancer control patients, which would not have happened if the excess smoking recorded for lung cancer patients had been due to bias in the observations.

This was one of the first case–control studies, and acceptance of its results required several years of debate about, amongst other things, the value of the case–control approach. This study produced results in 1950 [62]; the prospective study of British doctors, published 14 years later, gave substantially the same results [62], as shown in Table 3.7. The authors of these studies became very important epidemiologists in chronic disease, all receiving British knighthoods: Sir Richard Doll, Sir Austin Bradford Hill, and Sir Richard Peto, who all worked in Oxford and London. There is an excellent biography of Sir Richard Doll which describes much of this work [63].

Other examples and applications

Although their main contribution has been to aetiological studies, case–control studies are applicable to many other questions. For example, the effect of population-based interventions can be assessed; studies of screening for cancer have been done by comparing subjects who die from the disease in question with samples of the unaffected population [64,65]. The benefits of screening are shown by a less frequent history of screening in those who suffer the outcome which screening is designed to prevent, such as death or advanced disease, although the interpretation of these

Table 3.7 Comparison of results. The relationship between smoking and lung cancer in men, as shown by different British reports. Relative risk, or its close approximation odds ratio, is the basic measure of association given by these studies and shows the ratio of the frequency of lung cancer at each level of smoking compared with the frequency in non-smokers (see Chapter 4).

Relative risks of lung cancer by daily cigarette smoking from different studies			
Non-smokers (referent)	1.0	1.0	1.0	1.0
1–14	11.0	7.0	8.1	7.8
15–24	13.9	9.5	19.9	12.7
25+	27.0	16.3	32.4	25.1
Publication date:	1950	1952	1964	1976
	(1)	(2)	(3)	(4)

(1) Doll and Hill (1950): 3 years' study: 1298 subjects: case–control, incidence, odds ratio [60].

(2) Doll and Hill (1952): 5 years' study: 2714 subjects: case–control, incidence, odds ratio [61].

(3) Doll and Hill (1964): 13 years' study: 34 445 subjects: cohort, mortality, relative risk [46].

(4) Doll and Peto (1976): 25 years' study: 34 445 subjects: cohort, mortality, relative risk [62].

Source data from Doll R and Peto R., 'Mortality in relation to smoking: 20 years: observations on male British doctors', *British Medical Journal*, Volume 12, Issue 6051, pp. 1525–1536, © 1976 [62].

studies can be difficult [66]. For example, no randomized trial has yet been done to assess whether routine examination of the skin results in ultimate benefit, that is, a reduction in mortality from the most serious skin cancer, melanoma. However, case–control studies have shown that having had routine skin checks is associated with being diagnosed with smaller melanomas with a better prognosis [67], and with a lower risk of death [68].

Case–control studies deserve to be more widely used in assessments of such population interventions, and also in assessments of clinical issues and non-health issues. Thus, prognostic factors in breast cancer have been studied in a case–control comparison of long-term survivors with patients who had died [69]. To assess the risk of bankruptcy, financial and management features of companies that went bankrupt have been compared to a sample of companies that did not, in a case–control study [70].

Case–control studies can be quite large. In an expansion of the routine function of disease registries, in Canada, information has been collected routinely from newly diagnosed cancer patients and controls chosen from the population with a similar age and sex distribution, to give a database which can be analysed for many exposure factors and different types of cancer. An analysis of obesity using data on 21 000 cancer cases and 5000 population controls found a significant increase to cancer risk overall and increased risks for several individual cancers, and concluded that excess body mass accounted for 7.7 per cent of all cancers in Canada [71].

Poor quality case–control studies

Unfortunately there are many examples of badly performed case–control studies, which have led to erroneous results. There are more examples of poor quality case–control studies than there are of poor cohort studies. This is partly because the case–control design is more subtle and more difficult to apply than a cohort design, but also because case–control studies may appear deceptively easy. There has been a simplistic view that case–control studies are 'quick, simple, and cheap' compared to cohort studies, whereas in fact to mount a well-designed case–control study of an important question is often a complex and expensive endeavour. However, because of this impression, many case–control studies have been carried out with inadequate resources and poor design, and not surprisingly have given erratic results. The issues are those of appropriate study design and quality control of the information collected, which will be discussed in Chapters 5 and 6; and the issues of appropriate analysis, sample size, power, and publication bias, which will be discussed in Chapters 7 and 8.

Case-crossover aetiological studies

The equivalent of the crossover trial in an aetiological study is to look at factors related to an episodic event, comparing them to a similar time period for the same individuals that did not result in an event, often called a case-crossover design. Thus in a study to assess the role of mobile phone use in motor vehicle accidents, drivers were identified who had reported a motor vehicle accident, and 74 699 of these drivers who owned a mobile phone allowed access to their cellular phone records [72]. The study was done in Toronto, before there were any legal restrictions on mobile phone use while driving. The analysis consisted of assessing from these records whether the cell phone was being used immediately before the reported accident, as compared to use by the same driver in a set of control periods defined, for example, as the same time on the day before, the same time and the same day of the week before, and so on. The analysis showed an association, an increased relative risk of a motor vehicle accident if the cellular telephone call was between 1 and 5 minutes prior to the accident, with the risk decreasing as the time interval between the call and the accident increased, up to 16–20 minutes before. The relative risk was 4.8, and was no lower where a hands-free cell phone was used.

Cross-sectional surveys

Objectives

The basic purpose of a survey is to measure the prevalence (frequency at one point in time) of a condition. It is therefore appropriate to answer questions such as 'Is anaemia common in this community?' 'What is the prevalence of hypertension in elderly people?' 'How satisfied are patients with the health services?' Surveys also allow the assessment of associations, such as whether hypertension or a poor diet is more common in one social group than in another, and such comparisons can lend themselves to causal thinking. Thus a survey of two groups of villagers in Tanzania showed that those who consumed a fish-based diet had lower blood pressure than those who had a vegetarian diet [73]. The key properties of surveys are shown in Table 3.8.

Table 3.8 Key properties of surveys

Design	Surveys
Question asked	How common is this condition?
	Are conditions and exposures associated?
Applicability	Any exposure, condition, or association which is reasonably common and for which assessment at one point in time is sufficient
	Primary method of assessing prevalence
Major strengths	Representative samples of a population can be drawn
	Methods can be standardized, reliable and single blind
	Efficient in resources needed
	Cooperation may be high
	Can be repeated using similar methods
Major weaknesses	Lack of time dimension limits causal interpretations
	Inefficient for rare exposures or conditions

Advantages

The advantages of a cross-sectional survey arise primarily because of its relative simplicity, as the complications of retrospective data collection and prospective follow-up are both avoided. Thus the methods to be used can be extensively pre-tested, applied on a large scale, and made reproducible and at least single blind, in that the investigators need know nothing about the state of the individuals being assessed. Because of their simplicity, cooperation can be high, as little is demanded of the subjects.

Sampling methods

As the primary function of a survey is to assess prevalence, the methods obtained to draw samples from a defined population are crucial, and various randomized or systematic methods are available which have been discussed in detail in standard texts [74–76]. The use of such methods can ensure that the subjects surveyed are a representative sample of the community, and allows the repetition of the survey at other times or in other communities using identical methods and yielding comparable results. Thus, surveys can monitor changes in a population in time and assess differences between population subgroups.

Limitations

The main disadvantages of survey methods also arise from their simplicity. Because of their lack of a time dimension, the interpretation of their results in terms of cause and effect is very limited, and over-interpretation in this regard is a considerable danger. Their power in assessing prevalence, and therefore in assessing associations between different states, requires a reasonable prevalence of that condition in the population, otherwise they will be inefficient.

Extensions

Our definition of a cross-sectional survey is quite narrow; if a population is surveyed to find out which subjects have a poor diet, and these subjects are then compared to those with a better diet in terms of subsequent health care utilization, we classify the first part as a survey, but the second as a prospective cohort study. Thus, in two areas of Sweden, a health survey was carried out in 1963–65, and subsequent linkage of the data to mortality and cancer registration data up to 1987 allowed a prospective cohort analysis of the association between obesity and cancer risk [77].

Choice of study design

The major properties of the different study designs have been summarized in Tables 3.4, 3.5, 3.6, and 3.8. In deciding which approach to adopt to deal with a specific question, these properties can be used as a general guide, but the final decision on the appropriate method will be based on a detailed consideration of the issues to be addressed in the study, including the likely effects of bias, confounding, and chance on the interpretation of the results. These concepts will be explored in subsequent chapters.

Self-test questions

Answers in Appendix 1, p.396.

Q3.1 What types of study design are illustrated by the following situations? (Consider the groups being compared and the time relationship.)

(a) The frequency of deep venous thrombosis in people who have recently had a long-distance air flight is compared with the frequency in an age-matched sample of people who have not travelled.

(b) To assess a possible protective effect of exercise, past involvement in competitive sports is assessed for women who have hypertension and for a group of women of the same age who have not.

(c) Total mortality over the last 30 years is assessed in men employed in a uranium mine at some time during that period, and compared with the general population.

(d) To assess an effect of smoking, men admitted to hospital with myocardial infarction are compared with similar unaffected men in the community.

(e) In a continuation of the same study as in (d), the risk of future repetition of the heart attack (reinfarction) is compared between those who smoked and those who did not at the time of their first heart attack.

(f) Groups of breast-fed and non-breast-fed babies are identified at 6 months of age, and then surveyed at later times. To study the association with small stature, children in the lowest decile of height at age 10 years are compared with a sample of all the other children in regard to many factors.

(g) A dermatologist offers a new treatment for acne to all her teenage patients, and compares the results with those who chose to continue the traditional treatment.

Q3.2 Do you agree with the following conclusions?

(a) A study shows higher rates of diabetes in unemployed than in employed men. This shows that becoming unemployed leads to diabetes.

(b) A survey of residents in an aged care facility shows that smoking is much less frequent in 95-year-olds than it is in 85-year-olds. This shows that many people give up smoking between these ages.

(c) In a study of breast cancer patients, 40 per cent reported stressful life events in the last 2 years compared with only 25 per cent of age-matched controls. This shows that stress increases the risk of breast cancer substantially.

(d) A survey of workers in a clothing factory shows that the frequency of repetitive strain injury is lower than the rate reported in a general population survey. This shows that repetitive strain injury is not caused by this type of work.

Q3.3 What type of study is most useful to assess the various consequences of an environmental hazard, such as radiation exposure? What are its main disadvantages, in terms of an outcome such as cancer occurrence?

Q3.4 What are the prime advantages and disadvantages of a case–control study in assessing the causes of a newly recognized disease?

Q3.5 What are the main advantages of the randomized trial design?

References

1. Younis N, Broadbent DM, Vora JP, Harding SP. Incidence of sight-threatening retinopathy in patients with type 2 diabetes in the Liverpool Diabetic Eye Study: a cohort study. *Lancet* 2003; **361**(9353):195–200.

2. Stocks P, Karn MN. A co-operative study of the habits, home life, dietary and family histories of 450 cancer patients and of an equal number of control patients. *Ann Eugen* 1933; **5**:237–280.

3. Kendall GM, Muirhead CR, Darby SC, Doll R, Arnold L, O'Hagan JA. Epidemiological studies of UK test veterans: I. General description. *J Radiol Prot* 2004; **24**(3):199–217.

4. Muirhead CR, Kendall GM, Darby SC, Doll R, Haylock RG, O'Hagan JA, et al. Epidemiological studies of UK test veterans: II. Mortality and cancer incidence. *J Radiol Prot* 2004; **24**(3):219–241.

5. Baverstock K. The 2003 NRPB report on UK nuclear-test veterans. *Lancet* 2003; **361**(9371):1759–1760.

6. Packer CN, Stewart-Brown S, Fowle SE. Damp housing and adult health: results from a lifestyle study in Worcester, England. *J Epidemiol Community Health* 1994; **48**:555–559.

7. Kojima M, Wakai K, Tokudome S, Suzuki K, Tamakoshi K, Watanabe Y, et al. Serum levels of polyunsaturated fatty acids and risk of colorectal cancer: a prospective study. *Am J Epidemiol* 2005; **161**(5):462–471.

8. Elwood JM, Little J, Elwood JH. *Epidemiology and Control of Neural Tube Defects*. Oxford: Oxford University Press; 1992.

9. Hibbard ED, Smithells RW. Folic acid metabolism and human embryopathy. *Lancet* 1965; **1**:1254–1256.

10. Smithells RW, Sheppard S, Schorah CJ. Vitamin deficiencies and neural tube defects. *Arch Dis Child* 1976; **51**(12):944–950.

11. Smithells RW, Sheppard S, Schorah CJ, Seller MJ, Nevin NC, Harris R, et al. Apparent prevention of neural tube defects by periconceptional vitamin supplementation. *Arch Dis Child* 1981; **56**(12):911–918.

12. MRC (Medical Research Council) Vitamin Study Group. Prevention of neural tube defects: results of the Medical Research Council Vitamin Study. *Lancet* 1991; **338**(8760):131–137.

13. De Wals P, Tairou F, Van Allen MI, Uh SH, Lowry RB, Sibbald B, et al. Reduction in neural-tube defects after folic acid fortification in Canada. *N Engl J Med* 2007; **357**(2):135–142.

14. Foulkes WD, Brunet J-S, Sieh W, Black MJ, Shenouda G, Narod SA. Familial risks of squamous cell carcinoma of the head and neck: retrospective case-control study. *BMJ* 1996; **313**(7059):716–721.

15. Ghebreyesus TA, Haile M, Witten KH, Getachew A, Yohannes AM, Yohannes M, et al. Incidence of malaria among children living near dams in northern Ethiopia: community based incidence survey. *BMJ* 1999; **319**:663–666.

16. Freedman B. Equipoise and the ethics of clinical research. *N Engl J Med* 1987; **317**(3):141–145.

17. **British Medical Journal**. Fifty years of randomised controlled trials. *BMJ* 1998; **317**(7167):1167–1248.

18. **Doll R**. Controlled trials: the 1948 watershed. *BMJ* 1998; **317**(7167):1217–1220.

19. **Yoshioka A**. Use of randomisation in the Medical Research Council's clinical trial of streptomycin in pulmonary tuberculosis in the 1940s. *BMJ* 1998; **317**(7167):1220–1223.

20. **Fisher-Box J**. *RA Fisher: The Life of a Scientist*. New York: John Wiley and Sons; 1978.

21. **Fibiger J**. Om serumbehandlung af Difteri. *Hospitalstidende* 1898; **6**:309–325.

22. **Chalmers I, Clarke M**. Commentary: The 1944 patulin trial: the first properly controlled multicentre trial conducted under the aegis of the British Medical Research Council. *Int J Epidemiol* 2004; **33**(2):253–260.

23. **McCord J**. A thirty year follow-up of treatment effects. *Am Psychol* 1978; **33**(3):284–289.

24. **Smith AFM**. Mad cows and ecstasy: chance and choice in an evidence-based society. *J R Statist Soc Series A* 1996; **159**(3):367–383.

25. **Hill JD, Hampton JR, Mitchell JRA**. A randomised trial of home-versus-hospital management for patients with suspected myocardial infarction. *Lancet* 1978; **311**(8069):837–841.

26. **Thornley B, Adams C**. Content and quality of 2000 controlled trials in schizophrenia over 50 years. *BMJ* 1998; **317**(7167):1181–1184.

27. **ISIS-4 (Fourth International Study of Infarct Survival Collaborative Group)**. ISIS-4: A randomised factorial trial assessing early oral captopril, oral mononitrate, and intravenous magnesium sulphate in 58 050 patients with suspected acute myocardial infarction. *Lancet* 1995; **345**(8951):669–685.

28. **Shapiro S, Venet W, Strax P, Venet L, Roeser R**. Ten- to fourteen- year effect of screening on breast cancer mortality. *J Natl Cancer Inst* 1982; **69**:349–355.

29. **Altman DG, Schulz KF, Moher D, Egger M, Davidoff F, Elbourne D, et al**. The revised CONSORT statement for reporting randomized trials: explanation and elaboration. *Ann Intern Med* 2001; **134**(8):663–694.

30. **Hills M, Armitage P**. The two-period cross-over clinical trial. *Br J Clin Pharmacol* 1979; **8**:7–20.

31. **Schrader H, Stovner LJ, Helde G, Sand T, Bovim G**. Prophylactic treatment of migraine with angiotensin converting enzyme inhibitor (lisinopril): randomised, placebo controlled, crossover study. *BMJ* 2001; **322**(7277):19–22.

32. **Cook DJ**. Randomized trials in single subjects: the N of 1 study. *Psychopharmacol Bull* 1996; **32**(3):363–367.

33. **March L, Irwig L, Schwarz J, Simpson J, Chock C, Brooks P**. n of 1 trials comparing a non-steroidal anti-inflammatory drug with paracetamol in osteoarthritis. *BMJ* 1994; **309**(6961):1041–1046.

34. **Ukoumunne OC, Gulliford MC, Chinn S, Sterne JAC, Burney PGJ, Donner A**. Methods in health service research. Evaluation of health interventions at area and organisation level. *BMJ* 1999; **319**(7206):376–379.

35. **Adish AA, Esrey SA, Gyorkos TW, Jean-Baptiste J, Rojhani A**. Effect of consumption of food cooked in iron pots on iron status and growth of young children: a randomised trial. *Lancet* 1999; **353**(9154):712–716.

36. **English DR, Burton RC, Del Mar CB, Donovan RJ, Ireland PD, Emery G**. Evaluation of aid to diagnosis of pigmented skin lesions in general practice: controlled trial randomised by practice. *BMJ* 2003; **327**(7411):375–380.

37. **Bunker CB, Barnes JA, Mosteller F (Eds.)**. *Costs, Risks and Benefits of Surgery*. New York: Oxford; 1977.

38. **Ruffin JM, Grizzle JE, Hightower NC, McHardy G, Shull H, Kirsner JB**. A co-operative double-blind evaluation of gastric 'freezing' in the treatment of duodenal ulcer. *N Engl J Med* 1969; **281**(1):16–19.

39. **Goldacre B**. *Bad Science*. London: Fourth Estate; 2008.

40. **Arnold FA, Dean HT, Jay P, Knutson JW**. Effect of fluoridated public water supplies on dental caries prevalence. Tenth year of the Grand Rapids-Muskegon study. *Public Health Rep* 1956; **71**(7):652–658.

41. **Farquhar JW, Fortmann SP, Maccoby N, Haskell WL, Williams PT, Flora JA, et al**. The Stanford five-city project: design and methods. *Am J Epidemiol* 1985; **122**(2):323–334.

42. **Fortmann SP, Flora JA, Winkleby MA, Schooler C, Taylor CB, Farquhar JW**. Community intervention trials: reflections on the Stanford five-city project experience. *Am J Epidemiol* 1995; **142**(6):576–586.

43. **Soderstrom L, Woods WG, Bernstein M, Robison LL, Tuchman M, Lemieux B**. Health and economic benefits of well-designed evaluations: some lessons from evaluating neuroblastoma screening. *J Natl Cancer Inst* 2005; **97**(15):1118–1124.

44. **Smithells RW, Sheppard S, Wild J, Schorah CJ**. Prevention of neural tube defect recurrences in Yorkshire: final report (letter). *Lancet* 1989; **2**(8661):498–499.

45. **Selikoff IJ, Churg J, Hammond EC**. Asbestos exposure, smoking and neoplasia. *JAMA* 1968; **204**(2):106–112.

46. **Doll R, Hill AB**. Mortality in relation to smoking: ten years observations of British doctors. *BMJ* 1964; **i**:1399–1410.

47. **Doll R, Gray R, Hafner B, Peto R**. Mortality in relation to smoking: 22 years' observations on female British doctors. *BMJ* 1980; **i**:967–971.

48. **Hennekens CH, Speizer FE, Rosner B, Bain CJ, Belanger C, Peto R**. Use of permanent hair dyes and cancer among registered nurses. *Lancet* 1979; **1**(8131):1390–1393.

49. **Stampfer MJ, Colditz GA, Willett WC, Manson JE, Rosner B, Speizer FE, et al**. Postmenopausal estrogen therapy and cardiovascular disease. Ten-year follow-up from the Nurses Health Study. *N Engl J Med* 1991; **325**(11):756–762.

50. **Dawber TR**. *The Framingham Study: The Epidemiology of Atherosclerotic Disease*. Cambridge, MA: Harvard University Press; 1980.

51. **Wilson PW**. Established risk factors and coronary artery disease: the Framingham Study. *Am J Hypertens* 1994; **7**(7 Pt 2):7S–12S.

52 **Wadsworth M, Kuh D, Richards M, Hardy R**. Cohort Profile: The 1946 National Birth Cohort (MRC National Survey of Health and Development). *Int J Epidemiol* 2006; **35**(1):49–54.

53. **Poulton R, Caspi A, Milne BJ, Thomson WM, Taylor A, Sears MR, et al**. Association between children's experience of socioeconomic disadvantage and adult health: a life-course study. *Lancet* 2002; **360**(9346):1640–1645.

54. **Susser E, Terry MB**. A conception-to-death cohort. *Lancet* 2003; **361**(9360):797–798.

55. **Manolio TA, Weis BK, Cowie CC, Hoover RN, Hudson K, Kramer BS, et al**. New models for large prospective studies: is there a better way? *Am J Epidemiol* 2012; **175**(9):859–866.

56. **Collins R**. What makes UK Biobank special? *Lancet* 2012; **379**(9822):1173–1174.

57. **Allen N, Sudlow C, Downey P, Peakman T, Danesh J, Elliott P, et al**. UK Biobank: Current status and what it means for epidemiology. *Health Policy Technol* 2012; **1**(3):123–126.

58. **Bingham S, Riboli E**. Diet and cancer—the European Prospective Investigation into Cancer and Nutrition. *Nat Rev Cancer* 2004; **4**(3):206–215.

59. **Herbst AL, Ulfelder H, Poskanzer DC**. Adenocarcinoma of the vagina: association of maternal stilbestrol therapy with tumor appearance in young women. *N Engl J Med* 1971; **284**(16):878–881.

60. **Doll R, Hill AB**. Smoking and carcinoma of the lung. Preliminary report. *BMJ* 1950; **2**(4682):739–748.

61. **Doll R, Hill AB**. A study of the aetiology of carcinoma of the lung. *BMJ* 1952; **2**(4797):1271–1286.

62. **Doll R, Peto R**. Mortality in relation to smoking: 20 years' observations on male British doctors. *BMJ* 1976; **ii**:1525–1536.

63. **Keating C**. *Smoking Kills: The Revolutionary Life of Richard Doll*. London: Interlink Signal; 2009.

64. **MacGregor JE, Moss SM, Parkin DM, Day NE**. A case-control study of cervical cancer screening in north east Scotland. *BMJ* 1985; **290**:1543–1546.

65. **Selby JV, Friedman GD, Quesenberry CP, Jr.**, Weiss NS. Effect of fecal occult blood testing on mortality from colorectal cancer: a case-control study. *Ann Intern Med* 1993; **118**:1–6.

66. **Weiss NS, McKnight B, Stevens NG**. Approaches to the analysis of case-control studies of the efficacy of screening for cancer. *Am J Epidemiol* 1992; **135**(7):817–823.

67. **Aitken JF, Elwood JM, Baade PD, Youl P, English DR**. Clinical whole-body skin examination reduces the incidence of thick melanomas. *Int J Cancer* 2010; **126**(2):450–458.

68. **Berwick M, Begg CB, Fine JA, Roush GC, Barnhill RL**. Screening for cutaneous melanoma by skin self-examination. *J Natl Cancer Inst* 1996; **88**(1):17–23.

69. **Fentiman IS, Cuzick J, Millis RR, Hayward JL**. Which patients are cured of breast cancer? *BMJ* 1984; **289**:1108–1111.

70. **Taffler RJ**. Forecasting company failure in the UK using discriminant analysis of financial ratio data. *J R Statist Soc* 1982; **145**(3):342–358.

71. **Pan SY, Johnson KC, Ugnat AM, Wen SW, Mao Y**. Association of obesity and cancer risk in Canada. *Am J Epidemiol* 2004; **159**(3):259–268.

72. **Redelmeier DA, Tibshirani RJ**. Association between cellular-telephone calls and motor vehicle collisions. *N Engl J Med* 1997; **336**(7):453–458.

73. **Pauletto P, Puato M, Caroli MG, Casiglia E, Munhambo AE, Cazzolato G, et al**. Blood pressure and atherogenic lipoprotein profiles of fish-diet and vegetarian villagers in Tanzania: the Lugalawa study. *Lancet* 1996; **348**(9030):784–788.

74. **Moser C, Kalton G**. *Survey Methods in Social Investigation*. London: Heinemann; 1979.

75. **Bailey KD**. *Methods of Social Research*. New York: Free Press; 1978.

76. **Cartwright A**. *Health Surveys in Practice and in Potential: A Critical Review of Their Scope and Methods*. London: King Edward's Hospital Fund for London; 1983.

77. **Törnberg SA, Carstensen JM**. Relationship between Quetelet's index and cancer of breast and female genital tract in 47,000 women followed for 25 years. *Br J Cancer* 1994; **69**(2):358–361.

Chapter 4

The results obtained from studies of causation

When you can measure what you are speaking about, and express it in numbers,
you know something about it; but when you cannot measure it, when you cannot
express it in numbers, your knowledge is of a meagre and unsatisfactory kind:
it may be the beginning of knowledge, but you have scarcely, in your thoughts,
advanced to the stage of science.

—William Thomson, Lord Kelvin: *Popular Lectures and Addresses*; 1891–94

Introduction

In Chapter 3, we reviewed a classification of study design which separated the criteria used to select the groups of individuals to be compared, from the time relationships of the study. The logic of this system will appear clear when we discuss the results obtained from these studies. The format of the results and therefore the appropriate methods of interpreting them depend on the groups being compared. The extent to which particular problems and biases occur depends largely on the time relationships.

Cohort and intervention studies

The cohort design applies both to observational cohort studies and to intervention trials. In this design we are comparing groups of individuals who are classified by their exposure to the putative causal factor. The simplest situation is with two groups, 'exposed' and 'non-exposed'. This will often be the real situation; for example, we might compare women using oral contraceptives with women who do not use oral contraceptives, or patients on one therapy with patients on another. In other situations, the cohorts may be more numerous and may be ordered, such as groups of individuals characterized by the amount they smoke, or groups of patients with different severities of disease. The format of the results in any cohort study is the same. The same method of analysis is used for aetiological studies looking at individuals exposed to external agents in the environment, observational studies comparing the outcome of groups of patients given different therapies, and randomized trials. It makes no difference to the analysis whether the cohort study is prospective (where subjects were identified at the start of the study and followed forward in time), or retrospective, where the subjects are identified using records and their experience up to the current time provides the outcome data.

Table 4.1 Results of a cohort study of mothers with epilepsy, comparing those treated with valproic acid with those treated with another drug, in regard to the occurrence of major malformations in their offspring.

Exposure	Number of infants			Prevalence of malformation (%)
	Malformed	**Not malformed**	**Total**	
Valproic acid	44	671	715	6.15
No valproic acid	47	1663	1710	2.75

Source: data from Morrow J et al., 'Malformation risks of antiepileptic drugs in pregnancy: a prospective study from the UK Epilepsy and Pregnancy Register', *Journal of Neurology, Neurosurgery, and Psychiatry*, Volume 77, Issue 2, pp. 193–198, © 2006 British Medical Journal Publishing Group [1].

The simplest situation is illustrated by Table 4.1 which shows the results of a study in expectant mothers who had epilepsy during pregnancy, which was treated with one antiepileptic drug. The comparison is between those treated with one specific drug, valproic acid, and those treated with other single agents. Mothers with epilepsy who required no drug treatment and those who received two or more drugs are excluded, as they are likely to have less or more severe epilepsy. The data come from a prospective cohort study in the UK, based on enrolments of women during pregnancy from both general practitioners and specialists [1]. Being a study of pregnancy outcome, the follow-up period is fixed and relatively short, and the outcome of interest is the frequency of a major congenital abnormality in the offspring. The results therefore have a simple format. For each group of mothers, exposed and unexposed, we have the number of infants delivered, and the number of these infants who has an abnormality.

The results show the two proportions, or prevalence rates at birth. If there were no difference in outcome between the two groups—that is, if the 'null hypothesis' were true—the prevalence rates in the two groups would be the same, apart from random variations. It is logical to compare either the difference in the rates, or the ratio of the rates, and these considerations lead to important and widely used epidemiological measures. Box 4.1 shows the measures which can be derived.

Relative risk and relative odds

The '*relative risk*' or '*risk ratio*' is the ratio of the rate of disease among those exposed (mothers using valproic acid) to the rate in those not exposed (mothers taking other drugs), and being a ratio has no units. In this example, the relative risk is 2.24.

We can also consider a further measure, which is the '*odds ratio*'. The odds of a baby in the exposed group being malformed are 44:671 (approximately 1 in 15), compared to the odds in the unexposed group of 47:1663 (about 1 in 35). The ratio of these is the odds ratio, 2.32, which is similar but not identical to the relative risk. The odds ratio and the relative risk are similar where the frequency of the outcome is low; they diverge as the outcome becomes more frequent. For example, if the prevalence in the exposed group were 50 per cent (odds 1:1), and that in the unexposed group were 25 per cent (odds 1:3), the risk ratio is 2, but the odds ratio is 3. For both relative risk and odds

Box 4.1 Derivation of measures of association, from the results of the cohort study shown in Table 4.1.

Note: in this and subsequent tables, the calculations are shown with limited decimal places for clarity, but the calculations themselves are carried out from the basic data, to avoid rounding error

	RESULTS OF A COHORT STUDY (2)			
Exposure	**Number of infants**			**Prevalence of malformation (%)**
	Malformed	**Not malformed**	**Total**	
Valproic acid	44	671	715	6.15
No valproic acid	47	1663	1710	2.75
Whole population	91	2344	2425	3.75

(assuming sample is representative)

RR, Relative risk, or risk ratio, = $6.15 / 2.75 = 2.24$

OR, Odds ratio, = $(44/671)/(47/1663) = 2.32$

AR, Attributable risk, or risk difference = $6.15 - 2.75 = 3.41\%$

AP_{exp}, *Attributable proportion in exposed subjects*, = attributable risk/total risk in exposed = $3.41 / 6.15 = 55.3\%$

Also, $AP_{exp} = (RR - 1) / RR = (2.24 - 1) / 2.24 = 55.3\%$

AP_{pop}, *Attributable proportion in the population*:

For the whole population, risk = 3.75 per cent

Attributable proportion in the whole population = $(3.75 - 2.75) / 3.75 = 26.8\%$ (using full data to avoid rounding errors)

More generally, where p = the proportion of the population exposed, estimated from the study or from other sources, the attributable proportion in the population is given by

$$AP_{pop} = \frac{p(RR - 1)}{p(RR - 1) + 1}$$

Here $p = 715 / 2425 = 29.4\%$

So $AP_{pop} = 26.8$ per cent

Source: data from Morrow J et al., 'Malformation risks of antiepileptic drugs in pregnancy: a prospective study from the UK Epilepsy and Pregnancy Register', *Journal of Neurology, Neurosurgery, and Psychiatry*, Volume 77, Issue 2, pp. 193–198, © 2006 British Medical Journal Publishing Group [1].

ratio, the value of 1.0 corresponds to the situation of no association between exposure and outcome.

Risk difference (attributable risk)

The difference between the two rates is the '*risk difference*', and has the same units as the risk measure. It is sometimes called the '*attributable risk*', but this is less satisfactory as it assumes that there is a causal relationship. The risk difference gives, in absolute terms, the frequency of the outcome which is associated with the exposure. In this example, the attributable risk is 3.41 per cent. If there were no association present, the risk difference would be zero.

If we divide the attributable risk by the total risk in the exposed group, the result (assuming causation) is the proportion of disease in those exposed which is associated with the exposure; this may be called the '*attributable proportion in exposed subjects*'. Here it is 3.41/6.15 = 55 per cent. It is also known as the '*aetiological fraction*' in exposed subjects. If all the difference in risks is due to causation, this measures the proportion of the outcomes that would be prevented in exposed subjects if the causal agent were removed. The attributable proportion in the exposed is also given from the risk ratio as (RR − 1)/RR.

If for the population under study the proportion of subjects who are exposed is known, the proportion of total disease in the population which is associated with the causal factor can be calculated; this is the '*attributable proportion in the population*', or '*population aetiological fraction*'. In this example it is 27 per cent. Again, if all the difference in risks is due to causation, this measures the proportion of the outcomes that would be prevented in the population if the causal agent were removed.

The uses of risk difference and relative risk

The risk difference, unlike relative risk, describes the absolute quantity of the outcome which is associated with the exposure. It is therefore useful in considering the practical implications of studies, once a decision has been reached that the association represents causation. Thus a comparison of the attributable risks in terms of total mortality conferred by a number of environmental exposures gives an indication of how much mortality will be prevented by successful action on each one of the exposures, and such an approach has been useful in setting priorities for public health and health promotion campaigns. A similar consideration in terms of the long-term outcome of a complex disease such as diabetes, whose course may be influenced by a large number of factors, may be used to indicate what aspects of care, if dealt with successfully, will result in the greatest improvements in outcome. Attributable risk is therefore particularly useful in well-researched situations where the implications of soundly supported results are being considered. It is of less value in the preliminary stages of assessment of a possible causal relationship.

The great advantage of the relative risk estimate is the empirical finding that in many human disease situations, the relative risk of disease incidence or mortality associated with a particular exposure is fairly constant over a wide range of populations and groups of subjects, even where other factors differ. If the relative risk for a particular exposure is the same in two different populations, but because of differences in other factors the total risks of the outcome are different, then the attributable risks will be different. In comparing evidence from a number of sources concerning a particular causal relationship, it is more reasonable to expect consistency in terms of relative risk than of attributable risk. This property of consistency makes relative risk more valuable in evaluating whether a particular relationship is or is not likely to be causal. It is also rather easier to predict the effects of non-causal factors on the observed relative risk than on the observed attributable risk.

There is another important reason for concentrating on relative risk, and that is because this measure, unlike attributable risk, can be derived from any of the main study designs. As will be shown, case–control studies provide estimates of relative risk (by the odds ratio), but do not provide direct measures of attributable risk. For these reasons the relative risk is the more useful index to summarize the results of a study in order to discuss the interpretation of the association. In the rest of this book we will therefore concentrate on the interpretation of relative risk.

Preventive factors, and application to intervention studies; number needed to treat

If the factor under consideration is protective, the rate of outcome in the exposed group will be less than in the unexposed group, and therefore the relative risk will be less than one, and the risk difference will be negative. There is no difficulty with this apart from terminology.

Table 4.2 shows the result of a large-scale randomized trial in which patients with myocardial infarction (a heart attack) were treated with a new drug ('captopril'), and compared to a placebo group [2]. This was a very large trial with about 29 000 subjects in each group. As shown, there was a protective effect of the new drug, with a relative risk of 0.94, and a risk difference of −4.9 deaths per 1000 subjects. Rather than calling this a risk difference or, if we assume causality, an attributable risk of −4.9 deaths per 1000, a better terminology is to call it an *attributable benefit* of 4.9 deaths averted per 1000 subjects. We can also simply refer to this absolute benefit as the 'number of deaths averted per 1000 treated', which will be again 4.9. We can also invert that figure, and express the results of the trial in terms of the 'number of subjects treated with the new drug to prevent one death', often called the *'number needed to treat'* (NNT). This is 1000/4.9, or approximately 200. This is an easily understandable and readily applicable figure [3]. Thus the result of this study (assuming we interpret it as a causal relationship) is that treatment of these patients with this new drug resulted in a reduction in death rate, with one death averted for every 200 subjects treated. Whether this benefit is worthwhile will depend on how it is balanced by the disadvantages of the new drug, in terms of side effects, costs, and so on. (More correctly, one death is averted for every 200 offered treatment, as not all those randomized to captopril would have necessarily accepted it or taken the full dosages.)

Consider what would happen if the relative effect of the drug were the same, that is, a relative risk of 0.94, but the death rate of both the treated and the comparison groups were higher, as would happen if the treatment were offered to patients with particularly severe disease. If the relative risk is constant, and the mortality rate in the

Table 4.2 Results of a clinical trial: number needed to treat. Results of randomized trial of a drug treatment (captopril) in patients with suspected myocardial infarction; deaths in first 35 days. From ISIS-4 study [2]. As noted in Box 4.1, calculations avoid rounding errors, which is why the risk difference is −4.9, not −5.0 from the simple calculation shown.

Actual results

	Deaths	Survivors	Total	Death rate per 1000
Treated with captopril	2088	26940	29028	71.9
Placebo group	2231	26791	29022	76.9

$$\text{Relative risk} = 71.9/76.9 = 0.94$$
$$\text{Risk difference per 1000} = 71.9{-}76.9 = -4.9$$
$$\text{Deaths averted per 1000 treated} = 76.9{-}71.9 = 4.9$$
$$\text{Number treated to prevent one death} = 1000/4.9 = 202$$

Hypothetical results if relative risk remains the same, but baseline mortality rate doubles

	Deaths	Survivors	Total	Death rate per 1000
Treated with captopril	4176	24852	29028	143.9
Placebo group	4462	24560	29022	153.7

$$\text{Relative risk} = 143.9/153.7 = 0.94$$
$$\text{Risk difference per 1000} = 143.9{-}153.7 = -9.9$$
$$\text{Deaths averted per 1000 treated} = 153.7{-}143.9 = 9.9$$
$$\text{Number treated to prevent one death} = 1000/9.9 = 101$$

Source: data from ISIS-4 (Fourth International Study of Infarct Survival Collaborative Group), 'ISIS-4: A randomised factorial trial assessing early oral captopril, oral mononitrate, and intravenous magnesium sulphate in 58 050 patients with suspected acute myocardial infarction', *The Lancet*, Volume 345, Issue 8951, pp. 669–685, © 1995 Published by Elsevier Ltd [2].

non-treated group is doubled, the number of deaths averted per 1000 treated (the attributable benefit) is doubled, and the number treated to prevent one death (NNT) falls to about 100. The difference between 100 patients treated to avert one death, and 200, could well be important in terms of the comparison with ill effects and costs. Although in this example only the data on early mortality are shown, the overall results of this major study looking at longer-term mortality gave essentially similar results and from consideration of this plus other literature, the authors indeed concluded that the use of the captopril therapy would save about one life per 200 treated in average-risk patients, and about one per 100 treated in higher-risk groups.

Perceptions given by relative and absolute risks: framing

The association shown by studies can therefore be expressed as a ratio measurement, or a measurement on an absolute scale. Results which are actually the same can produce different impressions when presented in different ways, an effect referred to as 'framing', and the question of whether relative or absolute measurement of benefits or risks should be used can be controversial. Effects expressed as absolute benefits are often numerically smaller than when expressed as relative risks, and often have a lesser impact [4], for example, on influencing doctors to prescribe cholesterol-lowering drugs [5]. In a population survey, 80 per cent of people said they would accept a screening test when presented with data on relative risk reduction, while only 45 per cent would accept it when given equivalent data expressed as number needed to screen [6]. Both absolute and relative measures have value. The trial just described showed a very useful property of relative risk, in that this was fairly constant over the range of underlying absolute mortality rates. The absolute benefit measure, which can be expressed as the number needed to treat to avert one outcome, is very useful in regard to clinical and cost implications. For example, early randomized trials of an important new drug for breast cancer (the monoclonal antibody trastuzumab, Herceptin), showed that adding this drug in standard therapy gave a relative risk of 0.67, a one-third reduction in the average death rate [7]. The absolute mortality reduction was a reduction from 8.3 per cent mortality to 5.7 per cent with 3 years of follow-up, a risk difference of 2.6 per cent, giving a number needed to treat of 38 (1/0.026). Thus treating 38 eligible women with the new drug would result in one less death; as the cost was about US \$50 000 for each woman treated, the cost of averting one death would be about US \$2 million.

Understandably, these important new results led to considerable discussion in terms of appropriate drug costs and therefore drug approval and funding. Later work with longer follow-up give a similar relative risk, conferring a greater absolute mortality reduction, so the number needed to treat reduces.

Person-time as the denominator of rates

In the data for pregnancies in Box 4.1, the outcome measure is the proportion of malformed births. In cohort studies of other outcomes, the follow-up time is not fixed and may not be the same for each subject. Consider a cohort study in which men are classified by their level of exercise, and subsequently the occurrence of deaths from heart disease is recorded. Each subject contributes information from the time he enters the study until his death, until the end of the follow-up period, or until some specified time at which the data collection ends. Some subjects may leave the study before any of these end points; they are 'censored', or become 'lost to follow-up', but still contribute to the study up to the time at which their outcome status was last known. To assess the incidence rate, the number of heart disease deaths is divided by the total follow-up period: that is, the sum of the follow-up times for all individuals, expressed as person-time (person-years, man-months, etc.).

Example

One of the classic studies showing a relationship between physical exercise and coronary heart disease mortality was the prospective cohort study of longshoremen (dock workers) in San Francisco, California, USA [8]. Between 1951 and 1961, men who were assessed at a health screening clinic and were aged 35–74 were entered into the study; men first assessed at a younger age entered the study when they turned 35. The follow-up continued until death, attaining the age of 75, the end of the follow-up period in 1972, or the date of loss to follow-up. Less than 1 per cent were lost to follow-up. Thus the follow-up varied from very short, if an early death occurred, to 22 years. In total, 6351 men entered the study, contributing 92 645 man-years of experience; there were 598 deaths from coronary heart disease, giving a crude death rate of 598/92 645 = 64.5 deaths per 10 000 man-years. This total incidence rate in this example is the average for the whole follow-up period. If the rate of outcome varies greatly over the follow-up period this simple average will not be adequate, and more complex methods of analysis are necessary. As the issues of interpretation can be adequately dealt with using simple data, such methods are not discussed here but are presented in Chapter 8 (time-to-event methods).

More than one causal agent

Table 4.3 shows death rates from cardiovascular disease in cohorts of women defined by two exposures, smoking and contraceptive usage, from a large prospective cohort study [9]. Women exposed to neither oral contraceptives nor smoking had a cardiovas-cular death rate of 3.0 per 100 000 woman-years. Those who smoked but did not use oral contraceptives had a rate of 8.9/100 000, while those who used oral contraceptives but did not smoke had a rate of 13.8/100 000. We can call the women who were exposed to neither factor as the baseline or 'referent' group, and to consider attributable risks and relative risks as compared to this group. What rate would we expect in women who both used oral contraceptives and smoked?

To derive an expected rate, we must make an assumption about how the two expo-sures may interact; that is, we must assume a 'model' for this. There are an infinity of possibilities, but there are two that are simple and seem reasonably possible.

We could assume the effects add together, using absolute risks. Thus, women who are exposed to both agents will have the baseline risk of the unexposed group (3.0 per 100 000), plus the attributable risk associated with smoking (5.9), plus the attributable

Table 4.3 Two causal factors. Results of a prospective cohort study comparing women classified by smoking habit and oral contraceptive (OC) use in terms of deaths from circulatory system diseases. For effects of joint exposure, see text.

Exposure	Mortality from circulatory system diseases, per 100 000 woman-years	Relative risk	Attributable risk/10^5 woman-years
Non-smoker, no OC use	3.0	1.0	0 (referent)
Smoker, no OC use	8.9	3.0	5.9
Non-smoker, OC user	13.8	4.6	10.8
Smoker, OC user	?	?	?

Source: data from Royal College of General Practitioners, 'Mortality among oral-contraceptive users: Royal College of General Practitioners' Oral Contraception Study', The *Lancet*, Volume 310, Issue 8041, pp. 727–731, © 1977 Published by Elsevier Ltd [9].

risk due to oral contraceptive use (10.8). So, assuming an *additive* model, their expected cardiovascular mortality rate will be 3.0 + 5.9 + 10.8 = 19.7 deaths per 100 000 woman-years. The relative risk for the group exposed to both factors, compared to the unexposed, is 19.7/3.0 = 6.6. We can derive the same figure using relative risk estimates by combining what is called the *excess relative risk*, which is the relative risk minus one. The additive calculation therefore is the excess relative risk from smoking (3.0 − 1 = 2.0), added to the excess relative risk from oral contraceptive use (4.6 − 1 = 3.6) plus the baseline relative risk (1.0), which sums to give us 6.6 as the relative risk for subjects with both exposures, compared to those with neither.

The other simple hypothesis is that the risks multiply together, and use the relative risks from the table. As smoking increases an individual's risk by 3.0 times, and oral contraceptive use increases it by 4.6 times, then the joint effect of smoking and oral contraceptive use, assuming a *multiplicative* model, may increase the risk by 3.0 × 4.6, that is, 13.8 times. We multiply this 13.8 relative risk with the baseline absolute risk of 3.0 deaths per 100 000 woman-years to get an expected death rate for women with both exposures of 41.4 deaths per 100 000 woman-years.

Because this was a big study, we can compare these predictions with what actually happened. In fact, the cardiovascular death rate in women who both smoked and were exposed to oral contraceptives was 39.5 per 100 000 woman-years. The multiplicative model is the better fit to the data. We should be cautious, however, as the numbers of deaths in each group shown in Table 4.3 are small (2, 3, 5, and 19 in the four groups) and more information would be needed to be confident that the multiplicative model is a better fit to the data than the additive model. This example is based on an early report of this cohort study with follow-up from the start of the study 1968 to 1976. A later report from this study, based on follow-up to 1993, showed that the increased mortality from circulatory diseases is largely restricted to current and recent users of oral contraceptives [10]; and a further report from another cohort study of the topic showed that the increase in deaths from ischaemic heart disease associated with oral contraceptive use was confined to heavy smokers [11].

Case–control studies

The other major design is the case–control study, comparing a group of individuals who have experienced the outcome under study with a group who have not. For each subject in the study, their exposure to the factor under consideration is ascertained retrospectively. The results appear as a 2 × 2 table as shown in Table 4.4 and Table 4.5. In the case–control design, a sample of all available cases is taken ($a + c$), and independently a sample of unaffected subjects (controls) is drawn ($b + d$). As these two groups are sampled separately, rates of disease in the exposed or unexposed groups cannot be calculated, nor can relative risk be directly measured. However, the *odds ratio* can be obtained, and so it is the primary measure of association in case–control studies.

Note the simple algebra of the calculation of odds ratio; the number of exposed cases (a) is multiplied by the number opposite it on the diagonal of the table, and this result is then divided by the two other numbers multiplied together; because of this simple arithmetic, the odds ratio is sometimes referred to as the *cross-products ratio*.

Table 4.4 Simplest form of results for a case–control study. The odds ratio, or relative odds, is the key measure of association. Because of the sampling used, the total number of exposed subjects is not a + b, and the risk in exposed subjects is not a/(a + b); see text for explanation.

	Cases	Controls
Exposed	a	b
Unexposed	c	d
	a + c	b + d

Odds ratio = (a/b)/(c/d)
            = ad/bc the 'cross-products' ratio

Table 4.5 shows the results of a case–control study in which 1391 births with anencephalus, a severe and fatal abnormality, were compared to 5000 live births, the exposure being the mother's past history of a stillbirth [12]. The odds ratio is 4.13, showing a strong association. As OR is a close estimate of the risk ratio if the outcome is not

Table 4.5 Format of results from a case–control study assessing the relationship between a history of a previous stillbirth and the occurrence of anencephalus. Mothers of all notified babies with anencephalus in a defined population form the case series (*n* = 1391); an arbitrary number of 5000 mothers of liveborn babies were chosen as controls.

	Cases Numbers	Controls Numbers
Exposed (one or more previous stillbirths)	141	133
Unexposed (no previous stillbirths)	1250	4867
	1391	5000

(a) Odds ratio = (141 × 4867)/(133 × 1250) = 4.13

(b) Relative risk undetermined but will be similar to relative odds as other information shows that anencephalus is uncommon (about 1–2 per 1000 births).

Attributable risk undetermined.

Attributable proportion in exposed subjects $= \dfrac{4.13 - 1}{4.13} = 75.8\%$

Attributable proportion in population; if controls are representative of all unaffected births, then prevalence of exposure p = 133/5000 = 0.0266 and attributable proportion in the population

$$= \frac{p(RR - 1)}{p(RR - 1) + 1} = \frac{0.0266 \times 3.13}{(0.0266 \times 3.13) + 1} = 7.7\%$$

Source: data from Elwood JM, Raman S, and Mousseau G, 'Reproductive history in the mothers of anencephalics', *Journal of Chronic Disease*, Volume 31, Issue 6–7, pp. 473–481, © 1978 Published by Elsevier Inc [12].

frequent, the attributable proportion in exposed subjects can be estimated as $(OR - 1)/OR$, which gives 76 per cent; which is only meaningful if causation is assumed. The attributable proportion in the population can be calculated if the prevalence of exposure in the population is known, usually from another source. The proportions of cases and of control that are exposed are valid estimates, and may be useful in description; 10.1 per cent of cases were exposed, compared to 2.7 per cent of controls. The ratio of these proportions is not useful: the ratio of the odds of exposure in the two groups is the odds ratio.

What cannot be calculated from Table 4.5 is the actual rate of disease in either the exposed or unexposed groups, or the risk difference. If Table 4.5 is misinterpreted, by a failure to consider that the data come from a case–control study, it might be thought that the risk of this defect in births to mothers who had had a previous stillbirth was $141/(141 + 133) = 51$ per cent—an order of magnitude different from the true value, 4.4 per 1000, given in Table 4.6.

To see how these results were derived, Table 4.6 shows the source population, that of all births in certain cities in Canada over a 20-year period. There were 1391 births with anencephalus, all of which were included in the case–control study; and there were 1 193 600 live births, of which only 5000 were selected to form the control series. From Table 4.6, all the measures of risk can be calculated, as shown. Note that the relative odds and the relative risk are virtually the same: this is because the frequency of the disease is low, so the numbers of unaffected and of total subjects are not very different.

Now, return to Table 4.5 and see what measures can be calculated. The odds ratio estimate is valid, differing from that in the whole population only by sampling variation; knowing that the outcome being studied is uncommon allows us to use the odds ratio

Table 4.6 Relationships in a population. The relationships between anencephalus and previous stillbirths in all pregnancies in the population in which the case–control study shown in Table 4.5 was conducted.

	Anencephalus births	Unaffected births	Total births	Prevalence of anencephalus per 1000 births
Previous stillbirth	141	31 750	31 891	4.42
No previous stillbirth	1250	1161 850	1 163 100	1.07
	1391	1193 600	1 194 991	1.16

Relative odds $= (141/31\ 750)/(1250/1\ 161\ 850) = 4.13$

Relative risk $= (141/31\ 891)/(1250/1\ 163\ 100) = 4.11$

Attributable risk $= 4.42 - 1.07 = 3.35$ per 1000 births

Attributable proportion in exposed subjects $= 3.35/4.42 = 75.8\%$

Attributable proportion in population $= (1.16 - 1.07)/1.16 = 7.8\%$

Source: data from Elwood JM, Raman S, and Mousseau G, 'Reproductive history in the mothers of anencephalics', Journal of *Chronic Disease*, Volume 31, Issue 6–7, pp. 473–481, © 1978 Published by Elsevier Inc [12].

as an estimate of relative risk. What cannot be estimated just from the case–control data is the outcome rates in exposed and unexposed subjects, the relative risk, and the risk difference (attributable risk).

The attributable proportion in the exposed can be derived from the odds ratio, and is a good estimate of the result derived from all the data. The attributable proportion in the population can only be derived if we have data on the prevalence of the exposure in the population; in this example, the control group can be considered as a representative sample of the total population, so this proportion is given by the proportion of controls exposed. However, often this is not so; for example, if the controls have been matched to the cases on certain characteristics, they will not be representative of the population and an independent source of evidence will be necessary to give the proportion of the population which is exposed.

Use of the odds ratio

As has been already shown, the odds ratio is a very good estimate of relative risk in most situations, the exception being where the outcome is very frequent. For outcomes which are frequent, cohort designs will be efficient, as only a reasonable number of subjects will have to be followed to obtain an adequate number who experience the outcome under study. The great disadvantage of cohort studies is in attempting to study outcomes which are uncommon, so that many hundreds or thousands of individuals have to be followed before a reasonable number of them experience the outcome. It is in this situation that case–control studies are most useful. Therefore, in most situations for which case–control studies are advantageous, the difference between relative odds and relative risk will be trivial, and certainly much less important than other potential sources of error in the study. So in some literature odds ratios produced from case–control studies may be referred to as relative risks. Odds ratios are also valid measures in their own right, and more complex methods of analysis such as logistic regression (discussed in Chapter 7) use odds ratios as the primary measure of association, even in cohort studies.

Odds ratio from case–control studies: a more formal derivation

(For the more curious reader: others may wish to skip to the next section.) The differences between the results from a case–control study and those from the entire source population arise because the sampling fractions are different for the cases and for the controls. In the study shown in Table 4.5 and Table 4.6, the sampling fraction for the cases was 1.0, and that for the controls was $5000/1\,193\,600 = 0.00419$. Usually in a case–control study, the sampling fractions are unknown, but they will be often of this nature, in that the sampling fraction of the cases will be 1.0 or very high, and the sampling fraction of controls will be very low.

Table 4.7 summarizes the algebra of case–control studies, showing that in the odds ratio calculations the sampling fractions cancel out, and therefore the odds ratio is a direct estimate of the odds ratio in the source population, even if the sampling fractions are unknown. This simple algebra emphasizes a crucial point in the design of case–control studies: the sampling system used for cases must be 'without bias' in respect

Table 4.7 Algebraic justification for the calculation of odds ratio from a case–control study.

	Cases	Controls
Exposed	$a = fA$	$b = gB$
Unexposed	$c = fC$	$d = gD$
	$a + c = f(A + C)$	$b + d = g(B + D)$

odds ratio in population $= (A/B)/(C/D) = AD/BC$
odds ratio in study $= (a/b)/(c/d)$
$\qquad = (fA/gB)/(fC/gD)$
$\qquad = AD/BC$

Capital letters = numbers of individuals in the population (A, B, C, D)
Lower case letters = numbers of individuals in the study (a, b, c, d)
f = sampling fraction for cases = $(a + c)/(A + C)$
g = sampling fraction for controls = $(b + d)/(B + D)$
The essential design characteristic of case–control studies is that the fractions
f and g are the same for both exposed and unexposed subjects

to exposure, that is, the same sampling fraction f must apply to both exposed and un-exposed cases. If that is so, the ratio of the numbers of exposed to unexposed cases in the study will be the same as the ratio in the population. The same logic applies to the controls, which must also be sampled without bias in regard to exposure status, so that the (different) sampling fraction g applies both to exposed and to unexposed controls.

Different sampling schemes in case–control studies: why a case can also be a control; incidence density sampling

The traditional, and intuitively clear at first glance, process of selecting controls in a case–control study is to select them as a representative sample of the *unaffected* subjects from a particular population. In Table 4.8 we present a hypothetical set of data concerning an exposure in pregnancy and a malformation, which is based loosely on the data presented in Table 4.1, but quite deliberately shows a much greater prevalence at birth of the malformation. So in this hypothetical example, the exposure is associated with a relative risk of 4.23, but an odds ratio of 5.65. The substantial difference between these two measures is because the frequency of the malformation overall is quite high.

Now suppose we set up a case–control study in this situation. One design of case–control study would take as cases, a representative sample of malformed infants, and as controls, a representative sample of the *unaffected*, not malformed, infants. We could sample all the malformed infants (260) and an arbitrary sample of 400 of the unaffected infants (there is nothing magical about having an equal number, or a fixed ratio of controls to cases, and the actual size chosen will depend on practical issues such as cost). The numbers in subtable A are calculated by integer numbers given by a random sample of 400 controls. This sample yields an *odds ratio* of 5.61, which is a good estimate of the actual odds ratio of 5.65 in the population, but is clearly different to the relative risk.

Table 4.8 Different sampling schemes for controls in a case–control study. Subtable A shows the whole population data; both odds ratio and relative risk can be calculated. Subtable B shows controls drawn as a random sample of unaffected pregnancies; the results yield the odds ratio. Subtable C shows controls drawn as a random sample of all pregnancies; the results yield relative risk.

(A) Total population

Exposure	Malformed	Not malformed	Total	Prevalence of malformation (%)
Exposed	120	273	393	30.5
Unexposed	140	1799	1939	7.2
Total population	260	2072	2332	11.1

Odds ratio = 5.65

Relative risk (prevalence ratio) = 4.23

(B) Case–control design, sampling controls from non-affected only

Exposure	Malformed	Controls = not malformed
Exposed	120	53
Unexposed	140	347
Total population	260	400

Sample estimate of odds ratio $= (140 \times 347)/(53 \times 140) = 5.61$

(C) Case–control design, sampling controls from all pregnancies

Exposure	Malformed	Controls = not total pregnancies
Exposed	120	67
Unexposed	140	333
Total population	260	400

Sample estimate of relative risk $= (120 \times 333)/(67 \times 140) = 4.26$

A second type of case–control design would again sample all the 260 malformed infants as cases, but take as controls a representative sample of *all infants*. The distribution of the controls would therefore reflect the exposure frequency in the whole population, not just the unaffected babies. The cross products ratio from this design yields directly a sample estimate of *relative risk*, as the control sample represents the total population rather than only the 'non-case' population. As is seen, a good estimate of the relative risk is obtained, which is clearly different from the odds ratio.

The practical ways in which these studies would be carried out would make clear another seemingly complex issue. For the first design, comparing cases with non-cases, malformed infants would be entered into the study as cases as they are recognized; and a sample of non-malformed infants would be chosen, for instance, by selecting a number of such infants from the same hospitals each week and interviewing their mothers as non-diseased controls.

The second design is equally simple. Again, malformed infants would be classified as cases as they occur, but the comparison sample here would be a representative, perhaps random, sample of all births occurring in the birth population which yields the cases. In this sampling design, an affected 'case' infant is also eligible for selection as a control; if that affected infant appears in the representative sample of controls, it should be used as a control. Thus, the same individual can appear as both a case and a control. Although this seems obscure, it is simply analogous to the calculation of any measure of occurrence rate, such as prevalence or incidence rate. In these rates (as noted in Chapter 2), the number of affected individuals is the numerator, and it is divided by the total number of individuals at risk, which of course includes those who are affected. Affected individuals therefore appear in both the numerator and the denominator of a calculated frequency rate. Therefore in a case–control study designed to produce an estimate of the ratio of such rates, that is, a relative risk, the same individual can appear as a case and a control.

Many case–control studies are of the type which directly yields an estimate of the relative risk. A typical design for a case–control study of a chronic disease such as cancer is to enter individuals as cases as soon as they are diagnosed with the disease, and to obtain a control at that time from the entire population from which that case is sampled. The control series therefore provides a sample based on the population at risk at the time when the case became an incident case. The design can be referred to as *incidence density* sampling. The cross products ratio, as in subtable B of Table 4.8, gives an estimate of the relative risk. In this design, an individual can be sampled as a control, and then shortly afterwards could become a case and be eligible to be sampled as a case. This is quite appropriate theoretically.

Surveys

In principle, survey designs yield the same type of results as cohort studies; in cross-sectional surveys, all information on both exposures and outcomes is in terms of prevalence. The terms relative risk, relative odds, and so on may be used, remembering that in this situation these apply to ratios of prevalence rates, rather than ratios of incidence rates as in a prospective cohort design. The use of relative odds is also more limited because frequently in a survey the prevalences of conditions being studied are quite substantial, and therefore the relative odds may be substantially different from the relative risk. Thus in the survey comparing Tanzanian villagers with different diets, the prevalence of borderline or frank hypertension was 38.7 per cent in those with a vegetarian diet, and 12.5 per cent in fish-eaters, giving a prevalence rate ratio of 3.1; the odds ratio is 4.4 [13].

Table 4.9 shows the results of a cross-sectional survey of the prevalence of smoking in a sample of schoolchildren in England, and explores the association, at that point in time, between the parents' current smoking habit and the children's [14]. Where one or both parents smoked, the prevalence of 'ever smoking' in the children was 57.0 per cent; where neither parent smoked, it was 51.5 per cent. The relative risk, the prevalence ratio, is 57.0/51.5 = 1.11. The odds ratio can be calculated, as shown, but tends not to

Table 4.9 Results of a cross-sectional survey in which questionnaires were given to 8–9-year-old subjects in industrial areas of northern England; these results show the smoking history of the subjects, compared with their report on their parents' smoking. Note: for the attributable proportion calculation, rounding errors can be considerable. Thus RR = (3203/5621)/(1601/3109) = 1.1066; (RR − 1)/RR = 0.1066/1.1066 = 9.6 per cent although (1.11 − 1)/1.11 = 9.9 per cent.

Parent's smoking	Smoking in young children		Total	Prevalence, ever smoked (%)
	Ever smoked	Never smoked		
One or both smoke	3203	2418	5621	57.0
Neither smokes	1601	1508	3109	51.5
Total	4804	3926	8730	55.0

Prevalence ratio (relative risk) = $57.0/51.5 = 1.11$

Odds ratio = $(3203/2418)/(1601/1508) = 1.25$

The odds ratio is not a very useful measure, as the prevalence ratio can be calculated as easily, and it is substantially different from the prevalence ratio as the outcome is common.

Attributable risk or prevalence difference = $57.0 - 51.5 = 5.5\%$

Attributable proportion in exposed $= \dfrac{5.5}{57.0} = 9.6\% = \dfrac{(RR-1)}{RR}$

Attributable proportion in population $= \dfrac{55.0-51.5}{55.0} = 6.4\%$

$$= \dfrac{p(RR-1)}{p(RR-1)+1}$$

where $p = 5621/8730 = 0.64$

Source: data from Charlton A., 'Children's coughs related to parental smoking', *British Medical Journal (Clinical Research Edition)*, Volume 288, Issue 6431, pp. 1647–1649, © 1964 BMJ Publishing Group Ltd [14].

be used as it is different from the relative risk as the prevalence of the outcome is high. The attributable risk, and proportions, are calculated as shown and expressed in terms of prevalence.

General applicability of these analytical approaches

We have now presented a format of results for a cohort study, and for a case–control study. The cohort format applies to any study in which the comparison is between two or more groups defined by differences in the exposure. Thus for example, Sloan and colleagues [15] compared the assault and murder rates in Vancouver, Canada, and Seattle, USA, two generally similar cities which have different laws affecting access to firearms. This is a descriptive study, but as the comparison is between the 'exposure' to different legislative systems, the results can be expressed in the format of a cohort study, and show the great excess of assault and murder related to firearms in Seattle compared to Vancouver, contrasting with similar rates of assault and murder involving

Table 4.10 Descriptive study with results in a cohort format. These annual rates of assault and murder in Vancouver (Canada) and Seattle (USA) represent the outcome; the city of residence, and its legal system, is the exposure.

Crime	Annual rate per 100 000 population		Relative risk
	Seattle, USA	Vancouver, Canada	
Aggravated assault using:			
Firearms	87.9	11.4	7.7
Knives	78.1	78.9	1.0
Other means	320.6	330.2	1.0
All aggravated assault	486.5	420.5	1.2
Murder (homicide) using:			
Firearms	4.8	1.0	5.1
Knives	3.1	3.5	0.9
Other means	3.4	2.5	1.3
All homicide	11.3	6.9	1.6

Source: data from Sloan JH et al., 'Handgun regulations, crime, assaults, and homicide', *New England Journal of Medicine*, Volume 319, Number, pp. 1256–1262, © 1998 Massachusetts Medical Society. All rights reserved [15].

other weapons (Table 4.10). Relative risks are calculated, and the other measures shown in Box 4.1 can be derived.

Other surveys may equate to the case–control design, where the essential comparison is between groups with and without the outcome of interest, in which case the format of results applicable to case–control designs is applied.

Self-test questions

Answers in Appendix 1, p.397.

Q4.1 The trial of tuberculosis treatment shown in Chapter 2 showed four deaths from 55 patients treated by streptomycin, compared with 14 deaths from 52 controls. Calculate:

(a) The mortality rates in each group. What type of rates are these?

(b) The relative risk.

(c) The odds ratio.

(d) The attributable risk.

(e) The attributable benefit.

(f) The 'number needed to treat' for one death prevented.

Q4.2 In a cohort study of diet and heart disease in men, the study population is considered in two groups. In the high-fat diet group there were 12 500 man-years of observation and 48 deaths; in the lower-fat group there were 22 000 man-years of observation and 64 deaths. Calculate:

(a) The mortality rates in each group.

(b) The relative risk.

(c) The attributable risk of the high fat diet.

(d) What proportion of disease in the high-fat diet group is attributable to the high-fat diet?

(e) What proportion of disease in the whole population group is attributable to the high-fat diet?

Q4.3 If the incidence rate of asthma is 400 per 10 000 person-years in those who smoke, 100 in those who are exposed to air pollution, and 50 in those with neither exposure, what is the expected incidence in those with both exposures, assuming:

(a) an additive model.

(b) a multiplicative model.

Q4.4 In a case–control study of arthritis of the knee, there are 500 cases, and 180 have a history of a previous knee injury; of 800 controls free from knee arthritis, 120 had a history of injury. Calculate:

(a) The relative risk.

(b) The odds ratio.

(c) The attributable proportion in those with a previous injury.

Q4.5 If, in Q4.4, the cases were all newly diagnosed cases in a given community and the controls were a random sample of that community, each selected at the time a case occurred, what difference would that make to the answers to Q4.4 (a) and (b)?

Q4.6 If we assume that the effects seen in Table 4.10 represent an effect of the difference in gun laws, and if Canadian gun laws could be introduced to Seattle:

(a) What proportion of murders in Seattle, using firearms, would be prevented?

(b) How many people would be affected by the change for each firearm-linked murder prevented?

(c) What proportion of all murders in Seattle would be prevented?

References

1. **Morrow J, Russell A, Guthrie E, Parsons L, Robertson I, Waddell R, et al**. Malformation risks of antiepileptic drugs in pregnancy: a prospective study from the UK Epilepsy and Pregnancy Register. *J Neurol Neurosurg Psychiatry* 2006; **77**:193–198.

2. **ISIS-4 (Fourth International Study of Infarct Survival Collaborative Group)**. ISIS-4: A randomised factorial trial assessing early oral captopril, oral mononitrate, and intravenous magnesium sulphate in 58 050 patients with suspected acute myocardial infarction. *Lancet* 1995; **345**:669–685.

3. Cook RJ, Sackett DL. The number needed to treat: a clinically useful measure of treatment effect. *BMJ* 1995; **310**:452–454.

4. Edwards A, Elwyn G, Covey J, Matthews E, Pill R. Presenting risk information—a review of the effects of 'framing' and other manipulations on patient outcomes. *J Health Commun* 2001; **6**:61–82.

5. Bucher HC, Weinbacher M, Gyr K. Influence of method of reporting study results on decision of physicians to prescribe drugs to lower cholesterol concentration. *BMJ* 1994; **309**:761–764.

6. Sarfati D, Howden-Chapman P, Woodward A, Salmond C. Does the frame affect the picture? A study into how attitudes to screening for cancer are affected by the way benefits are expressed. *J Med Screen* 1998; **5**:137–140.

7. Romond EH, Perez EA, Bryant J, Suman VJ, Geyer CE, Jr, Davidson NE, et al. Trastuzumab plus adjuvant chemotherapy for operable HER2-positive breast cancer. *N Engl J Med* 2005; **353**:1673–1684.

8. Paffenbarger RS, Hale WE. Work activity and coronary heart mortality. *N Engl J Med* 1975; **292**:545–550.

9. Royal College of General Practitioners. Mortality among oral-contraceptive users. Royal College of General Practitioners' Oral Contraception Study. *Lancet* 1977; **310**:727–731.

10. Beral V, Hermon C, Kay C, Hannaford P, Darby S, Reeves G. Mortality associated with oral contraceptive use: 25 year follow up of cohort of 46,000 women from Royal College of General Practitioners' oral contraception study. *BMJ* 1999; **318**:96–100.

11. Vessey M, Painter R, Yeates D. Mortality in relation to oral contraceptive use and cigarette smoking. *Lancet* 2003; **362**:185–191.

12. Elwood JM, Raman S, Mousseau G. Reproductive history in the mothers of anencephalics. *J Chronic Dis* 1978; **31**:473–481.

13. Pauletto P, Puato M, Caroli MG, Casiglia E, Munhambo AE, Cazzolato G, et al. Blood pressure and atherogenic lipoprotein profiles of fish-diet and vegetarian villagers in Tanzania: the Lugalawa study. *Lancet* 1996; **348**:784–788.

14. Charlton A. Children's coughs related to parental smoking. *BMJ* 1984; **288**:1647–1649.

15. Sloan JH, Kellermann AL, Reay DT, Ferris JA, Koepsell T, Rivara FP, et al. Handgun regulations, crime, assaults, and homicide. *N Engl J Med* 1988; **319**:1256–1262.

Chapter 5

Selection of subjects for study

On the 20th of May, 1747, I took twelve patients in the scurvy, on board the
Salisbury at sea. Their cases were as similar as I could have them. They all in general
had putrid gums, the spots and lassitude, with weakness of their knees. They lay
together in one place ... and had one diet common to all .... Two of these were
ordered each a quart of cyder a-day. Two others took twenty-five gutts of elixir
vitriol three times a day .... Two others took two spoonfuls of vinegar three times
a day .... Two of the worst patients ... were put under a course of sea water ....
Two others had each two oranges and one lemon given them every day .... The
two remaining patients, took the bigness of a nutmeg three times a-day, of an
electuary recommended by an hospital surgeon .... The consequence was, that the
most sudden and visible good effects were perceived from the use of the oranges
and lemons.

—James Lind: *A Treatise of the Scurvy*, 1753

Introduction

How the subjects are selected in analytical and intervention studies is critical. Good
selection procedures strengthen the study, but problems also may be introduced by
the methods used to select subjects for the study. In observational cohort studies, we
need to select subjects who are or have been exposed to the putative causal factor, and a
suitable comparison group who are unexposed or less exposed. In a case–control study,
we select subjects in whom the outcome has occurred (cases) to compare with subjects
in whom the outcome has not occurred (controls). In intervention studies, we select
subjects who are suitable and willing to have either the intervention being assessed or
the alternative(s), which may be no intervention. Part 1 of this chapter will cover the
general principles, and Part 2 will show the application of these principles to each type
of study.

Part 1. Principles of subject selection

Target, source, eligible, entrant, and participant populations

As the derivation of subjects in a study is sometimes quite complex, we shall use five
terms to describe the selection process (Figure 5.1):

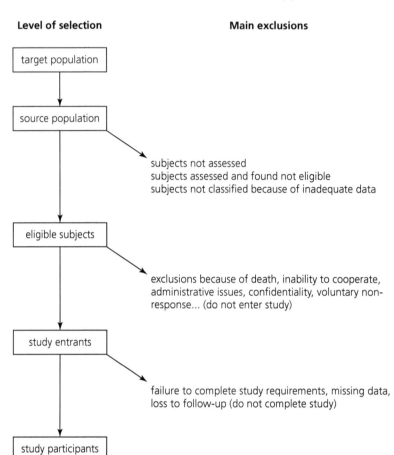

Figure 5.1 Formation of different levels in subject selection.

1. *Participants*—the individuals who complete the study, or parts of it, and contribute information to it; the results are derived from the data relating to these participants.

2. *Study entrants*—all those who enter the study. Ideally, all become participants, but usually some study entrants do not complete the procedures or provide the data requested. The correct handling of subjects who enter but who do not complete the study is an important issue, particularly in intervention trials, and will be discussed specifically in that context. Some individuals may complete part of a study (e.g. they may complete a clinical examination, but not provide a blood sample), so they will be participants for some analyses, but only study entrants for others.

3. *Eligible population.* The study entrants are derived from the eligible population—those individuals who have been defined as eligible for entry into the study. Some eligible subjects may not become study entrants: because they are not invited although eligible, or they are unable to participate because of death, illness, administrative or confidentiality issues, or they do not wish to participate.

4. *Source population.* The eligible population is a subset of the source population. The source population is determined by practical considerations, and might consist of patients in a hospital or an individual doctor's practice, members of a particular community, a workforce, or some other group. For some studies, the source population can be strictly defined and enumerated, and the proportion eligible can be calculated; in other studies, the source population cannot be measured exactly, although it still needs definition. Within the source population there will be four groups of subjects; those who are eligible, those who are adequately assessed and found not to be eligible, those who cannot be classified because of inadequate information, and those who are not assessed because of lack of resources, unavailability, or other reasons.

5. *Target population.* To have practical value the study results must be applicable to subjects other than those in the original source population; for example, a study of medical treatment needs be relevant to future patients. The population to which we aim to apply the results is the target population, or rather target populations; unlike the other entities in the scheme, the target population is not fixed, and its definition can be modified by information from outside the study results.

In terms of subject selection, these five levels give five successively smaller subsets of subjects, each derived from the one preceding it (Figure 5.2). In terms of the application of the study results, they are five successively larger populations, for each of which a further generalization of the results derived from the participants is needed.

As an example, consider a clinical trial assessing different treatments for acute myocardial infarction (heart attack), carried out in a major hospital. The study *participants* are those patients who enter the study, are randomized, and provide outcome data; their outcome information is used in the results. Some subjects may be study *entrants*, but for some reason their outcome information is not available, so they are not full participants, as they do not contribute to the key analysis.

The *eligible* population consists of all patients with the appropriate diagnosis seen at the hospital in a defined time period, within pre-set limits of age and perhaps other factors, and without the various clinical contraindications that will be defined in the trial protocol. The study will be of little value unless we can assume that the results based on the study participants will apply to this eligible population. If many subjects enter but do not complete the trial, many others do not give their consent to enter the trial, and if many are excluded for reasons other than those stipulated in the trial protocol, there will be substantial differences between the eligible and participant populations; then, we would question whether the results apply to the eligible population.

LEVELS OF SUBJECT SELECTION (2)

Figure 5.2 The different groups of subjects to be considered in interpreting studies.

The *source* population for this trial of treatment for myocardial infarction consists of the patients admitted to the hospital, or to the particular clinical unit, over a certain period of time. In principle, all such patients should be assessed to see if they are eligible for the study.

The *target* population is much wider, and will include patients seen in other geographical areas, perhaps even other countries, and certainly include patients seen at a future time. The definition of the target population will reflect the eligibility criteria, but also the characteristics of the source population. For example, studies assessing whether children who had convulsions related to fever (febrile convulsions) also had an increased risk of further convulsions showed results ranging from 60 per cent subsequent risk down to 2–5 per cent [1]. The studies showing high risks were based on hospitals or speciality clinics, relating to children referred to them, whereas the studies with low subsequent risks were of children identified through community-based or primary care sources, who are likely to have less severe initial disease. Similarly, the remission rate in patients with leukaemia varied from 44 to 85 per cent, depending on the eligibility criteria applied [2].

The methods used to select the subjects who participate in a study can affect not only how the results of the study can be applied, but also whether the results of the study are in fact valid. To go further, it is important to distinguish two important aspects of study validity.

The distinction between internal and external validity

All these studies involve a comparison between, at the simplest level, two groups of subjects. Thus, in a cohort study or intervention trial we are comparing 'exposed' with 'non-exposed' subjects. The *internal validity* of a study is a measure of how closely the observed result (the difference in outcome between these two groups) is indeed due to a causal effect of the exposure, as compared to alternative explanations. These alternative explanations are that the observed difference in outcome between the groups is due to *bias* in the way the observations are made, to differences between the groups in terms of other relevant factors (*confounding*), or to *chance* variation. These will each be discussed in detail in subsequent chapters.

Animal experiments are used to test the cancer-causing potential of a chemical, and the accepted best design uses random allocation, placebo control, and blind assessment. Using laboratory rats bred from the same genetic strains and kept under identical conditions of diet, environment, and handling, some animals are randomly allocated to receive the chemical, while others receive an inert placebo substance. Post-mortem examination of all animals at the end of their natural lifespan is done to determine the prevalence of cancers, these examinations being performed 'blind' by a pathologist who is unaware of which animals have been given the chemical. Thus the possibility of the observations of cancer occurrence being biased can be dismissed, the likelihood of there being some other difference between the animals who received the chemical and those who did not is small, and if adequate numbers are used, the possibility of chance variation will be small. We conclude that the study has *high internal validity*: an observed difference in cancer occurrence between the exposed and unexposed animals is most likely due to the chemical, from a cause and effect relationship. However, assuming that the result will apply to humans takes us beyond the internal considerations, and is more difficult.

In contrast, consider a study of the relationship between regular exercise and heart disease, in which a group of men who report that they take regular exercise is compared to a group of men who do not, the outcome of the study being determined by the diagnoses of heart disease made by the subjects' doctors over the following few years.

A difference in the recorded frequency of heart disease between these groups could be due to differences in ascertainment; for example, if there were differences in the frequency with which subjects visit their doctors, or differences in the doctors' diagnostic criteria or in their record-keeping. A difference in outcome could also occur because of other differences between the two groups of men that could affect their frequency of heart disease, such as variations in cigarette smoking or diet. Further, the test groups are fairly small, so the possibility of the difference seen having arisen through chance variation might be considerable. In such a study, we would recognize that the result—the observed difference between the groups—may not be a valid measure of the effect of exercise: the study has low internal validity.

The *external validity* of a study refers to the ability to apply the results of the study to a wider population. The earlier-mentioned rat experiment has high internal validity; we can agree that that chemical, as given in the experiment, does cause cancer in these rats; but we would not use the results, without further evidence, to conclude that the chemical causes cancer in humans. An epidemiological study of the same topic, for example, comparing workers who use the chemical in their job to workers who do similar jobs but without such exposure, could give a result with much higher external validity. (In practice, decisions on the likely cancer-causing potential of chemicals are based on a review of both animal and human studies.)

Obviously, the best studies have both high internal validity and high external validity; but such studies may be difficult or impossible to do. Often the design considerations which help to increase the internal validity of a study may work against its external validity (such as studying the disease in animals). Difficult choices in study design often have to be made. Going back to the example of the comparison between exercising and non-exercising men, one could argue that this study might have acceptable external validity, as it is after all looking at the topic in free-living individuals. However, the internal validity of that study is so low that its external validity is irrelevant. It is important to realize that *external validity is useful only if the internal validity of a study is acceptable*; studies with very low internal validity have very little value. Studies that have high internal validity may have some value, even if the external validity is low.

So, we need to pay attention both to internal validity and to external validity; but of these two, internal validity is the more important.

In evaluating or designing a study, each step in the chain from target population to study participants should be examined. We should ask whether the losses seen at each point produce differences between the groups of individuals being compared which may compromise the internal validity of the study, or produce a limited or atypical group of study participants, which may compromise the external validity of the results.

Selection bias and its effects

Selection bias can be regarded as any potentially misleading effect caused by the way subjects are selected to participate in a study. The selection processes can have three effects: it can affect both the internal validity and the external validity of a study, and can result in changing the hypothesis being assessed (Box 5.1).

Box 5.1 Three effects of selection bias on a study

Selection Bias

Selection bias can have three types of effects on a study. It may:

    Affect the internal validity

    Affect the external validity

    Modify the hypothesis being tested.

Effects on internal validity

First, selection effects can influence the *internal validity* of the study; but this happens only if the selection process has different effects on the different groups being compared. As a very simple example, suppose we want to compare boys' and girls' reading ability in a school. We have a well-designed test, but the study has to be voluntary. If children with poor reading skills tend to avoid doing the test (very likely), our overall estimate of reading ability will be too high. The boy-to-girl comparison will still be valid if the non-response issue is the same in the two groups; but if the lower response from poor readers is seen more in boys, the overestimation of ability will be greater in the boys, and we may conclude that boys' ability is higher than girls'—because that may be true for participants in our study, even if it is not true in the eligible population (all the students).

Selection factors affect internal validity only if they have *different* effects on the groups of subjects being compared within the study; this is the important distinction from the effect on external validity discussed next. As we have seen, internal validity is the more important concept, so the primary objective in designing appropriate selection procedures is to preserve internal validity.

Effects on external validity

Second, selection issues can affect the *external validity* of the study. If a trial of two treatments for myocardial infarction is restricted to patients who are male, aged under 55, and have a particular pattern of infarction, the results can be directly applied to a target population which shares these features, but extension beyond needs to be justified by other evidence. Thus the selection criteria control the nature of the target population, and so limit its external validity. As these selection restrictions apply to all the groups being compared, they should not impair the internal validity. So, in the studies of subsequent convulsion frequency in children who have had febrile convulsions, each individual study may have been internally valid, but their results depend greatly on the selection criteria for the subjects included.

Effects on the hypothesis being tested

Selection bias can have a further, and very interesting, effect on a study: it can mean that the study as performed tests a different hypothesis to that originally envisaged.

Consider a case–control study of the causes of 'rheumatoid arthritis'. The selection procedure used to identify cases may mean that the study actually assesses possible causative factors for 'rheumatoid arthritis that is sufficiently severe to lead to hospital treatment', which may be a hypothesis considerably different from that originally envisaged.

This issue is closely related to that of misclassification. External validity will be highest where the cases in the case–control study, or the exposed group in a cohort study, are representative of all cases or of all exposed individuals in the source population. However, frequently the attempt to maintain high external validity introduces the risk of inaccuracies in the definition of these study groups, so that they include non-cases or non-exposed individuals. For example, in the case–control study of rheumatoid arthritis there are choices between the two extremes of entering all individuals in a defined community (the source population) who have any type of diagnosis of rheumatoid arthritis, or of entering only those who have rheumatoid arthritis defined by specific criteria and supported by specific laboratory and radiological investigations. The latter procedure will lead to less misclassification, but if full investigation is performed only on patients with severe disease, the participants will be less likely to be representative of all individuals with rheumatoid arthritis. The balance between these two options will depend on the particular circumstances of the investigation.

Example

In the 1970s, several case–control studies (e.g. [3]) compared women with endometrial (uterus) cancer with control groups selected on various criteria, and showed a much higher frequency of the use of oestrogens, prescribed mainly for the control of menopausal symptoms, in the endometrial cancer cases. A subsequent case–control study, however, showed no association; the controls for that study were chosen as women who had been investigated for endometrial cancer, but found not to have it. It was argued that using such a control group would ensure that no controls had unrecognized endometrial cancer, that is, misclassification was avoided. However this method means that the comparison is between women with endometrial cancer and other women investigated because of similar symptoms, such as uterine bleeding. If oestrogens cause both endometrial cancer and also other conditions that lead to bleeding, both these groups would have increased oestrogen use. A further study compared women with endometrial cancer with three other groups: women being investigated for gynaecological symptoms including bleeding, gynaecological patients with other diagnoses not related to bleeding, and a community-based group. Both the women with cancer and those with gynaecological symptoms had much more oestrogen use than the community-based group [4].

A similar issue applies to case–control studies assessing psychological parameters and previous life events in relation to breast cancer. Some studies were done by studying women attending breast clinics for the investigation of symptoms. This allowed interviews to be done prior to diagnosis, avoiding the response bias that might arise after the diagnosis. Factors that are more common in the women who subsequently are diagnosed with breast cancer than in the women without cancer have then been interpreted as causal factors for breast cancer. However, the comparison being made is not between women with breast cancer and women representative of the general population, but between women with breast cancer and women with other breast problems. A positive association with breast cancer could arise because the factor prevents other breast conditions that would lead to attendance at that clinic; one such factor is oral contraceptive use, which decreases the risk of some benign breast conditions.

Methods of reducing selection biases

Selection effects are of two kinds. First, effects of incomplete participation; and second, effects produced by the selection criteria. The investigator should have knowledge and control over the selection criteria, but usually has only partial control of participation.

Reporting, and optimizing, participation and response

The reporting of participation in a study is important, but is often unclear or inconsistent. We define some useful terms here, but there is considerable variation in the terms used in the literature. It is useful to distinguish *participation rate* from *response rate*.

The *participation rate* is defined as the number of study participants divided by the number of eligible subjects, and shows how much loss there is from the ideal of all eligible subjects providing results. It is particularly useful to compare the participation rates of the different groups of subjects in the study, as differences may affect the internal validity of the study.

The *response rate* is the number of study participants divided by the number of eligible subjects who were identified, contacted, and asked to participate: it is a measure of the completeness of voluntary response by the subjects. As such, it is useful and indicates one important part of the selection process. As it does not account for losses by mortality, failure to locate, exclusion by doctors, and so on, it should not be used as the only or main estimate of participation, although it often is in publications, perhaps because it is often impressively high. The participation rate is of course always lower than, or at the maximum equal to, the response rate. For example, in a large international case–control study of brain cancers [5], 3255 subjects with glioma (the main type of brain cancer) were approached for interview, and 2765 were interviewed, giving a response rate of 86 per cent, which is very satisfactory. However, another 1066 cases were excluded and not asked for an interview, as they could not be found, had died or were too ill, or their doctors refused permission, so the participation rate is only 64 per cent, derived by 2765 divided by the number of eligible cases, 4301. However, some other studies on this topic report only the response rate, not the participation rate, so may be misleading.

Ideally, all studies should report on both the participation and response rates. In a survey, 355 epidemiological studies published in 10 major journals in 2003, information on participation was given in only 32 per cent of cohort studies, 44 per cent of case–control studies, and 59 per cent of surveys. The information given was sparse; for example, participation and subject response rates could both be calculated in only 16 per cent of reported case–control studies [6]. Participation rates declined over the period 1970 to 2003.

Obtaining high response rates in surveys and questionnaires is a major subject in its own right. A systematic review in 2009 (a Cochrane review) included 481 randomized trials evaluating 110 different ways of increasing response to postal questionnaires, and 32 trials involving 27 methods for computer-based questionnaires [7]. Successful methods were many, including monetary and non-monetary incentives, a promotional message on the envelope, hand-written addresses, and stamped instead of franked return envelopes. Response rates were reduced when sensitive questions were included. For Internet studies, responses were increased by including a picture, and decreased by the word 'survey' in the subject line. Of course, the various trials reviewed were all in different contexts, and not all factors would be relevant to all questionnaires.

Effects of selection in different study designs

Randomized trials

The stronger study designs are those that preserve internal validity by making the selection criteria apply equally in each of the groups being compared. So, in a randomized intervention trial (Figure 5.3, type (a)) only subjects who are eligible and have given their consent to the study, including consent to randomization and to each of the interventions being offered, enter the study. The selection criteria are identical to the point of randomization, so the factors influencing participation act prior to randomization, and so will affect the intervention and comparison groups equally. From the point of randomization, all subjects are included in the analysis (an 'intention-to-treat' analysis), irrespective of whether they accept the prescribed intervention and complete the follow-up procedures or not (as discussed more fully in Chapter 7). As the selection criteria apply to each of the groups equally, selection issues will not affect internal validity. However, the external validity of this design may be quite limited, as the strict eligibility criteria and the requirement for consent prior to randomization may make the participant group less representative of the eligible and source populations.

Observational studies

The effects of selection on internal validity become more severe as the design departs from the ideal of the randomized trial. Figure 5.3, types (b), (c), and (d), shows designs in which the differences in selection appear at the levels of the participant, eligible, and source populations respectively. As an illustration, consider the design of a prospective cohort study comparing women using oral contraceptives with those using other methods of contraception, in terms of later disease. The ideal design would be a randomized trial, but this is ethically impossible. The next strongest design is one in which a suitable source population is identified and eligibility criteria are set which are identical for exposed and unexposed women; this is design (b). For example, the eligible population could be defined as all women attending a defined group of doctors who start a new contraceptive method (oral contraception or other method); an example of this design will be described subsequently. By having the same eligibility criteria for both groups, some similarity is ensured; however, the

SELECTION LEVELS IN DIFFERENT DESIGNS

Figure 5.3 Study designs showing different selection schemes. From (a) to (d), the pathways for selection of groups to be compared become more different, and so the possible influence of selection on internal validity increases. (a) is a randomized trial design; (b), (c), and (d) are varieties of non-randomized intervention, cohort, or case–control designs. Partic. = participants.

eligible groups of oral contraceptive users and non-users may differ in other factors that affect their outcome rates, and the participation rates for users and non-users may differ. The analysis of the study needs to take account of these possible differences between the groups.

If the eligibility criteria for oral contraceptive users and for the comparison subjects are not the same, greater differences will be introduced, and this becomes design (c). For example, oral contraceptive users might enter the study from the time of their first use of an oral contraceptive, but it may be convenient to enrol comparison subjects using other contraceptive methods whether they were just starting on these methods or had used them for some time. This difference in eligibility criteria could introduce further differences between the groups being compared, giving greater effects on internal validity.

Another design would be of type (d), where the source populations are different. For example, the oral contraceptive users might be identified as women who had received their contraceptive prescriptions from a certain clinic, while comparison subjects might be taken as women using other methods of contraception, identified in other ways. The source populations are therefore different, and factors affecting this difference in source populations, such as factors influencing whether women go to a particular clinic, can then contribute to the differences between the exposed and un-exposed groups.

The same types of consideration apply to case–control studies. It is therefore helpful in assessing or designing studies to define the participant, eligible, source, and target populations, as this may illustrate where problems of validity may arise.

Selection of subjects for comparative studies

A few clear principles apply to the selection of subjects for all comparative studies, whether intervention trials, cohort studies, or case–control studies. While the details are specific to each study design, the principles apply to all these studies.

In comparative studies, there are two groups of subjects: the group of prime interest—the cases in a case–control study, the exposed group in a cohort study, and the intervention group in a trial—and the comparison group. There are four principles relating to the selection of the group of prime interest, shown in Box 5.2.

1. The groups should be what they are designed to be; that is, the group of prime interest should truly be cases, or exposed, or an intervention group. If we include in a cohort defined as exposed some subjects who are in fact not exposed, we will underestimate the true size of the association between exposure and outcome. This 'dilution' effect—*misclassification* of exposure in a cohort study, or case status in a case–control study—will usually reduce the size of the association seen, that is, bias the results of the study towards the null value. The direction of this effect is important. In interpreting a study that shows a strong association, this dilution is less important. In interpreting studies that show no association, however, perhaps a true association exists and there has been sufficient misclassification to disguise it. This is further discussed in Chapter 6.

2. The group of prime interest should be ascertained from the beginning of the factor's operation; that is, a case group should be selected from newly incident cases, and an exposed or intervention group from the beginning of the

---

Box 5.2 Criteria for the groups of prime interest in a comparative study. Total fulfilment of all criteria is rarely possible

Qualities of the 'exposed' Group in a cohort study and the 'case' group in a case–control study

1. Should be truly 'exposed' or a 'case'.
2. Should be newly exposed, or be a newly incident case.
3. Should be representative of a defined eligible population.
4. Should be available for study so that necessary information can be collected in the same way as it is for the comparison subjects.

exposure or intervention. Consider a study to look at the frequency of muscular pain in workers doing repetitive jobs in a factory. The simplest design is to go to the factory, examine the workers, and find out how many of them have muscular problems. This will almost certainly underestimate the problem, as it includes only workers who have started the job and have continued it until the time of the study. If instead, we study all workers who start on the job, we might find that many of them develop muscular problems and then change their job or leave the workforce entirely. Similarly, a case–control study of a severe chronic disease like cancer is best based on newly diagnosed patients, incident cases, to avoid missing severe cases and oversampling the long survivors, which will happen if a prevalence sample is used, such as patients currently under treatment.

3. The exposed or case subjects should be representative of a defined eligible population. As we have seen, this defined eligible population is the essential link between the exposed or case group in the study and the comparison group.

4. The subjects must be chosen so that the necessary other investigations can be carried out; that is, the assessment of outcome in a cohort study, of exposure in a case–control design, and of related factors in either. These other investigations should be carried out in a similar manner in the control groups chosen, and with similar completeness. So, if the controls in a case–control study are selected from the electoral roll and contacted through a listed phone number, the cases in that study should also be on the electoral roll and have a listed number.

A little consideration will show that feature 4 just listed relates primarily to dealing with bias in observations; features 3 deals mainly with dealing with differences between the groups in regard to other factors, that is, confounding; and features 2 and 1 relate to the points we have just reviewed, that the selection of subjects may affect both the internal and external validity of the study, and may modify the hypothesis under test. Good study design requires a balance between these four features; often a strategy to improve one of these features may compromise another.

Selection of the comparison subjects

The essential characteristics of the comparison group, whether it be the unexposed group in a cohort or intervention study, or the unaffected group in a case–control study, follow logically from, and are equivalent to, the criteria for the exposed or case groups (Box 5.3).

1. The controls must be representative of the group they are designed to be. In cohort studies, that means they should be unexposed or minimally exposed. In many case–control designs, controls are defined as free of the outcome of interest, and so should be selected to fit that definition. Alternatively, the design may call for the controls to be a sample of the whole population, as discussed in Chapter 4. Misclassification, as with the exposed or case groups, will have the effect of biasing the measured association towards the null value,

---

Box 5.3 Criteria for the comparison groups in a cohort or case–control study. Total fulfilment of all criteria is rarely possible

Qualities of the comparsion group in a cohort or case–control study

1. Should be truly 'non-exposed' or 'non-diseased'.

2. Should be available for the study so that necessary information can be obtained in the same way as it is for the exposed or case subjects.

3. Should be representative of a defined eligible population, analogous to that for the 'exposed' or 'case series'; this can be modified in that comparison subjects may be chosen specifically to be similar to the exposed or case series with regard to particular factors.

---

and cannot exaggerate the true association. A small degree of misclassification may therefore be acceptable, particularly if to avoid it would compromise other parts of the research design.

2. The control group should be chosen so that the relevant information can be collected by the same methods used for the exposed or case series.

3. A useful general concept is that comparison subjects should be representative of the unaffected (or of all) members of the same eligible population that provided the exposed or case subjects. While this general statement is usually applicable, the choice of appropriate comparison subjects is a complex issue and the ideal characteristics cannot be fully described in a simple inclusive statement. Therefore we shall explore this issue more fully, in the context of the different study designs.

Assessment of selection issues in a completed study

We have seen how the selection of subjects for a study can influence both internal and external validity, and affect the hypothesis under test. In assessing a study, it is useful to examine the component populations, and a simple scheme is shown in Table 5.1. The general questions, applying to the whole study, are relevant to external validity and to the hypothesis; the questions concerning differences between the groups being compared are relevant also to internal validity.

Part 2. Application of the principles of selection of subjects to each type of study, and examples

In this section, we will discuss in more detail the issues in selection of subjects for studies, with examples of all the major study designs: a small clinical, and a larger community-based, randomized trial; two related prospective cohort studies, and a retrospective cohort study; and a small hospital-based and a larger community-based case–control study.

Table 5.1 Selection of subjects. An outline scheme to assist in the consideration of issues of subject selection in a particular study. The questions should be considered generally, and specifically in regard to the comparability of the relevant groups: exposed and unexposed in cohort and intervention studies; affected and unaffected in case–control studies.

General questions	Comparison of the groups
What is the definition of the eligible population?	Are the definitions comparable?
How do the participants relate to the eligible population?	
What is the participation rate?	Compare the groups
What are the reasons for losses, and how frequent is each?	Compare the groups.
	Are differences likely to affect internal validity?
	Do the losses compromise external validity?
What is the source population?	Is it the same for each group?
How do the source and eligible populations relate?	Is the relationship similar for each group?
	Is the main result likely to apply to the source population?
What is the target population?	Is the main result applicable to this target population?

Randomized intervention trials

Selection of subjects and randomization

In the most used design for randomized trials, subjects are identified (from the source population), checked as fulfilling the eligibility criteria (becoming eligible subjects), and then invited to join the study. Those who give informed consent (study entrants) are then randomly allocated into the intervention and comparison groups.

In an alternative design, eligible subjects are identified and randomization is then done; those randomized to be offered the intervention are then approached for consent and participation, while those randomized to the comparison group receive their normal care, and may indeed be unaware that the trial is proceeding. This design has been used in large-scale interventions comparing a new intervention with routine care, as consent is required only for those who will be offered the new intervention. Thus, in the first trial of breast cancer screening in the 1960s, some 64 000 women were randomized into two equal groups; one group was offered screening and their consent to screening was sought, while the other group continued with normal care without any need for consent [8].

Progress after randomization and intention-to-treat analysis

Ideally, all those randomized to the intervention are offered it and accept it, and the comparison group do not. In practice, this is rarely likely to happen without some compromises. Some subjects randomized to the intervention may not accept it (even if they gave consent earlier), or clinical contraindications arise, or there are administrative difficulties; and some of those who start may not continue it for very long. There is therefore some misclassification produced, which will reduce the difference between the intervention and comparison groups. Despite this, the appropriate analysis compares the ultimate outcome in the original total groups defined by the randomization. Only this comparison maintains the advantages of the randomized design; this is the '*intention-to-treat*' analysis. If comparisons are based only on the subjects who accept the intervention, or complete it, the comparisons are open to all the difficulties of comparing non-randomized cohorts. Thus in the breast cancer trial noted earlier, death rates were compared between all women in the control group and all women in the group randomized to be offered screening, although only about two-thirds of them accepted the offer.

Contamination

Ideally, no members of the control group(s) are influenced by the intervention. However, this may not apply, especially if the intervention (or components of it) is available to the control group. For example, in a trial of health education, an intervention group may be selected by randomization and offered a new education programme; but the comparison group, which is not offered the intervention, may make similar changes themselves. This is referred to as '*contamination*' or '*dilution*'. In the MRFIT (Multiple Risk Factor Intervention Trial) in the United States, 12 866 men at high risk of coronary heart disease were randomly allocated to a special intervention programme or to normal care [9]. Men allocated to the intervention programme showed substantial reductions in blood pressure, cholesterol levels, and smoking. However, substantial, although lesser, reductions were also seen in the group randomized to normal care. The trial results showed only a small and non-significant reduction in mortality from heart disease in the intervention group. This was an 'open' trial; that is, both the participants and their own doctors were aware of the trial. For men in the control group, the information from the assessments made was sent to their own doctors, although without any recommendations for action. The changes seen in the normal care group could have been produced by several factors: enrolment in the trial, even although they were randomized to the normal care group; to those volunteering for the trial being already motivated to change; to the impact of the new knowledge of risk factors from the examinations carried out in the trial; or to the doctors of men in the normal care group making their own intervention recommendations. Carrying out the trial in a more rigorous fashion without giving feedback on the results of the regular examinations to men in the normal care group was regarded as unethical. A large US randomized study of screening for prostate cancer offering regular prostate-specific antigen tests (PSA) was compromised because the men in the control group also had a high frequency of such testing; in a European trial, where the PSA test was less generally used, the rate of testing in the control group was low, so the trial was better able to assess the effect of testing [10,11].

Time of first exposure

As the interventions are under the control of the investigators, the issue of being newly exposed should be well defined. Sometimes prior exposure to a similar intervention (e.g. the same drug) is expected to influence the effect of the exposure under test, and so lack of prior exposure may be used as an eligibility criterion.

Similarities between groups

Both the intervention and comparison groups, being derived by randomization, will be representative of the participant population. The random selection procedure, if done on adequate numbers, will result in two groups that are likely to be similar in terms of any particular factor that could influence the outcome. The exposure is added independently to one group and so should not be associated with other factors influencing the outcome. Thus it is reasonable to assume that the frequency of outcome seen in the comparison group would also be seen in the exposed group if the exposure had not occurred or had no effect; in other words, there should not be substantial confounding effects. This ideal does depend on adequate numbers, and even randomized groups may differ from each other by random variation. This is discussed fully in Chapter 7.

Blinding of outcome assessments

In a randomized design, the methods of ascertaining outcome and other relevant factors can be identical in the two groups. There is the special opportunity, rarely provided in the other designs, to use single-blind and double-blind techniques. That is, study designs where the subjects are not aware of which intervention they are receiving, or where those making the observations of outcome are aware of this (*single blind*), or, the ideal, both of these *double-blind*). This is obviously easiest with drug trials, and more difficult with trials of other interventions. (In a *triple-blind* design, in addition those analysing the data have only a code indicating which intervention has been given, without knowing what the code means.)

Representativeness

A limitation is that the strict eligibility criteria and management protocols may mean that the participants in a randomized trial may not be representative of a wider group, the source and the target populations; thus, the results of the trial may not be easily applied to a wider population. A related limitation is that trials may be designed primarily to address scientific issues, rather than the questions faced by decision-makers providing health care. In contrast, *pragmatic* or *practical* clinical trials [12] are designed to address important clinical or management issues, to include a diverse population of participants recruited from a range of health care settings, and to collect data on a wider range of health outcomes, adding patient-centred outcomes, such as symptom control and quality of life measurements, and economic outcomes to the more traditional clinical outcomes.

Data monitoring and stopping the trial

In many large and long-term trials, the results are monitored as they come in by a *data monitoring committee* which is independent from the principal investigators of the trial, and can operate in a 'triple-blind' fashion. This is to fulfil the ethical ideal of stopping the trial as early as possible so that a conclusion can be reached and the optimum treatment can be offered to all participants in the trial and to other people. The decision of whether or not to stop a trial can be complex and is often controversial. Stopping a trial too late delays results and will mean that more participants of the trial are given the inferior treatment; but stopping a trial too early can make interpretation difficult and may lose the scientific value of the trial not only for all its participants but for people in general. With appropriate monitoring, including the use of specific statistical methods designed for interim analyses, trials can be stopped if there is clear evidence of benefit before the predetermined study size is reached; the trial of the benefits of folic acid in preventing birth defects is an example [13]. This issue is discussed further in Chapter 8.

Summary

The prime advantages of a randomized trial are that both groups are drawn from the same participant population, and that the randomization is likely to lead to comparability in regard to other factors, and to similarity in how the observations of outcome are made. These characteristics, numbers 2, 3, and 4 in the generic list in Box 5.2, are given prominence over feature 1, so that the analysis by comparing randomized groups may accept a degree of misclassification due, for example, to incomplete participation of those randomized.

The 'CONSORT' report format for randomized trials

The CONSORT (Consolidated Standards of Reporting Trials) statement is a recommended way of describing the results of randomized trials [14]. It follows the principles set out already, and emphasizes the need to document all exclusions or departures from the protocol after randomization. The use of the format has been shown to improve reporting [15]. The CONSORT scheme is shown in Figure 5.4, and is described at http://www.consort-statement.org where amendments and new publications are given. As can be seen, it deals with the trial from the randomization onwards, and so addresses issues of internal validity; it does not deal with questions of external validity. Extensions to cluster trials, pragmatic trials, and many other issues are given on the website.

Registration of trials

Another emphasis has been on ensuring all trials that are performed are reported, so that all the results can be assessed, to avoid publication bias [16]; this is discussed further in Chapter 9. Investigators are encouraged to register their trial and submit the protocol when the trial is designed. Many leading medical journals will now only publish the results of trials which have been registered in advance, and which are reported according to the CONSORT criteria. Most countries, many specialist organizations, and the World Health Organization through its International Clinical Trials Registry Platform (ICTRP) (http://www.who.int/ictrp/en/) support this concept.

Example: a small randomized trial—treatment for acne

This was a trial of an innovative laser treatment for facial acne [17]. Figure 5.5 shows the conduct of the trial, following the CONSORT scheme. Eligible patients were selected

CONSORT FLOWSHEET FOR RANDOMIZED TRIALS

Figure 5.4 The CONSORT (Consolidated Standards of Reporting Trials) recommended flowchart to describe a randomized trial.

Reproduced from *The British Medical Journal*, Schulz KF et al, 'CONSORT 2010 statement: updated guidelines for reporting parallel group randomized trials,' Volume 152, Number 11, pp. 726–732, © 2010, British Medical Journal Publishing Group, with permission from BMJ Publishing Group Ltd [14].

from one hospital clinic or recruited by a public advertisement, and had to be aged between 18 and 45 years and have mild to moderate facial inflammatory acne, assessed on a scoring system accepted by dermatologists. Because previous treatments could affect the trial, minimum time intervals were set, for example, patients had to have had no oral antibiotic treatment during the last 4 weeks, but no treatment by isotretinoin (a vitamin A derivative), which has a much longer effect, during the last 52 weeks.

Of 62 patients assessed for eligibility, 15 did not meet the entry criteria and a further 6 chose not to participate, giving 41 patients who were randomized. A 3-to-1 randomization scheme was used, resulting in 31 patients allocated the new laser treatment and 10 allocated 'sham' treatment, where the disconnected laser handpiece was moved across the face in an identical manner used in active treatment. All patients wore opaque goggles to protect their eyes, so they were likely 'blind' to the treatment

A SMALL CLINICAL RANDOMIZED TRIAL

Figure 5.5 CONSORT flowchart for a randomized trial of laser treatment compared with sham treatment for inflammatory acne.

Reprinted from The Lancet, Volume 362, Issue 9393, Seaton ED et al., 'Pulsed-dye laser treatment for inflammatory acne vulgaris: randomised controlled trial,' pp. 1347–1352, © 2003 Elsevier Ltd, with permission from Elsevier, http://www.sciencedirect.com/science/journal/01406736 [17].

received. Four of the 31 patients allocated laser treatment discontinued it for reasons shown in Figure 5.5, and one of the 10 patients allocated sham treatment discontinued it, giving 27 and 9 respectively who completed the study. However, follow-up examinations were done on all patients initially randomized, allowing the comparison of the primary outcome, based on a clinical assessment of the acne after 12 weeks, to be made on an intention-to-treat basis, using all 41 originally randomized subjects. There was a substantial improvement in acne in the laser group, with no change in the sham treatment group. Some other secondary end points could only be assessed on those who completed the study, which is less satisfactory, although here the number of subjects discontinuing the trial is small.

In the paper, information is given comparing the laser and sham treatment groups in regard to demographic factors, previous treatments, and characteristics of the initial acne. The internal validity of the results is good. The eligibility criteria were clinically relevant, so the results should be applicable to similarly defined patients elsewhere. However, there is no guarantee that the patients seen at this particular clinic are representative of any wider group, and verification of that would logically come from repetition of the study with other populations.

Example: a large pragmatic randomized trial—maternity care

A much more complex trial is one comparing two methods of providing maternity care in Scotland [18]. The objective was to assess, for women who are not at high risk, whether a specialist-led care system (which was the norm at that time) produced any different results from a new system of care led by general practitioners and midwives; an important management question, and so a pragmatic trial. As shown in Figure 5.6, this required a great deal of set-up work, starting with getting 51 general practices to agree to participate in the study by assessing women and excluding them if there were indications of high risk, and obtaining the support of all the specialist obstetricians in the area.

From the 2642 women assessed as eligible, 475 were excluded because they were already beyond 18 weeks of pregnancy or had already seen an obstetrics specialist. A further 402 women did not consent to the study, leaving 1765 who were randomized into two approximately equal groups. A small number of women withdrew after randomization but could be included in the analysis. There were further exclusions because of missing clinical records. A survey to assess the patients' opinions of their care had a good response rate, 78 per cent, but even so, the results for that part of the trial are based on smaller numbers.

This was a complex design, but there is little doubt that the randomized trial design did ensure that the women using each of the two systems of care were comparable, and the general design of the study ensures that the results are relevant to the community and health care system in which the study was done. The study showed that the new general practitioner and midwife care system produced better continuity of care, fewer antenatal hospital admissions, a modest reduction in routine clinic visits, and a lower frequency of some of the commoner complications of pregnancy. The levels of satisfaction of both groups of women with their care were very similar, and high. The authors concluded that general practitioner and midwife care was an acceptable alternative to obstetrician-led care, which was the norm at the time.

Observational cohort studies

Exposed subjects

In an observational cohort study, the groups compared are the exposed group(s) and comparison group(s). The 'exposed' group should truly be exposed, as misclassification by exposure status, including subjects who are in fact unexposed, dilute the comparison and bias the results towards the null value. However, often an indirect indicator of

A LARGE COMPLEX RANDOMIZED TRIAL

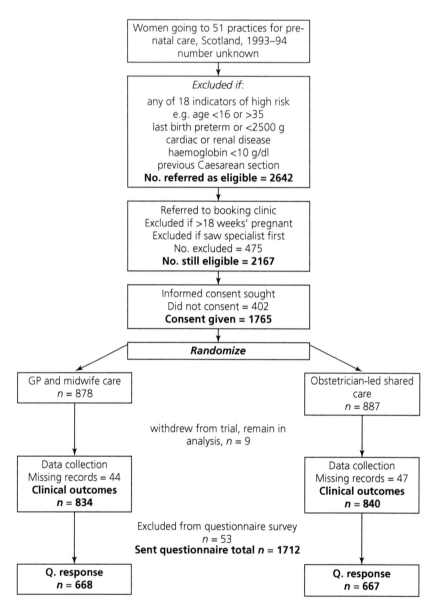

Figure 5.6 Derivation of groups in a randomized trial comparing two systems of prenatal care for low-risk women in Scotland.

Source: data from Tucker et al., 'Should obstetricians see women with normal pregnancies? A multicentre randomised controlled trial of routine antenatal care by general practitioners and midwives compared with shared care led by obstetricians,' *The British Medical Journal*, Volume 312, Issue 7030, pp. 554–559, © 1996, British Medical Journal Publishing Group [18].

exposure is used and this conservative bias accepted. Thus, to assess the health effects of exposure to asbestos an 'exposed' group of subjects who have worked in an environment where asbestos was used may be chosen, even though many of them may have had little or no personal exposure. The results will show the effects of the average exposure of this group; a real effect may be missed or underestimated if there are many people in the group who have no exposure.

Changes over time

The exposure may change over time. In the study of asbestos, initial cohorts of exposed and unexposed workers may be defined, but as the study follow-up proceeds, some exposed workers will cease exposure and some unexposed workers will begin exposure, introducing further misclassification. If such variations are large, special types of analysis will be necessary, such as defining each subject on the basis of total length of exposure. This method was used in a study of oral contraceptive users discussed later in this chapter.

New exposures

Study subjects should ideally be newly exposed to the causative agent under study. As noted previously, a 'prevalence' survey of currently employed workers may underestimate a problem that leads some workers to quit. This relates to the definition of the exposure; for example, in studying disease in workers exposed to a particular chemical, we could assume that a substantial amount of exposure would be necessary before any detectable increase would occur, and therefore define exposure as a minimum of, say, 5 years' work in an occupation with exposure to the chemical. So we define 'newly exposed' as having just passed that 5-year minimum period, and the study follow-up period starts at that time for each subject. Subjects who leave the workforce or change jobs before they have 5 years' exposure would not enter the study.

Unexposed subjects—controls

Similarly, the comparison group of subjects who are defined as unexposed, should actually be unexposed. Misclassification, by including some actually exposed subjects, will bias the measured association towards the null value, but cannot exaggerate a true association. A modest degree of misclassification may therefore be acceptable, particularly if to avoid it would compromise other valuable parts of the research design.

Comparability of data collected

The exposed and unexposed subjects should be chosen so that the appropriate investigations, the assessment of outcome and of related factors, can be carried out in a similar manner in all subjects, and with similar completeness.

Options for control groups in cohort studies

The main options in the design of cohort studies are summarized in Table 5.2.

Table 5.2 Design of cohort studies. Some methods of selection of exposed and comparison groups in cohort and intervention studies. The list is not meant to be exhaustive.

Design	Exposed group	Comparison group	Applicability
Randomized			
Randomized trial	Random selection from eligible population: intervention applied	Random selection from same eligible population: intervention not applied	Only for ethical interventions of likely benefit
Unmatched internal controls			
One or more outcomes, confounders not fully known	Exposed subset of an eligible population	Representative sample of unexposed members of same eligible population; no individual matching	Preferable if multiple outcomes; confounders controlled in analysis
Matched internal controls			
Specific outcome, main confounders known	Exposed subset of an eligible population	Unexposed subjects matched for other factors which influence outcome	Only if outcome specified and main confounders known in advance
External controls			
	Exposed subjects, or all members of a population with high exposure	All or sample of another population with no exposure or lower exposure	If internal controls not possible

The purpose of controls

It is helpful to concentrate on the *purpose* of the control group. In a cohort study, we measure the frequency of the outcome in exposed subjects. The function of the control group is to estimate what that rate would be in those same subjects, had they not been exposed (a counterfactual situation). The frequency observed in the exposed group will depend on the effects of the exposure factor, but also on the other characteristics of that exposed group that influence the outcome. An appropriate comparison is therefore a group of subjects who share, as far as possible, all the other factors which influence the outcome, apart from the exposure; or for whom the effects of these other factors can be measured and adjusted for.

The optimum

The best way to achieve this is by a randomized trial. However, often random allocation and an intervention design are not possible. In the randomized trial design, the control group has two properties; it is a representative sample of the original eligible population, and it is likely to be similar to the exposed group in regard to other relevant factors. Procedures for selecting controls in non-randomized studies can be logically determined by starting from one or other of these properties.

Representativeness

The control series can be chosen as *a representative sample of the unexposed* members of the eligible population from which the exposed subjects are also drawn—design (b) in Figure 5.3. Thus all potential controls, if they had been exposed, should be eligible for inclusion in the exposed group. This approach ensures comparability of the exposed and unexposed groups in regard to characteristics that define the eligible population.

Self-selection

In an observational cohort study the subjects themselves, or, in the case of therapy, their medical advisers, may have chosen their exposure. This self-selection will usually mean that the exposed and unexposed groups differ in regard to other factors. For example, smokers and non-smokers differ in regard to other aspects of lifestyle such as alcohol use and diet; a non-randomized comparison of patients who have been given different treatments will often be made difficult because the patient's clinical findings and current prognosis will influence the treatment given.

Matching

If we know a great deal about the factors that influence the outcome under study, we could choose a comparison group that is *deliberately made similar to the exposed group* in terms of the other factors that determine outcome. This results in a matched design, in which for each exposed subject, one or more unexposed subjects are chosen because they share the other characteristics that affect the frequency of the outcome variable. Thus to study the long-term outcomes of amniocentesis, Baird and colleagues [19] identified a cohort of 1296 liveborn infants whose mothers had had amniocentesis during that pregnancy, and compared them in terms of later disabilities to 3704 control liveborns whose mothers were matched for sex, maternal age, area of residence, and time of birth. No differences were found except for an increase in haemolytic disease due to isoimmunization. Matching can give a powerful design, but its disadvantages are several. It is not often that we know all the factors that influence the outcome under study. For this design we not only have to know them but we have to be able to measure them, and we have to be able to find matched comparison subjects who share those characteristics with the exposed subjects. Matched designs although elegant in theory, are therefore often difficult to employ in practice; matching is discussed more fully in Chapter 7.

Internal and external control groups

The designs described so far involve *internal control groups*: that is, controls derived from the same source population as the exposed subjects (e.g. the same community, workplace, or medical practice). A rather weaker design uses an *external control group*, from a different source population. While the source populations for the exposed and unexposed groups are not the same, they must both relate to a common target population. Thus, the health effects of asbestos could be assessed by comparing workers who use asbestos with workers in the same industry, who have generally similar jobs, but do not use asbestos—an *internal* control group. The effects of asbestos could also be assessed by comparing the death rates of workers in jobs using asbestos with the death rates for the whole population in that area or country—an *external* control group. If the effects are large this may be an adequate design, but is weak as there may be many other differences between the groups being compared. For example, if workers in an industry with asbestos exposure have a higher stomach cancer rate than the general population (external controls), that may indicate a hazard; but if the stomach cancer risk is the same for workers exposed to asbestos as for other workers in that same industry (internal controls), it suggests asbestos is not the cause of the increase in stomach cancer, but some other exposure in that industry may be.

Example: a large prospective cohort study of long-term effects of oral contraceptives

In the 1960s, the contraceptive pill was a new drug, used by very large numbers of women, and its long-term effects were unknown. To study such effects required a long-term cohort study capable of assessing multiple end points and of giving results that would be widely applicable. Such a study would be a large, expensive, and long-term commitment, not easily repeated; therefore the design needed to optimize both internal and external validity. We will review one such study set up in the UK.

Eligible subjects

This study was based on 17 of the largest clinics run by the Family Planning Association (FPA) [20] (Figure 5.7). Over 17 000 women entered the study between 1968 and 1974. Eligible subjects were aged 25–39, had given consent, and also had to be married and a white British subject; these criteria were primarily to ensure adequate follow-up, and would probably be unacceptable restrictions in a modern study.

Exposed and unexposed groups

The exposed groups were current oral contraceptive users with at least 5 months' use. The two 'unexposed' groups were women using a diaphragm or an intrauterine device currently and for at least 5 months, without past exposure to oral contraceptives. The 5-month duration criterion was to exclude substantial numbers of women who would change their method of contraception within a few months after starting.

First exposure

The exposed and comparison groups were not defined from the time of first exposure, but were a prevalent sample of contraceptive users. This was a practical compromise: the ideal, to identify new users of any of the three methods and enter them when they had accumulated 5 months' use, would have been much more difficult, especially as women who changed their use after only a short time could not enter the study. As a result, the study cannot assess short-term effects of oral contraceptive use.

PROSPECTIVE COHORT STUDY (2)

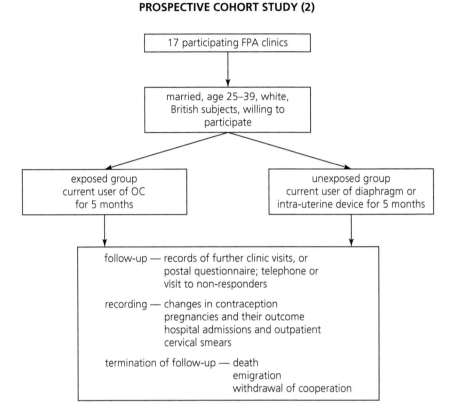

Figure 5.7 Design of a prospective cohort study of oral contraceptive (OC) use: based on Family Planning Clinics [21,22].

Source: data from Vessey MP et al., 'Neoplasia of the cervix uteri and contraception: a possible adverse effect of the pill,' *The Lancet*, Volume 322, Issue 8356, pp. 930–934, © 1983; [21] and Hannaford PC et al., 'Mortality among contraceptive pill users: cohort evidence from Royal College of General Practitioners' Oral Contraception Study,' *The British Medical Journal*, Volume 340, c927, © 2010 British Medical Journal Publishing Group [22].

Follow-up and definition of outcomes

Follow-up information was based on the FPA clinic records, and follow-up forms sent directly to the patient, supported by telephone calls or home visits where necessary. The loss to follow-up was only around 0.4 per cent per year, and was similar in the different contraceptive groups. The primary outcome measures were mortality and morbidity recorded as inpatient or outpatient hospital visits. Follow-up ceased at death, emigration from the UK, or at the subject's request.

Internal and external validity

This good follow-up was achieved by the eligibility criteria which selected women with a stable lifestyle, and applied to both the oral contraceptive and comparison groups;

but this advantage in internal validity was achieved at the cost of external validity. The women in the FPA study are not representative of all oral contraceptive users in the UK, and exclude, for example, women of non-white origin and younger unmarried women who may have different sexual behaviours. However, any major biological associations assessed in this study might well apply to other groups. Thus some external validity has been sacrificed to facilitate follow-up and to achieve good internal validity.

Outcomes, and value of two control groups

This study continued to 2010. There was no effect of oral contraceptive use on total mortality, non-reproductive cancers, or on breast cancer, where the relative risk (RR) was 1.0, with 95 per cent confidence limits (see Chapter 8) of 0.9–1.1. There were increased deaths from cervical cancer (RR 3.4), but decreased death rates from ovarian and endometrial cancers (RRs both 0.5) [20]. The conclusion was that oral contraceptives had a net beneficial effect on cancer risks.

The use of two comparison groups, users of a diaphragm or of an intrauterine device, was very valuable. Thus, it was shown that the incidence of cervical cancer and dysplasia was lower in women who used a diaphragm than in either of the other two groups, suggesting a protective effect of diaphragm use rather than an increased risk from the other methods. To assess whether cervical cancer was increased in oral contraceptive users, the relevant comparison was between oral contraceptive users and users of an intrauterine device, excluding diaphragm users entirely from that analysis [21].

Another cohort study

Another cohort study of oral contraceptive users in the UK was set up in 1968 by the Royal College of General Practitioners (RCGP), with 1400 volunteer general practitioners and over 46 000 participants [22]. Participating general practitioners selected the first two women in each month for whom they prescribed an oral contraceptive, either for the first time or as a repeat prescription. For each, an age-matched (within 3 years) control was selected as the next woman identified from the practice records who had never used an oral contraceptive. Both users and non-users had to be married or living as married, and thus were likely to be sexually active. Follow-up over 39 years has shown a reduced overall death rate in oral contraceptive users compared to non-users (RR 0.88), and decreases in ovarian cancers and some other cancers, and in heart disease; there was a small but not significant increase in the incidence and mortality of cervical cancer [22,23]. In the RCGP study, the external validity may be somewhat greater than in the FPA study, as the eligibility criteria are less limiting, even though the participating general practitioners are unlikely to be representative of all general practitioners. However, the internal validity may be weaker: as the non-users included women who were not using any method of contraception, differences between them and oral contraceptive users in other features related to sexual activity may be substantial.

Retrospective cohort studies

The prospective cohort studies described needed many years of follow-up to produce results. Retrospective cohort studies can reduce the length of time required for follow-up. Powerful studies can be carried out efficiently using computer-based record linkage techniques if high-quality databases are available.

Example of a retrospective cohort study: mobile phones and cancers

Thus study was designed to assess possible links between the use of cellular (mobile) telephones and cancer [24,25] (Figure 5.8). In Denmark, cell phone services started in 1982 and were provided by two operating companies. After scientific and ethical review, both companies made their records available for the study, and it was possible to link the lists of subscribers to a central population register which had information on mortality and date of emigration, and in turn to link this to the Danish cancer registry which records information on all cancers diagnosed. This demonstrates the immense potential for research of the use of linkable population registries, which in Denmark include a unique 10-digit personal identification number that assists accurate linkage between the registers. In many other countries such links are impossible either because the registries do not exist, or because legal issues prevent the linkages being established; in fact a similar proposed study using subscriber lists for cell phone customers in the United States had to be abandoned after a legal challenge.

Eligible subjects

Thus the investigators were able to identify 723 421 subscribers to cell phone accounts. They excluded 200 507 business (corporate) subscribers, as these subscriptions cannot be linked to an individual, leaving 522 914 non-corporate subscribers. The assumption is that the non-corporate subscriber is the user of the cell phone, which is obviously not always true. Further exclusions were because of errors in name or address of the telephone user, addresses which were not residential, duplicates, subscriptions initially identified but which were outside the eligibility period chosen, people under age 18, and residents in Greenland and the Faroe Islands. The study needed only access to the registers, and the subjects were not asked for consent and were not informed if they were included. The study was publicly announced, and the two telephone companies issued a notice that subscribers could contact them if they wished to be excluded; only 53 people actively excluded themselves in this way. The final cohort was of 420 095 cellular telephone subscribers, representing 80.3 per cent of the non-corporate subscribers initially identified. Linkage to the cancer registry then allowed the calculation of incidence rates for various cancers, which were compared to the incidence in the whole country as an external comparison population. There was information on the year of first subscription, age at first subscription, the type of telephone system, and the duration of subscription, allowing 'internal' comparisons between different subscriber groups. Special attention was paid to brain tumours, which were analysed with respect to site within the brain and pathological subtype. There is no information on individual features of use, for example, the intensity of use, or on which side of the head the cell phone was normally used.

Follow-up

The eligible cell phone subscriptions started between 1982 to 1995 and cancer incidence was analysed for each subscriber from the start of their subscription up to 1996

A RETROSPECTIVE COHORT STUDY

Figure 5.8 Design of a retrospective cohort study: a national study of cancer occurrence in mobile phone subscribers in Denmark [24].

Reproduced from Johansen C et al., 'Cellular telephones and cancer—a nationwide cohort study in Denmark,' *Journal of National Cancer Institute*, Volume 93, Issue 3, pp. 203–207, © 2001 Oxford University Press, with permission from Oxford University Press [24].

in a first report [24] and extended to 2007 [25]; follow-up through record linkage can continue.

Outcomes

The results showed no indication of an increased risk of cancer in total or in any tumour type, even in subjects with the longest duration of exposure, which was the only measure of intensity of exposure in the study. A strength of the study is its precision, as the study is extremely large, with 17257 cases of cancer, and 356 brain cancers, by 2007. There was no increase in risk seen for those with the longest period of phone subscription (13 or more years), and no dose-response, that is, no higher risks with longer subscriptions, or for tumours in the parts of the brain closer to the ear.

Internal and external validity

The comparison to general population data is rather weak in terms of external validity, as phone subscribers may differ from the general population in many features, but the internal comparisons between different levels of use are stronger. The exclusion of corporate subscribers may exclude subjects with the most intense usage, such as sales people. The follow-up period is a limitation, although the study is being be extended as follow-up time increases.

Selection of subjects for a case–control study

The selection of subjects for a case–control study follows the same principles, outlined in Box 5.2. Here we are selecting groups on the basis of outcome, selecting a case group who have already suffered the outcome, and a control group.

Defining cases in case–control studies

Defining a case

The cases should truly be cases. The inclusion of some individuals who do not have the outcome within the case group will dilute the case group and bias the results of the study towards the null value. However, as we have seen earlier, this ideal has to be balanced with the logistical difficulties of ascertaining a representative case group. Suppose the diagnosis of the disease requires complex procedures. Then, to ensure that all those classified as cases do have the disease may involve restricting the study to subjects who have had the opportunity to go through such diagnostic tests. This will exclude individuals who have the disease but have not been investigated so thoroughly. The restricted case series may not be representative of the disease in the wider community; it may be slanted towards individuals with more severe disease or to those with better access to health care. It may help to categorize cases by the certainty of their definition; thus in a case–control study of venous embolism and hormone replacement therapy, the association seen was stronger for the cases with a definite rather than a possible diagnosis [26].

Newly diagnosed (incident) or prevalent cases

Ideally the cases should be recently diagnosed. A series of prevalent cases, such as all cases being currently seen in a clinic or existing in a community, will exclude those subjects who have developed the disease and then left the area, died, or recovered, and will tend to contain a higher proportion of cases with a longer duration of disease. If the case series are patients with the disease of interest seen in hospital, selected as all who are being seen in the hospital, rather than only newly diagnosed patients, the case series will exclude patients not under follow-up, being those with particularly bad outcomes who may have died or been admitted elsewhere, and sometimes those with particularly good outcomes who need not return for further care.

Institutional or community cases

Often in case–control studies of disease there is a choice between a case series chosen from one or more hospitals or practices, or one derived from a community. Hospital series are acceptable if a very high proportion of those developing the disease will come into hospital for diagnosis or treatment, for instance, most cancers. If that is not so, the hospital-based cases may differ substantially from those in the community; for example, although melanoma is a cancer, many patients are diagnosed and treated in community practice and may never enter hospital; and for many diseases such as diabetes and asthma, only more severely affected patients need hospital care. This selection effect may be accepted in view of the logistic advantages of basing a study on hospital cases, but considerable care is then needed in the generalization of the results.

Defining the control group in a case–control study

Definition of a control

Choosing control groups in case–control studies is more complicated than in cohort studies. In the most frequently used design, subjects in the control group are chosen to be non-cases; truly without the outcome of interest at the time the study is performed. The objective is that by comparing representative samples of cases to controls who do not have the outcome, the study will provide an estimate of the odds ratio in the underlying population. Misclassification, that is, including in the control group some who are actually cases, will have a dilution effect and bias the results of the study towards the null value. If the prevalence of the outcome under study is small (such as cancer), only a few controls are likely to have the disease and the effect of this misclassification will usually be too small to be important. Where the outcome is relatively common in the underlying source population (such as hypertension or depression), this effect could be considerable, and it may be necessary to assess potential controls to exclude disease. The benefits of doing this must be compared to the likely fall in participation rate produced by such an assessment, added to the logistic, cost and ethical issues.

However, as noted in Chapter 4, there is an alternative design for a case–control study, in which the controls are selected not to be representative of subjects without the case condition, but designed to be representative of the whole eligible population at risk (which includes the cases)—incidence density sampling. In this design, the format of the results directly produces a relative risk estimate, and a case subject is also eligible for sampling as a control.

Institutional or community controls

Table 5.3 illustrates some commonly used designs. A major choice is between selecting cases and controls from the community, or from a health care facility or similar 'institutional' source. One strong design uses a case series that is a total or representative sample of all affected subjects drawn from a specified source population, and a control group that is chosen as a representative sample of unaffected members, or of all members, of that same source population.

A community-based design has the advantage that if all cases of the disease of interest can be ascertained in the community, the case series can be fully representative. Moreover the information from the control group may be much easier to interpret, as the controls will be healthy subjects representative of that community. The source population is also more closely related to other target populations, which will make the further generalization of the results more straightforward.

In a study based on a health care facility, for example, comparing patients with a particular disease to patients with other conditions in the same hospital, a danger is that these other conditions may be related (positively or negatively) to the exposure under consideration. A useful protection with hospital-based case–control designs is to use control subjects with a range of other diagnoses, as it is unlikely that the exposure under consideration will be related to all of them. Patients with diagnoses likely to be associated (positively or negatively) with the exposure factor under assessment should not be eligible as controls. Thus in a case–control study of venous embolism and hormone replacement therapy, data were presented for nine diagnostic categories of

Table 5.3 Design of case–control studies. Some methods of selection of case and control groups in case–control studies. The list is not meant to be exhaustive. Some options in case–control studies

Design	Case group	Control group	Applicability
Unmatched community-based	All or representative sample of all affected subjects in source population	Representative sample of unaffected (or of all) members of same source population; no individual matching	Preferable for multiple exposures or if confounders not known; confounders controlled in analysis
Unmatched institution-based	All or representative sample of all affected subjects in eligible population	Sample of unaffected members of same eligible population; no individual matching	Preferable for multiple exposures or if confounders not known; confounders controlled in analysis
Matched community- or institution-based	Affected members of eligible population	Unaffected subjects chosen to be similar to cases on certain specified matching factors; from same eligible population	Only if exposure specified and main confounders known in advance

hospital controls, showing considerable variation in the frequency of use of hormone replacement therapy [26]. Also, the applicability of the results to the target population may be more difficult to assess in a hospital-based study.

From this discussion, the advantages of community-based case–control studies would seem considerable, but against these must be balanced the greater difficulty of carrying out such studies, and particularly of ensuring a high response rate in the control series. It is more difficult to obtain a high degree of cooperation from subjects in the community as they have less incentive to be involved in the study than have patients who have been treated. Further, some studies may require clinical information on comparison subjects that may not be easy to obtain from subjects chosen from the community.

Frequency and individual matching

It is valuable to achieve general comparability between cases and controls by balancing the numbers chosen in terms of gender, age group, and perhaps a few other demographic factors, such as place of residence or hospital. This is referred to as *frequency matching* and is mainly for efficiency, as will be discussed in Chapter 7. Controls can instead be chosen to be *individually matched* to the case series in regard to specified confounding factors, which are associated with both outcome and exposure. This is useful under certain circumstances, discussed in Chapter 7, but adds complexity to the study. In an individually matched design, the matching of the control subjects takes precedence over their other characteristics but beyond this, institutional or community sources of controls may be used.

Comparability of data

Finally, the control subjects need to be chosen so that the information on exposure can be obtained in a similar manner as in the case group. This may involve modification of the case or the control criteria.

Example: a hospital-based case–control study—cell phones and brain cancers

One of the first studies of cell phone use and brain cancer was a hospital-based case–control study [27] (Figure 5.9). This was designed to efficiently enrol cases and controls for what is a fairly rare disease. The cases were patients aged 18–80 years, diagnosed with a primary brain cancer during the past year, and attending one of five hospitals in New York, Providence, and Boston, in the USA. Controls were chosen as inpatients in the same hospital, selected by checking each day's admissions and selecting the first patient who met the eligibility criterion of English language use and were of a suitable age, sex, race, and month of admission; thus using approximate frequency matching to give control groups similar on these factors to the case group, although cases and controls were not individually matched. Because there had been previous reports suggesting links between cell phone type radiation and lymphoma and leukaemia, such patients were excluded from the control group. The controls had diagnoses that fell into five major categories, and the use of cell phones is described for these five categories in

A HOSPITAL-BASED CASE—CONTROL STUDY

CASES

Figure 5.9 Selection of subjects in a hospital-based case–control study of the association between the use of cell phones and brain cancer [27].

Source: data from Muscat JE et al., 'Handheld cellular telephone use and risk of brain cancer,' *Journal of the American Medical Association*, Volume 284, Issue 23, pp. 3001–3007, © 2000 American Medical Association. All rights reserved [27].

the study results. Cases and controls were then interviewed while in hospital by health professionals; this system had the advantage of giving high response rates, but time pressures and other circumstances may not be ideal, and the health professionals knew the diagnoses. Of the 668 patients with brain tumours identified, 469 were interviewed, giving a participation rate of 469/668, 70 per cent. In the paper, 97 patients were regarded as ineligible, so a response rate is calculated as 469/571, 82 per cent, but this is less useful as the distinction between ineligibility and non-response seems unclear, with illness appearing in both. The response rate in controls is given as 90 per cent, without details on exclusions other than stating that 'half the non-respondents were refusals and half were unsuccessful interviews'. So, the participation rates of cases (and probably of controls) are acceptable. However it is impossible to assess if the control group is representative of the general population in terms of cell phone exposure, and the validity of the information collected at interview could be biased as the interviewers were aware of the diagnosis of the subjects.

Example: a community-based case–control study—breast cancer and oral contraceptives

In a case–control study of breast cancer in New Zealand assessing primarily oral contraceptive use, the investigators concentrated on obtaining population-based series of both cases and controls [28] (Table 5.4). The cases were defined as all New Zealand resident women aged 25–54 who were diagnosed with breast cancer between 1983 and 1985, identified from the national cancer registry. Cancer is the one disease for which most countries have a registry, that is, a system where pathology records of newly diagnosed patients with cancer are collected, and linked to clinical and other information. In many countries, including New Zealand, the notification of new cases to a central registry is a legal requirement, so records are virtually complete. However, the use of such information for research studies is strictly controlled and dependent on ethical reviews, which can be slow and complex.

The idea was to have controls representative of the whole population. The most complete available population listing was the electoral register, but this does not cover the entire population, and does not give age. As controls were selected from the electoral register, breast cancer cases who were not on the electoral register had to be excluded to maintain comparability. Information from cases and controls was collected by telephone interviews; so, both cases and controls had to have a listed telephone number. Thus the choice of controls compromises to some extent the sample of cases used.

Of 739 cases, women with newly diagnosed breast cancer within the age range, 189 were excluded by not being on the electoral roll, not having a listed telephone number, or having had previous breast cancer, giving 550 eligible subjects. The approach to the breast cancer patients required consent from their doctor, fitness to be interviewed, an interview not more than 8 months after diagnosis, and the patient's consent. There were 433 women who participated, representing 79 per cent of the 550 eligible subjects (response rate), but only 59 per cent of the original source population (participation rate). The least of the investigators' problems was failure of the subjects to agree to interview, with only 14 refusals; there were more women excluded because their doctor did not give permission for them to be approached.

The control group sampling was further complicated by the lack of age information on the electoral roll. The investigators had to take a random sample of women from the electoral rolls, exclude those for whom a telephone number could not be found, and then write to the women asking for their participation (ethical committees rules out making a direct telephone contact); they could determine age only if she responded, and previous breast cancer only when the interview was carried out. The eligible population cannot be precisely determined, but the best estimate is 1110 and the estimated participation rate is 81 per cent. This is a minimum estimate, as amongst the women not traced there are likely to be some who would have been ineligible because of age. Exclusions of controls because of illness or death were fewer than for cases, and of

Table 5.4 A case–control study. The source, eligible, and participant populations in the case a case–control study of breast cancer in New Zealand [28].

THE CASE SERIES IN A CASE–CONTROL STUDY

Source population	All New Zealand women aged 25–54 diagnosed with breast cancer between 1 July 1983 and 30 June 1985
Eligible population	Women aged 25–54, with histologically confirmed breast cancer notified to the NZ National Cancer Registry or to the Auckland Breast Cancer Study group between above dates (*n* = 739); no previous breast cancer; on current electoral roll; whose telephone number was found
n = 550	Exclusions = 189, eligible population = 550
Participant population	Had to have permission from their physician (28 not given)
	Be identified in time to allow interview 4–8 months from diagnosis (49 too late)
	Still alive (8 had died)
	Well enough (4 too ill)
	Exclusions (14 other exclusions)
	Agreed to participate (14 refused)
n = 433	Participant population 433; exclusions 117 all participants gave usable information on oral contraceptive use
Participants/eligible = 78.7%	
Participants/source = 58.6%	

THE CONTROL SERIES IN A CASE–CONTROL STUDY

Source population	All New Zealand women aged 25–54 and without diagnosed breast cancer
Eligible population	Women on electoral register, aged 25–54, with a telephone number, with no history of breast cancer: selected by
n = 1110	Random sampling from register; estimate of number = 1110
Participant population	Still alive (10 had died)
	Well enough (4 too ill)
	In New Zealand (12 overseas)
	No language difficulty (13 excluded)
	Agreed to participate (99 refused)
	Traced (75 not traced, of whom some were likely to be outside the age range)
n = 897	Participant population 897; exclusions 213
Participants/eligible = 80.8%	
Participants/source = unknown	

Source: data from Paul C et al., 'Oral contraceptives and breast cancer: a national study,' *The British Medical Journal*, Volume 293, Issue 6549, pp. 723–726, © 1986 [28].

course a doctor's permission was not required. The voluntary response rate of eligible controls was 897/996, 90 per cent; this is lower than that of the cases, although is still very high. The lower response would be expected as the control subjects have less motivation to take part in a health study than do the case subjects who have had a serious disease.

In both these case–control designs, the emphasis is on setting eligibility criteria and exclusion processes that are the same for the case and the control series, to preserve internal validity. Both studies have considerable difficulties that could compromise the results. It is likely for instance that the case series interviewed in the brain cancer study represents a more complete series of cases than the case series interviewed in the breast cancer study. However the control series in the breast cancer study is more likely to be representative of the general community.

Self-test questions

Answers in Appendix 1, p.399.

Q5.1 Define the target, source, eligible, and participant populations in the following study. To assess the role of magnetic fields in causing childhood leukaemia, children with leukaemia treated in a major referral centre were identified, those in a terminal stage of illness were excluded, and others were interviewed with a 60 per cent response.

Q5.2 Suppose that in the study described in Q5.1, an association is found with a history of measles in the first year of life (odds ratio = 2.5). Summarize the concepts of internal and of external validity in regard to this result.

Q5.3 What effects can selection bias have on the results of a study?

Q5.4 In selecting a case series for a case–control study, 1000 subjects with the disease in question are identified, and 800 fulfil the eligibility criteria of disease categorization and age. Of these, address information is incomplete on 50, and for 100, their doctors do not give permission for them to be approached. All the remaining subjects are approached for interview, and 400 consented; however, amongst those interviewed, 10 per cent have missing data on the key variables for the analysis. Summarize the selection process, calculating the participation rate, voluntary response rate, and the ratio of the participants to the eligible and to the source population.

Q5.5 In a randomized trial of smoking cessation, smokers are randomly allocated to be offered an intervention or not. After 1 year, the frequency of smoking cessation in those randomized to no intervention was 20 per cent. Of those randomized to the intervention group, only half accepted the intervention, and their cessation rate was 50 per cent. The cessation rate in those randomized to the intervention but who did not accept the programme offered was 10 per cent. What is the most appropriate summary result from this study?

Q5.6 What four criteria should be fulfilled by the exposed group in a cohort study?

Q5.7 In a case–control study, cases are identified through general practices (family doctors) and interviewed by telephone. What selection principles apply to the controls?

Q5.8 What is meant by a single-blind or double-blind trial?

Q5.9 In the context of a cohort study of workers exposed to a particular chemical, how could an internal and an external control group be defined?

References

1. **Ellenberg JH, Nelson KB**. Sample selection and the natural history of disease. Studies of febrile seizures. *JAMA* 1980; **243**:1337.

2. **The Toronto Leukemia Study Group**. Results of chemotherapy for unselected patients with acute myeloblastic leukaemia: effect of exclusions on interpretation of results. *Lancet* 1986; **1**:786–788.

3. **Ziel HK, Finkle WD**. Increased risk of endometrial carcinoma among users of conjugated estrogens. *N Engl J Med* 1975; **293**:1167–1170.

4. **Hulka BS, Grimson RC, Greenberg BG, Kaufman DG, Fowler WC, Jr, Hogue CJ, et al**. 'Alternative' controls in a case-control study of endometrial cancer and exogenous estrogen. *Am J Epidemiol* 1980; **112**:376–387.

5. **INTERPHONE Study Group**. Brain tumour risk in relation to mobile telephone use: results of the INTERPHONE international case-control study. *Int J Epidemiol* 2010; **39**:675–694.

6. **Morton LM, Cahill J, Hartge P**. Reporting participation in epidemiologic studies: a survey of practice. *Am J Epidemiol* 2006; **163**:197–203.

7. **Edwards PJ, Roberts I, Clarke MJ, DiGuiseppi C, Wentz R, Kwan I, et al**. Methods to increase response to postal and electronic questionnaires. *Cochrane Database Syst Rev* 2009; **3**:MR000008.

8. **Shapiro S, Venet W, Strax P, Venet L, Roeser R**. Ten- to fourteen- year effect of screening on breast cancer mortality. *J Natl Cancer Inst* 1982; **69**:349–355.

9. **Multiple Risk Factor Intervention Trial Research Group**. Multiple risk factor intervention trial: risk factor changes and mortality results. *JAMA* 1982; **248**:1465–1477.

10. **Schroder FH, Roobol MJ**. ERSPC and PLCO prostate cancer screening studies: what are the differences? *Eur Urol* 2010; **58**:48–52.

11. **Cuzick J, Thorat MA, Andriole G, Brawley OW, Brown PH, Culig Z, et al**. Prevention and early detection of prostate cancer. *Lancet Oncol* 2014; **15**:e484–e492.

12. **Tunis SR, Stryer DB, Clancy CM**. Practical clinical trials: increasing the value of clinical research for decision making in clinical and health policy. *JAMA* 2003; **290**:1624–1632.

13. **MRC (Medical Research Council) Vitamin Study Group**. Prevention of neural tube defects: results of the Medical Research Council Vitamin Study. *Lancet* 1991; **338**:131–137.

14. **Schulz KF, Altman DG, Moher D**. CONSORT 2010 Statement: updated guidelines for reporting parallel group randomised trials. *BMJ* 2010; 340:c332.

15. **Moher D, Jones A, Lepage L**. Use of the CONSORT statement and quality of reports of randomized trials: a comparative before-and-after evaluation. *JAMA* 2001; **285**:1992–1995.

16. **Elliott TR**. Registering randomized clinical trials and the case for CONSORT. *Exp Clin Psychopharmacol* 2007; **15**:511–518.

17. **Seaton ED, Charakida A, Mouser PE, Grace I, Clement RM, Chu AC**. Pulsed-dye laser treatment for inflammatory acne vulgaris: randomised controlled trial. *Lancet* 2003; **362**:1347–1352.

18. **Tucker JS, Hall MH, Howie PW, Reid ME, Barbour RS, Florey CD, et al**. Should obstetricians see women with normal pregnancies? A multicentre randomised controlled trial of

routine antenatal care by general practitioners and midwives compared with shared care led by obstetricians. *BMJ* 1996; **312**:554–559.

19. **Baird PA, Yee IML, Sadovnick AD**. Population-based study of long-term outcomes after amniocentesis. *Lancet* 1994; **344**:1134–1136.

20. **Vessey M, Yeates D**. Oral contraceptive use and cancer: final report from the Oxford-Family Planning Association contraceptive study. *Contraception* 2013; **88**:678–683.

21. **Vessey MP, Lawless M, McPherson K, Yeates D**. Neoplasia of the cervix uteri and contraception: a possible adverse effect of the pill. *Lancet* 1983; **322**:930–934.

22. **Hannaford PC, Iversen L, Macfarlane TV, Elliott AM, Angus V, Lee AJ**. Mortality among contraceptive pill users: cohort evidence from Royal College of General Practitioners' Oral Contraception Study. *BMJ* 2010; **340**:c927.

23. **Hannaford PC, Selvaraj S, Elliott AM, Angus V, Iversen L, Lee AJ**. Cancer risk among users of oral contraceptives: cohort data from the Royal College of General Practitioner's oral contraception study. *BMJ* 2007; **335**:651.

24. **Johansen C, Boice JD, Jr, McLaughlin JK, Olsen JH**. Cellular telephones and cancer—a nationwide cohort study in Denmark. *J Natl Cancer Inst* 2001; **93**:203–207.

25. **Frei P, Poulsen AH, Johansen C, Olsen JH, Steding-Jessen M, Schuz J**. Use of mobile phones and risk of brain tumours: update of Danish cohort study. *BMJ* 2011; **343**:d6387.

26. **Daly E, Vessey MP, Hawkins MM, Carson JL, Gough P, Marsh S**. Risk of venous thromboembolism in users of hormone replacement therapy. *Lancet* 1996; **348**:977–980.

27. **Muscat JE, Malkin MG, Thompson S, Shore R, Stellman S, McRee D, et al**. Handheld cellular telephone use and risk of brain cancer. *JAMA* 2000; **284**:3001–3007.

28. **Paul C, Skegg DCG, Spears GFS, Kaldor JM**. Oral contraceptives and breast cancer: a national study. *BMJ* 1986; **293**:723–726.

Chapter 6

Error and bias in observations

Mathematics may be compared to a mill of exquisite workmanship, which grinds you stuff of any degree of fineness; but, nevertheless, what you get out depends on what you put in; and as the grandest mill in the world will not extract wheat-flour from peascod, so pages of formulae will not get a definite result out of loose data

—T.H. Huxley: *Geological Reform*; 1869

Introduction

This chapter falls into two parts. First we will discuss general principles of identifying and minimizing error (inaccuracies) in observations, and in the second part we will look at how to measure and adjust for such errors.

Part 1. Sources of error and of bias

Assessing causation

In the previous chapters we have seen that in cohort studies and intervention trials, the subjects are defined by their exposure or intervention, and then the outcome is assessed. In case–control studies, the subjects are selected by their outcome, and their exposure is assessed. In both types of study, other relevant factors will also be assessed. The way in which the subjects are chosen sets the study design, influences the hypothesis being tested, and determines the external validity. For example, a study of treatment of rheumatoid arthritis may be relevant only to patients of a certain age who have a particular form of rheumatoid arthritis.

In the next stage of assessing scientific work, either our own or that of others, we accept what has been done in terms of the subjects included in the study and the design used. We can then ask this central question: do the results support a causal relationship between the exposure and the outcome, within the confines of the particular study?

If any association is shown within the study, it must be due to one (or more) of four mechanisms: *observation bias, confounding, chance,* or *causation.* In this chapter, we shall deal with observation bias and observation error. Observation bias is most relevant to the measurement of the dependent variable in the study, that is, the outcome in studies of a cohort design and the exposure in studies of a case–control design.

Measured factors

The central issue is the relationship between the *true value* of the factor being assessed (outcome or exposure) and the value of the variable that represents that factor in the study. In the study of treatment for rheumatoid arthritis, a relevant outcome would be an improvement in the function of the affected joints. How this improvement can be best assessed is a major question in the study design; possibilities include X-ray appearances, physiological measures such as hand grip, and questionnaire assessments of degree of functional impairment. Expert knowledge is obviously required, and attention must be paid to the acceptability, reproducibility, and relevance of the measures considered. The variable measured in a study is often considerably far removed from the biological factor or event that is defined in the causal hypothesis.

Consider a case–control study assessing whether high vitamin C consumption is protective against heart disease. The causal hypothesis relates the occurrence of heart disease to the intake of vitamin C over a long time period many years before the clinical diagnosis. The variable used to represent this factor in the retrospective study may be the responses to a questionnaire on diet at a defined period in the recent past, converted through a formula into an estimate of vitamin C consumption at that time. The variable appearing in the results as 'exposure' is considerably different from the biological 'exposure' in the hypothesis.

A good example is given by studies assessing the association between gastric cancer and infection with *Helicobacter pylori*, a bacterium that can survive within the stomach. The causal hypothesis relates to the occurrence of stomach cancer being increased in subjects who have had *H. pylori* infection, perhaps over a long time period many years before the clinical diagnosis of this tumour. In a case–control study, with recently diagnosed cases of stomach cancer and controls, the easiest way to assess *H. pylori* infection is to use a laboratory test for the presence of the bacterium at the time of the study. Many such studies have been done, usually showing an association with a modest relative risk of around 2–4. However, past exposure to *H. pylori* may not persist, and so such tests give only an inaccurate estimate of past exposure. Patients with certain immunological characteristics are much more likely to clear the bacteria from their stomach mucosa and so produce a negative test. This misclassification of exposure can be minimized by studying only the subgroup of cases with immunological features likely to lead to persistence of the bacteria; one study using this method of control for misclassification showed increases in the observed odds ratio from 3.7, based on all cases, to 18.3, based on cases in which false-negative tests were unlikely [1].

Sources of error

Several influences can cause differences between the true value of the factor being assessed and the *recorded value* of the variable chosen to represent it; these are shown in Figure 6.1. If we assume the true value is the usual value over a relevant time in an individual subject, the measurement used may have within-subject variation including true random variation, and also biological variations, such as circadian or seasonal variations. All methods of measurement will have some error as a function of the method used (the instrument), such as a question, clinical examination, or biochemical test; and error related to the person who conducts the testing and records the data. Data have to be recorded, and often raw data are converted in some way to give the final variable representing the factor under consideration. To minimize error, methods of measurement and recording need to combine precision, reliability, and practicality, and the conduct of the study needs careful planning and monitoring. The details are specific to each topic and may be very complex: the accurate assessment of exposures such as diet, electromagnetic fields, or social deprivation, and of outcomes such as cardiac function, mental state, or improved health, are all major topics in themselves. Errors of assessment may be *random*, meaning that their average value will approach the true average as more and more measurements are taken: often illustrated by a target or dartboard with dots representing the observations, showing a scatter, but one centred on the bull's eye. Errors may be *systematic*, so that taking more measurements does not remove the error, such as when the measurement used is always higher than the true value: shown on the dartboard by a scatter that is not centred on the centre of the board.

SOURCES OF ERROR AND BIAS

true value of factor

1. random variation
2. biological variation

true value of factor at the point of measurement

3. performance of the instrument used to measure the factor
   bias due to the influence of the subjects being assessed
   bias due to the influence of the observers
4. recording of the results
5. computation of the results

value of the variable used in the study

Figure 6.1 Sources of error and of bias in the observed value of a variable compared with the true value of the factor it represents.

Error or bias: non-differential and differential misclassification

However, in comparative studies, the important issue is whether the errors, whether random or systematic, *differ between the groups being compared*.

In studies comparing groups of people defined by exposures and outcomes, error in assessment is important if it results in *misclassification*. Consider a case–control study of heart disease, using a questionnaire to assess previous vitamin C intake, defining exposure as consumption less than some defined amount. Some subjects who are truly exposed (and would be reported as exposed if an accurate measure of vitamin C intake were used) will be instead classed as non-exposed, on the basis of the less accurate assessment; and some truly non-exposed subjects will be reported as exposed. The critical issue is whether this misclassification error occurs to the same extent in the case and in the control groups, giving *non-differential misclassification,* or whether it happens more (or less) in the case group, giving *differential misclassification.* These two situations have very different consequences, with differential errors being more difficult to deal with. Non-differential and differential misclassification can be regarded as error and bias, respectively.

Thus, the key principle for any comparative study is that the *methods used will be applied in the same manner and with the same care to all the subjects in the study, irrespective of the group to which they belong.* If this is done, then we will accept that a degree of error exists, but may be able to conclude that there is little possibility of systematic differences between the groups being compared, so that the error is *non-differential.*

Consider a study of breast cancer cases and controls where we want to assess weight. We may have data from simply asking the women their weight in an interview; we may also have measured weight on the medical record for the cases. Although the medical record weight may be more accurate, the interview response weight is more useful as it has been assessed in the same way for cases and for controls. Using the interview weight for controls and the medical record weight for cases is likely to give differential misclassification.

Non-differential misclassification and its effects

Misclassification, even if non-differential, is of course important. The greater the error, the more 'noise' there is in the system, and therefore the more difficult it is to detect a true difference between the groups being compared. In the extreme situation, if the measurement used is so inaccurate that its value has no relationship to the true value of the factor being assessed, we will not detect any differences between groups of subjects even if large differences exist. Thus, if physiotherapy is actually beneficial in improving joint function, a reasonably accurate method of assessing joint function will show this improvement, while a very inaccurate method will show no difference between treated and untreated groups of patients.

The effect of non-differential error is to make the observed association closer to the null value than is the true situation. Thus if a study shows a strong association, this association cannot be produced by error in the measurements used; on the other hand if a study shows no association or a weak association, error in the observations may be disguising a much stronger association. This applies to dichotomous outcomes or exposures (only two categories); with several categories the effects can be more complex.

Studies of disease causation often produce only weak associations, with small relative risks. This can happen if the exposure variable measured is only an inaccurate estimate of the true biological factor concerned. Where the factor assessed is a closer estimate of the true biological agent, relative risks will be higher. The inhalation of certain types of wood dust is a cause of cancers in the nose and nasal sinuses; if we compare employees in an industry which uses wood with the general working population, we find a moderately increased relative risk, perhaps of 2–3; if we compare workers employed on dusty processes which use wood with the general working population, we find a much higher relative risk, perhaps 10 or more, while if we assess workers who personally have had exposure over many years to particular types of wood we find a relative risk of 100 or more. Thus in a study in France, a relative risk of 303 was found for workers with over 35 years' exposure to hardwoods, while softwoods showed no increased risk [2]. The closer we come to the biological causal factor, the higher the relative risk will become.

Differential misclassification: observation bias

Differential misclassification is misclassification that is different in its size or direction in one of the groups under study than in the others. This can be referred to as *observation bias*, in contrast to (non-differential) *error*. This is a much more serious problem, as observation bias can influence the results of a study in any direction. Most importantly, it can produce an association when there is no true difference between the groups being compared. So if a study shows an association, observation bias is a possible explanation of the association seen; and it is the first issue we should consider, and perhaps rule out, before going on to consider other explanations for the results, including causation.

Examples of differential misclassification

Family history of arthritis

In a study to assess whether rheumatoid arthritis has a familial link, patients with the disease (cases) were asked whether their parents had had arthritis, and their responses compared to those of unaffected controls [3]. The results showed that the frequency with which parents were affected was much higher for the rheumatoid arthritis patients than for controls, with a high relative risk (Table 6.1). In a second comparison, another group of patients with rheumatoid arthritis were asked about arthritis in their parents, and independently the unaffected siblings of these rheumatoid arthritis patients were asked the same questions. The answers of course relate to the same parents, and therefore should be identical; however, these results also show a higher frequency of parental arthritis reported by the rheumatoid arthritis patients than by their unaffected siblings

Table 6.1 An example of subject recall bias. Results of case–control studies comparing patients with rheumatoid arthritis (RA) with unaffected controls in terms of whether their parents had arthritis, as reported by these respondents. Study A shows a strong positive association between RA and arthritis in parents. Study B also shows a positive association which, as it compares responses of RA patients and their unaffected siblings with regard to the same parents, must be due to variation in reporting. Knowledge of the results of study B will influence the interpretation of study A [3].

	Patients with RA	**Controls**	**Odds ratio**
(A) Arthritis in parents			
Neither	3	111	1.0 (referent)
One	10	74	5.0
Both	6	16	13.9
	19	201	
(B) Arthritis in parents			
Neither	11	20	1.0 (referent)
One	23	17	2.5
Both	6	3	3.6
	40	40	

Source: data from Schull WJ and Cobb S, 'The intrafamilial transmission of rheumatoid arthritis-III. The lack of support for a genetic hypothesis,' *Journal of Chronic Disease*, Volume 22, Issue 4, pp. 217–222, © 1969 Published by Elsevier Inc [3].

(Table 6.1). This result must be due to observation bias: subjects affected by a disease are more likely to know of family members with the same disease.

Family history of congenital abnormalities

In a study of family history, the mothers of babies with central nervous malformations were asked about whether there had been similarly affected babies in their own, or their partner's, family (Table 6.2). The results showed that these had occurred more in the maternal than in the paternal relatives. Such observations have led to hypotheses of complex sex-linked inheritance patterns. However, when control mothers (mothers of normal babies) were asked the same questions (Table 6.2), they also reported more malformations in their families than in the fathers' families, which must be due to biased reporting. Indeed, the relative risks were the same [4]. The bias is produced by mothers generally knowing more about births in their own family than in their partner's family.

These examples show that if the information is biased, the associations seen may be strong. There is no point in applying statistical tests to biased data; the fact that the associations are statistically significant gives no protection against observation bias.

Table 6.2 Recall bias in a genetic study. Table A compares the reported frequency of central nervous system malformations (CNSM) in cousins of an index series of 547 cases of these defects, and shows higher frequencies of CNS defects in maternal compared with paternal relatives (relative risk = 2.4). However, Table B shows the reported frequencies of CNSM in cousins of control births which did not have CNS defects, and shows a similar maternal–paternal difference (relative risk = 2.4) [4].

	Total	With CNSM	% affected
(A) Cousins of index subjects			
Mother's siblings' children	2327	26	1.12
Father's siblings' children	2627	12	0.46
(B) Cousins of control subjects			
Mother's siblings' children	1231	9	0.73
Father's siblings' children	1333	4	0.30

Source: Carter CO et al. 'A family study of major central nervous system malformations in South Wales,' *Journal of Medical Genetics*, Volume 5, Issue 2, p. 81–106, © 1968 [4].

Outcomes in a clinical trial

Issues of outcome measurement in a randomized trial comparing antibiotics and placebo in the treatment of otitis media in children in Pittsburgh, Pennsylvania, USA, resulted in a major conflict referred to as the 'Cantekin affair'. The first report of this trial, published in *The New England Journal of Medicine*, showed a doubling of the frequency of clinical resolution of the disease with antibiotic treatment, based on an outcome determined mainly by clinical examination [5]. However, other investigators in the trial thought that the ear examinations were open to observation bias, and submitted another analysis concluding that no benefit was seen, based on tympanometric measurements [6]. They concluded that the clinical examination results for each ear were not done independently, and that they were not compatible with more objective measurements. In fact, the difference was more quantitative than qualitative: the clinical examination showed a larger effect, while the results based on tympanometry also showed a benefit, but smaller, and not statistically significant in the analysis published. Both groups of investigators agreed that no benefit was shown if a further end point, hearing tests, was used. There were allegations that some of the clinical investigators had been influenced by drug company funding. This conflict led to several investigations, which had criticisms of both main parties, and raised issues about the peer-review and publication processes [7,8].

Methods to minimize bias

The most important sources of bias are variation in the subject's response to the method of assessment, and variation in the observer's response (Figure 6.1). The main principle in avoiding bias is to ensure that the same methods are used, under the same circumstances, by the same observers, for all subjects involved in the study, and to employ double- or single-blind techniques as far as possible.

Definitions of exposure and outcome variables

The outcome or exposure measures used must not only be relevant to the hypothesis, but be chosen to be objective, reproducible, and robust; that is, likely to be little influenced by variations in the method of testing. We must guard against mistakes in both directions, however; while an outcome which is extremely difficult to measure and open to highly subjective interpretation may be of little value, there is also the danger of choosing an outcome simply because it can be measured easily, even if it is not directly relevant to the hypothesis under test, or may even result in a distortion or change in that hypothesis. For example, we may want to know if a health education programme results in subjects changing their diet (behaviour), but as this is very difficult to measure, we may choose to use something much simpler, such as the subjects' responses to factual questions about diet (knowledge), or their opinions about changing it (attitudes). The hypothesis under test in our study has now changed. The study may still be worthwhile: but we must not assume, unless we have good evidence, that an improvement in knowledge or attitudes will result in a change in behaviour. This has been referred to as a '*substitution game*' [9]; we may want to know if a new drug for asthma produces major improvements such as fewer hospital admissions or even fewer deaths, but may only measure easy and short-term outcomes like improvements in respiratory capacity.

Intervention studies: double- and single-blind methods, and beyond

Double-blind studies

The best method is to avoid bias in measurements is to ensure that neither the subject nor the observer is aware of which group the subject is in, so that the study is *double-blind*. This is easiest to do in a prospective intervention trial. Thus to evaluate the effect of a new drug on the relief of symptoms from rheumatoid arthritis, a placebo drug can be made up which looks and tastes the same as the new drug, and the study is designed so that neither the subject nor the person making the observations of outcome is aware of whether the subject is taking the active drug or the placebo. Such a design should avoid most sources of subject and observer bias. Care has to be taken that the double-blindness is in fact preserved, and not broken either inadvertently through administrative lapses or through the active drug having some feature or side effect that makes its presence obvious. In the trial of treatment for acne described in Chapter 5 [10], the laser treatment process involved moving the laser instrument over the face, with the patient wearing opaque eye protection. For the controls, the same process was followed but with the instrument disconnected, to achieve patient-blindness. The treatment outcome was assessed by a standardized examination with counting and classification of lesions, with the assessors unaware of which treatment had been given, to achieve observer-blindness. It is stated that the treatment is usually not perceptible; but two patients reported discomfort and would have been aware they were receiving active treatment, so blindness cannot be assured.

Single-blind studies

In many other prospective designs, double-blindness is not possible. If, for example, a comparison is being made between surgery and medical therapy for coronary artery disease, it is impossible to achieve double-blindness. A *single-blind* assessment, where the observer is unaware of the treatment given to the subject may be possible. While the normal medical carers of the patient will be aware of the patient's treatment, outcome measures could be chosen as items which can be verified by an independent group of assessors on the basis of electrocardiograms, X-rays and so on, or those in which observer bias is not an issue, for example, total mortality. In the 1948 tuberculosis trial described in Chapter 2, those assessing the X-rays were kept unaware of the treatment the patient had received [11].

Example of a randomized trial without blind assessment

A randomized trial comparing specialist- and general practitioner-led prenatal care was described in Chapter 5 [12]. There was potential observation bias in this trial; it could not be single- or double-blind. Most of the clinical outcome information was based on routine clinical records, so the validity of recording may differ in the two groups. For example, fewer women in the general practitioner care group were recorded as having hypertension, proteinuria, or pre-eclampsia. This could be the real situation, despite the randomization, but could also indicate relative under-diagnosis or under-recording. The two groups had similar numbers of women with previously undiagnosed hypertension recorded at the time of admission in labour, giving some protection against this bias. An important section of the results is the self-report on satisfaction. This could be biased as of course the women are aware of only the care system they have experienced. An important aspect is that the response rate to this questionnaire was quite good (78 per cent), and was virtually identical in each of the two groups.

Triple-blind studies

The term 'triple-blind' has been used where the analysis of the trial is carried out by investigators with information on which study group each subject is in, without knowing which treatment was allocated to each group, which is often easy to achieve and desirable. It is particularly important in interim analyses, which may modify the conduct of the study and even terminate it early. Thus in a cluster-randomized trial comparing vitamin A supplementation with a placebo for women in Ghana, with mortality as the outcome, neither the women participants, the fieldworkers running the study, the doctors confirming and classifying the deaths, nor the statisticians and others on the monitoring committee, were aware of the treatment allocated to any individual [13].

To add to the confusion, some authors separate blindness of the investigators who deal with entry to the study and treatment from those investigators who determine outcome; then, adding patient-blindness and data analyst-blindness produces a 'quadruple-blind' study; an example is a trial of prevention of renal dysfunction after cardiac surgery [14]. Less seriously, some have referred to higher levels of blinding as studies where, even after analysis, no one knows what the results mean.

Observational cohort studies: bias in outcome assessment

In cohort studies, the subjects are selected in terms of their exposure, and the bias question applies mainly to the outcome data. In observational cohort studies, the subjects are usually aware of their exposure and the outcome may be assessed by the subjects' response to questionnaires or by routine clinical records. In such a situation, single- or double-blind outcome assessment may be impossible. It may be useful to compare the exposed and comparison groups in terms of the frequency with which routine examinations are done or outcomes are reported, who reports them, and the completeness and consistency of the observations. Comparability in these process measures will support comparability in the results. Another useful ploy is to look for specificity of the result, by showing that outcomes that are irrelevant to the causal hypothesis are similar in the groups being compared.

Example: biased outcome assessment

A critical issue is whether the exposure would influence the outcome assessed. In a retrospective cohort study comparing professional musicians with other workers in a large insurance system, the musicians were found to have a higher risk of hearing loss based on routine records; but this may be biased, as musicians may be more likely than other workers to complain about or be assessed for hearing loss, perhaps for compensation reasons [15,16]. A study where samples of musicians and others were tested objectively in the same way would be more convincing. Outcomes where legal issues may be involved may be difficult, such as studies of post-traumatic stress disorder.

Further examples

Two cohort studies of oral contraceptive use were described in Chapter 5 [17,18]. In both these studies, the outcome data were based on routine medical and clinical records. These could have been biased directly by knowledge of the method of oral contraceptive use, if certain conditions were looked for more carefully in women using a certain type of contraceptive method, and also indirectly, in that women using oral contraceptives might have visited a general practitioner or clinic more, or less, frequently than other women. For example, in the Royal College of General Practitioners' study, 18 per cent of all diagnoses were recorded on the prescription date of the oral contraceptive, suggesting that some complaints might have come to the general practitioner's notice only because the patient had to visit for the prescription [17]. Observation bias will be less likely if the assessment methods are more objective. In the Family Planning Association study, the association between oral contraceptive use and venous embolism was stronger where the evidence for the diagnosis was more objective [19], making bias less likely as an explanation. In this study, the morbidity information used was restricted to hospital referrals, partly in order to avoid problems of observation bias.

Case–control studies; recall bias in exposure assessment

In case–control studies, the main bias issue applies to the documentation of past exposure. In most case–control studies, information is obtained by interviewing cases and controls. The central issue is *recall bias* (or response bias); a differential response to questions between cases who have been diagnosed with disease, and controls who have not. A good study design will ensure use of a well-designed standardized interview, a consistent approach by well-trained interviewers, and a supportive and non-judgemental atmosphere for the interview. However, a difference in the ability or willingness to report past events is likely, even if unconscious on the part of the subject. Where the study concerns sensitive issues, this recall bias may be more marked.

Example of recall bias

For example, a meta-analysis (by methods to be described in Chapter 9) has brought together data on 83 000 women with breast cancer from 53 studies in 16 countries, relating breast cancer to a previous spontaneous or induced abortion [20] (Table 6.3). These included cohort studies and case–control studies in which record linkage methods used information on abortion that had been recorded before the occurrence of the breast cancer: these studies may have random error in the data on abortions, but differential bias can be excluded. There were also case–control studies using retrospective interviews, where the data on abortions were collected from the women after the diagnosis of breast cancer in the cases; these studies are open to bias as well as random error. For spontaneous abortion, both types of study showed no association. For induced abortion, no increased risk was seen in cohort studies or in the case–control studies with the information on abortions recorded before breast cancer occurred. But the case–control studies using retrospective interviews showed a modest but statistically significant association with induced abortion which, given that no association

Table 6.3 Effect of recall bias. Results from a combined analysis of studies of breast cancer and both spontaneous and induced abortion [20].

Time of recording of data on abortion	Number of studies*	Odds ratio for association of breast cancer with:	
		Spontaneous abortion	Induced abortion
Prior to diagnosis of breast cancer	12/13	0.98	0.93
After diagnosis of breast cancer	40/39	0.98	1.11

*Number of studies of spontaneous /induced abortion, respectively

Source: data from Collaborative Group on Hormonal Factors in Breast Cancer, 'Breast cancer and abortion: collaborative reanalysis of data from 53 epidemiological studies, including 83 000 women with breast cancer from 16 countries' *The Lancet*, Volume 363, Number 9414, pp. 1007–1016, © 2004 Elsevier Ltd. All rights reserved [20].

was seen in the other studies, is due to recall bias. The women who have been diagnosed with breast cancer must have reported induced abortions more readily than the control women [20].

Value of subsets of cases

A degree of blinding may be accomplished by doing the study on subjects with symptoms considered suggestive of the outcome under test, but who have not received a specific diagnosis. In the early study of lung cancer and smoking mentioned in Chapter 3 [21], there were some patients thought to have lung cancer at the time of interview, but for whom the final diagnosis was not lung cancer. The interview data showed that the smoking histories of these patients were similar to the controls, and differed from the histories in confirmed cases, which gives evidence against recall bias.

Choice of control groups

A control group may be chosen from subjects who have conditions of similar severity or nature to that of the cases; thus in a retrospective study looking at events during pregnancy in mothers of infants born with a specific congenital defect, the control group could be chosen as mothers of babies with a range of other defects, who would be expected to be influenced by the same factors affecting recall.

Blindness in assessment

Observer variation is difficult to control in a case–control study, as it is not easy to keep the observer unaware of the status of the interviewee. Simple precautions such as ensuring that cases and controls are assessed by the same observer or group of observers, by the same methods used under the same circumstances, are of help. Single-blinding may be attempted, with interviewers being unaware of whether they are talking to a case or a control subject; to do this, someone else may need to set up the interview. However, the interviewee may easily tell the interviewer their diagnosis.

Assessing bias

Some data may be helpful in judging whether subject or observer bias may be a problem, such as the length of time taken for examinations or interviews, the interviewer's assessment of the cooperation of the subject and the degree of difficulty experienced with some of the key questions, and asking the subjects at the end of the interview whether they are aware of any relationship between their condition and some of the factors asked about. Similarly, the examiners or interviewers can be asked to record whether they became aware of the case or control status of the subject before or during the assessment. Such recordings give the possibility of analysing subsets of data for subjects who were aware or were not aware of the key hypothesis, and those in whom the observer did or did not know their status. Questions for which cases and controls would be expected to give similar answers may be useful.

If the study relies on a small number of interviewers, the results for each interviewer should be examined. In a large survey of women in the United States carried out by four different interviewers, no interviewer variation was seen for questions requiring recall of specific events, but the responses to questions involving subjective and person information or requiring further probing from the interviewer varied between interviewers. As a result, results on the impact of support networks on psychological symptoms varied depending on which interviewers' data were used [22].

Example

In the case–control study of breast cancer in New Zealand described in Chapter 5 [23], the information was collected by a standardized telephone interview, after an initial approach by letter. The interviewer did not know whether the interviewee was a cancer patient or a comparison subject, which provides some protection against interviewer bias. However, the subjects themselves were well aware of whether they had been treated for breast cancer or not. A standardized, non-emotive, and systematic interview technique is the best protection against bias. The bias could also be overcome if information on the exposure of interest, in this case oral contraceptive use, were obtained from other independent sources, such as medical records (as applied in the study of abortions in Table 6.3). The investigators did assess general practitioners' records for women who reported recent use of prescribed contraceptives, and concluded that there was 'close agreement' between this information and that given by the women themselves. However, doing this in practice is often difficult, and it is unlikely that such sources will give comparable information on all the relevant confounding factors.

Practical issues in reducing bias and error

The design of methods of investigation that minimize error and bias is a large subject in its own right; we will only summarize some of the main approaches. Important issues include the *definition* of the items to be recorded, the choice of *methods of measurement*, the *standardization* of procedures, and *quality control* of all aspects of data gathering and processing (Table 6.4). It is essential in any research study to define precisely the factor being assessed, even when it appears simple; consider the definitional issues involved in items such as tumour stage, cardiac failure, pain relief, social class, diastolic blood pressure, high-fat diet, or cellular atypia.

The 'instrument' used to assess the factor must then be chosen: this general term includes any means of assessment, such as a clinical examination, laboratory test, questionnaire, or review of medical records. The way in which the instrument is to be applied must be standardized: by whom, when, how, and under what circumstances.

As an example of a difficult item to measure, the prevalence of stress disorder in 641 Australian Vietnam veterans was assessed. The lifetime prevalence of combat-related post-traumatic stress disorder assessed by a standardized interview format was 12 per cent, but when assessed by an interview which gave the interviewer the opportunity to interact more with the subject, was 21 per cent. Moreover, with the latter instrument, the prevalence found when the interviewer was a trained counsellor was up to twice as high as with non-counsellor interviewers, and for the counsellors, was considerably greater for a female interviewer than a male [24].

Quality control procedures should be used to monitor the information collected throughout the study, and to produce data that will attest to its quality. These processes

Table 6.4 Bias and error. An outline scheme to assist in the consideration of issues of observation bias and error. The questions should be considered for the whole study, and specifically with regard to the comparability of the relevant groups: exposed and unexposed in cohort and intervention studies; affected and unaffected in case–control studies.

What is the definition of the factor being assessed?	Is it the same for each group?
	Is it appropriate to the hypothesis?
What is the method of assessment?	Are the methods of assessment similar for each group?
Instrument used	
Observer making the assessment	Are the subjects, or the observers, aware of the grouping of the subjects when the assessment is made?
circumstances of use	
Subjects' circumstances	How accurate and reliable is the method of assessment?
Subjects' knowledge and cooperation	
When is the observation made?	Is it the same for each group?
In calendar time	
In relation to the hypothesis	
How are the data handled?	Are the methods the same for each group?
Recording, coding	
Computation	

of definition, standardization, and quality control are relevant not only to the collection of information, but also to recording, coding, and computer entry. Quality control should include systematic checks for gross errors such as variables which are irreconcilable such as males with menstrual problems, contradictory such as non-matching age and date of birth, or outside an expected range; systematic checks for inconsistencies, such as addresses or diagnoses from different sources; and rechecking of all or a sample of examination, interview, coding, and data entry procedures.

Assessment of bias and error in a completed study

In Table 6.4, a checklist is given for the assessment of bias and error. The questions can assess whether the variable recorded is a valid measurement of the factor that is relevant to the hypothesis under test. For each aspect of this measurement, a general question relates to the accuracy of the measurement, that is, primarily to *error*; and a more specific question deals with differences in the assessment between the groups under test, and therefore relates primarily to *bias*. Bias is the more serious problem as it may affect internal validity; we concentrate on whether the methods used have been applied identically to all subjects in the study, and whether the subjects' responses to these methods are likely to have been similar. Error will always be present, but may be a serious problem, causing the results of this study to be influenced towards a null result.

Often the assessments can be made only in a qualitative and subjective manner. We need to make a reasoned judgement as to whether the results can be accepted as valid. Good evidence on the validity, reproducibility, or consistency of the observations made is helpful, and so opportunities for such assessments should be taken when designing a study.

Part 2. Measuring and adjusting for observation error and bias

Most often, we can only assess if substantial error or bias in observations is likely. If we have some comparison data, we may be able to estimate the amount of error and of bias in the data of a study, and if we can do that, we can calculate the effects on the study results.

Measuring the consistency of information

It is important not only to collect data of good quality, but to be able to demonstrate its quality. The first criterion is *consistency*: data collected on more than one occasion or by more than one method or observer should be consistent. Opportunities to assess consistency should be built in to the design of a good study. Within an interview or clinical examination, key questions or assessments can be repeated at different points in the procedure, and key factors can be assessed in more than one way. All or a sample of subjects can be reassessed; the likelihood of a true change over time must be considered in interpreting the results. Observer and instrument variation can be assessed on all or a sample of subjects, comparing data collected independently by a number of observers or by different methods. Some variables can be included in the study, chosen not because they are of intrinsic interest but because they should be stable over time, between interviewers, between subjects, and so on, and so variation in their recorded values can be used to assess the consistency of the information.

A quantitative measure of consistency: kappa

Kappa is a measure of association used to assess consistency between sets of measurements, for example, where two methods have been used on the same subjects or two equivalent samples (two observers, two occasions, or two procedures) [25]. Table 6.5 shows a study of risk factors for melanoma (a skin cancer), for the same subjects, completing two questionnaires between 1 and 3 years apart [26]. For the question 'Have you ever had freckles?' of the 646 respondents, 593 responded in the same way on each questionnaire (255 as yes, 338 as no), giving an overall proportion with consistent responses, a, of 593/646 = 0.918.

However, even if there were no relationship between an individual's responses to the two surveys, substantial agreement would be expected by chance alone: this amount can be calculated as shown. The logic is that as 0.433 of all subjects gave a 'yes' response on the first survey, and 0.438 on second, if the two responses were unrelated, the

Table 6.5 Use of a re-interview technique to assess consistency of data. For questions related to the aetiology of melanoma, subjects were re-interviewed after a period of 1–3 years, and the data on consistency were used to adjust the risk estimates in a case–control study [26].

Question: 'Have you ever had freckles?'

		Second survey:					
		Yes		**No**		**Total**	
		Number	*Prop.*	**Number**	*Prop.*	**Number**	*Prop.*
First	Yes	255		25		280	0.433
survey	No	28		338		366	0.567
	Total	283	*0.438*	363	*0.562*	646	*1.000*

Observed agreement   = (255 + 338)/646 = 0.918

Expected agreement by chance = (0.433 × 0.438 + 0.567 × 0.562) = 0.508

Kappa, κ, = (observed agreement − expected agreement)/(1−expected agreement)
            = (0.918 − 0.508)/(1 − 0.508)   = 0.833

Prop. = proportion of all subjects

Source: data from Westerdahl J et al., 'Reproducibility of a self-administered questionnaire for assessment of melanoma risk,' *International Journal of Epidemiology* Volume 25, Issue, pp. 245–251, © 2006, Oxford University Press [26].

expected proportion giving 'yes' responses on both occasions would be 0.433 × 0.438 = 0.190. Similarly, the expected proportion responding 'no' on both surveys is 0.567 × 0.562 = 0.319. The total expected agreement is the sum of the expected agreement for each category: here it is 0.508. If we take the excess of agreement over expected agreement by chance (0.918 − 0.508), and divide it by the potential excess, which is (1 − 0.508), we obtain a statistic known as kappa, κ:

$$\kappa = \frac{(a-e)}{(1-e)}$$

where a is the proportion of subjects giving consistent responses, and e is the proportion with consistent responses expected by chance alone. Kappa has a range of + 1 (complete agreement), to 0 (agreement equal to that expected by chance), to negative values (agreement less than that expected by chance). Here kappa is 0.83, which indicates good consistency.

Interpretation of kappa

The kappa calculation assumes that the true results are the same for the two surveys. We need to consider if the true result might vary over time or because of other changes. A major limitation is that the interpretation of kappa is subjective. In general, kappa values above 0.80 are regarded as showing very good agreement, 0.60–0.80 good agreement, 0.40–0.60 moderate, and values under 0.40 fair to poor agreement [27]. The consistency of some common clinical assessments has been shown to be quite low, with kappa values of 0.3–0.7. The kappa value varies with the prevalence of the condition, being difficult to interpret where the prevalence is very low or very high [28]. If the prevalence is very low, kappa may be low even if the consistency is high; an example is shown later (see Table 6.6).

Example

Consistency results can be useful to show the best of several methods of assessment. For example, to assess routine skin screening in Australia, subjects were asked if they had had an examination of their skin by a doctor in the last 3 years and, in another question, in the last 12 months. The responses were checked against the doctors' records. The kappa value comparing the questionnaire to the medical records for the 3-yearly question was 0.87, showing very good agreement, but for the question on 12 months was only 0.27. This difference was attributed to *telescoping*, that is, patients tend to remember events as being more recent than they were: many subjects reported an examination within the last 12 months when in fact it had been more than 12 months in the past. This comparison showed that an analysis based on reported 3-yearly screening would be better for further studies [29].

Variance of kappa

The variance of kappa can be calculated and used to test whether the observed agreement is statistically significantly better than that expected by chance alone. Confidence limits can be calculated (see Chapter 8 for a general explanation of confidence limits, and Appendix 2, Table A2.10 for their calculation).

More than two categories

If the factor assessed has more than two categories, kappa can be calculated by assessing the probability of chance agreement in each cell of the $n \times n$ table. An example using three categories is shown in Appendix 2, Table A2.10. There are more complex methods; with three or more categories, results may be in adjacent categories or show greater differences, and assigning 'weights' to account for different degrees of disagreement gives a *weighted* kappa [30,31].

Other methods, intra-class correlation coefficient

The kappa method is described here because it is mathematically simple, and the effects of non-differential misclassification can be adequately explained by its use. Several other methods are computationally more complex although similar in concept [31]. One widely used measure is the *intra-class correlation coefficient*, which is derived from an analysis of variance. It is the ratio of the variance attributed to the different observation methods (e.g. two or more observers or episodes of observation) to the total variance. Like kappa, the range is from 1 to 0. A value of 1 means that all the variance in the data is equal to the variation between subjects and none of it is due to variation between observers, which means that there is no misclassification.

Using kappa to adjust for non-differential misclassification

As we have seen, where there are two categories of outcome or exposure, non-differential misclassification will cause the observed association to be closer to the null value, as compared to the true association.

For a study of any design with a 2 × 2 format, comparing diseased and non-diseased subjects, or exposed or unexposed, for non-differential misclassification there is an approximate relationship between the observed and the true odds ratios and the value of kappa [32]:

$$OR_o = \kappa(OR_T - 1) + 1$$

where OR_o is the observed odds ratio and OR_T is the true odds ratio. So, at the extremes, if kappa is 1.0, perfect assessment, the observed OR equals the true OR; and if kappa is 0, that is the measure of exposure is no better than chance, the observed OR is 1.0 irrespective of the true association.

For example, if the true odds ratio in a case–control study is 3.0, and the measure of exposure used has a kappa value of 0.8 compared to the true measure of exposure, the observed odds ratio will be about 0.8 (3.0 − 1) + 1 = 2.6.

If we know kappa (from a study of consistency of data), we can adjust an observed odds ratio to give an estimate of the true odds ratio. The formula is:

$$OR_T = (\kappa + OR_o - 1) / \kappa$$

The study shown in Table 6.5 was related to a case–control study showing an odds ratio of 1.51 between having had freckles and developing melanoma. Using the kappa value of 0.83 gives an estimated true odds ratio of (0.83 + 1.51 − 1)/0.83 = 1.61, modestly increased.

Adjustment for non-differential error in continuous exposure measures

Information on the reproducibility or validity of an exposure measurement is often expressed as the correlation between measurements over the range of the variable. For a continuous measure, such as caloric intake, number of cigarettes smoked per day, or level of blood pressure, the extent of non-differential misclassification can be expressed as the *validity coefficient, v,* being the correlation between the observed measure of the exposure and its true value [31]. The relationship between the observed odds ratio OR_O related to a unit change in the measured variable and the true odds ratio OR_T is given by the square of this validity coefficient:

$$OR_o = OR_T^{v^2}$$

or

$$OR_O = \exp(v^2 ln OR_T)$$

and

$$OR_T = \exp\left(ln OR_O / v^2\right)$$

Suppose a study shows an odds ratio of 1.50 with a unit increase in obesity, as measured in a field survey, and the correlation between that measurement of obesity and the true value, assessed by comparing the field measurement to an ideal measurement on an adequate sample of subjects, is 0.7.

Then, the true odds ratio is $exp(ln1.5 / 0.49) = 2.29$.

Often the validity coefficient will be unknown, as the true value of the quantity may be difficult or impossible to measure (e.g. exposures in the past). Often all that is available is information from repeated measurements. The correlation between two measures of an exposure is the *reliability coefficient, r*. Under ideal conditions this is equal to the square of the validity coefficient, so r can be substituted for v^2 in the earlier given equations. However, in practice such a measure should be assumed to be the upper limit, or most optimistic, estimate of validity.

For example, suppose a study assessing a relationship of adult disease to alcohol consumption in the teenage years yields an odds ratio of 2.0. There is no method of measuring the true value of this variable; but repeated measures using the same questionnaire will give a reliability coefficient. If this were 0.80, the revised estimate of the true odds ratio would be $exp(ln2.0 / 0.80) = 2.38$.

Further effects of non-differential misclassification

Effects if there are more than two categories

If the exposure is in more than two categories, the effects of non-differential misclassification may be more complex. If there are categories of unexposed, moderately exposed, and highly exposed, and the true situation is that the risk increases across that gradient, the effect of misclassification will be to reduce the observed association in the highly exposed group (as it will contain more individuals who are not actually highly exposed), but it could either increase or decrease the observed risk in the moderately exposed category. The trend in risk over the ordered exposure categories will then be affected, and the estimated trend could be either decreased (towards the null) or increased.

Associated errors

A further situation in which non-differential error can produce biases are away from the null is where the errors in the ascertainment of the exposure and of the outcome are not independent. For example, in a survey using a few interviewers and subjective data, interviewer differences in assessing exposure and outcome may produce related effects. Such situations need special caution, but the effects will be specific to the situation.

Misclassification of confounders

The ability to adjust for the effects of confounding (see Chapter 7) will depend on the accuracy of measuring the confounder; non-differential misclassification of a confounding variable will reduce the degree to which the confounding can be controlled.

Effects on the numbers of subjects needed in a study

One situation in which the calculation of observed values from assumed true values is useful is in the estimation of the size of a projected study. As will be discussed in Chapter 8, this estimation depends on the odds ratio that is assumed to apply. As the observed odds ratio will be closer to the null than the true ratio because of misclassification, it is prudent to take this into account, by using the projected observed odds ratio when calculating sample sizes.

Assessment of the accuracy of information: sensitivity, specificity, and predictive value

Now we will go beyond just considering consistency. Consider the situation where we have a method of assessment that can be regarded as definitive, often termed a '*gold standard*'; then the accuracy of any other method can be assessed against it. While this is relevant to the assessment of bias, it is the central issue in the assessment of the accuracy of diagnostic tests and screening tests. The results of a screening or diagnostic test can be compared against the final diagnosis achieved after full investigation. A measure of overall consistency is not so useful here, as the consequences of a positive and of a negative result will be very different. The terminology used here is easiest to describe in terms of screening and diagnosis.

Sensitivity

Sensitivity and specificity together describe the performance of a test against the 'true' result, so can be calculated only where the true result is known for all subjects. The sensitivity of a test is its accuracy in identifying truly affected subjects; it is the proportion of affected subjects with a positive test result. Table 6.6 shows the results of a screening test for a congenital abnormality compared to the final diagnosis [33]. There were 22 affected babies, of which 17 (77 per cent) had a positive (abnormal) screening test—these 17 are *true positives*. The sensitivity is 77 per cent; the other 23 per cent gave a negative (normal) test result, and were *false negatives*.

Specificity

Specificity is the accuracy in identifying subjects who are truly unaffected; here there are 6421 unaffected babies, of who 96.2 per cent had a correct, normal, screening test result (true negatives): the other 3.8 per cent were *false positives*. Note that although this proportion is low, the number of false positives was 245, much more than the number of true positives, 17; this is because the prevalence of true positives in the whole tested population is very low (22/6443, 0.34 per cent; this is a common situation with screening tests).

Weakness of kappa

A kappa statistic is of little value here. It only assesses overall consistency, whereas the implications of sensitivity and specificity are quite different. Also, the simple kappa statistic is not useful where prevalence is low. In Table 6.6, overall 96 per cent of subjects are classified correctly, but the low prevalence means that the likelihood of correct

Table 6.6 Assessment of accuracy of data by comparison with a fully accurate method: the validity of antenatal screening for neural tube defects by a measurement of α-fetoprotein in maternal serum at 16–22 weeks' gestation compared with the presence of a neural tube defect assessed after delivery. The test is only the first step in the screening process; the ultimate result was that terminations were carried out on 16 affected and two unaffected pregnancies. For open neural tube defects, the sensitivity was 17/18 (94 per cent) [33].

		True result		Total
		Affected	Unaffected	
Screening result	Abnormal	17	245	262
	Normal	5	6176	6181
	Total	22	6421	6443

Sensitivity = proportion of affected subjects giving a positive test

= 17/22 = 77%

Specificity = proportion of unaffected subjects giving a negative test

= 6176/6421 = 96.2%

Predictive value positive = proportion of subjects with positive tests who are affected

= 17/262 = 6.5%

Source: data from Wald N et al., 'Antenatal screening in Oxford for fetal neural tube defects,' *British Journal of Obstetrics and Gynaecology*, Volume 86, Issue 2, pp. 91–100, © 1979.

classification by chance is also high (95.6 per cent). Calculation of the kappa value gives a result of 0.11, which is not very informative.

Predictive value

In routine screening and diagnostic applications, only subjects giving a positive (abnormal) result in the first test will be investigated further; thus the *predictive value positive* will be the most easily measured parameter. It is a very relevant one, showing the proportion of all those testing positive who do have the condition being sought. Here, 262 subjects had positive tests, and required further investigation; 17, 6.5 per cent, were confirmed as positive. The predictive value increases with both the sensitivity and the specificity of the test, and for given levels of these, also increases with the true prevalence of the condition in all those tested. The *predictive value negative*, the proportion of all those with a negative test who in fact are disease free, may need specific research to measure it, as all people who test negative (or a representative sample) will need to be further assessed. In the example, the predictive value negative is 6421/6443, 99.66 per cent. But note that, because of the low prevalence of disease, this impressive specificity still means that there are 245 mothers with false-positive results, compared with only 17 true positives; all 262 need further investigation.

SNOUT and SPIN

A test that is very sensitive will miss few cases of disease: it has a high negative predictive value, that is, a negative result is reliable. This has been described in clinical terms by the mnemonic SNOUT; if a Sensitive test is Negative it rules OUT disease. Equally, a test that is very specific means that few people without disease will have positive tests; so the positive predictive value is high, that is a positive test is reliable. The mnemonic is SPIN: if a SPecific test is Positive, it rules IN disease. The ideal balance depends on the purpose of the test. For example, to test donated blood for HIV virus, we need to know that a negative test result will give virtual certainty of the safety of the sample. The test has to be highly sensitive, to rule out a hazard. However, if we were testing an individual patient for HIV, it is important to avoid giving a false-positive report, so the test has to be very specific [34].

Cut-off points

Defining a screening or diagnostic test involves both the technique and the cut-off point used. For a given test and a given prevalence of abnormality in those tested, if the cut-off point is made more extreme (e.g. a higher concentration of alpha-fetoprotein in serum), the sensitivity will fall (as more affected subjects will give a normal test) but the specificity will rise (as fewer unaffected subjects test positive). The optimum balance between sensitivity and specificity depends on the consequences of each. Cut-off points apply also to non-quantitative tests. For example, the diagnosis of cancer usually depends on the degree of abnormality in a pathology specimen, and many diagnoses will depend on the definition of abnormality in an X-ray or a clinical examination. The same principle applies: lowering the cut-off, by setting a lesser degree of variation from the normal as the diagnostic criterion, will classify more subjects or specimens as abnormal, increasing sensitivity and decreasing specificity.

Further methods

Studies of diagnosis and screening use many other methods, such as *likelihood ratios* and *receiver operating characteristic* (ROC) curves. An ROC plot is a graph of the sensitivity of the test against 1 minus the specificity; that is, the true-positive rate against the false-positive rate; the terminology refers back to radar signal detection and separating signals from noise. These will not be discussed here.

Use of sensitivity and specificity to calculate the effects of non-differential or differential misclassification

Information on sensitivity and specificity can be used to estimate the effects of misclassification, either non-differential or differential, on study results, in any study design. We will discuss this in the context of case–control studies.

Non-differential misclassification

The odds ratio seen in a case–control study is related to the true odds ratio in a way that depends on sensitivity, specificity, and the prevalence of exposure prevalence in the control group. The arithmetic required to adjust observed results using known values of sensitivity and specificity is simple, if rather tedious. The sensitivity and specificity estimates are applied to the observed data to produce estimated 'true' data giving the numbers of exposed and unexposed cases and controls, and then the 'true'

Table 6.7 Calculation of estimated 'true' results, adjusted for misclassification: hypothetical example of observed results of a case–control study with independent information on the sensitivity and specificity of the exposure measure.

Observed results of study

	Cases	Controls	
Exposed	200	100	
Unexposed	300	400	
Total	500	500	Odds ratio = 2.67

For each of the case and control groups:

estimated 'true' number of exposed subjects = $[O - (1 - \text{spec})N]/(\text{sens} + \text{spec} - 1)$

where O = observed number, N = total, sens = sensitivity, spec = specificity.

Estimated number of unexposed subjects by subtraction from total.

Non-differential misclassification: sensitivity and specificity equal in cases and controls

	Cases	Controls
Sensitivity	0.86	0.86
Specificity	0.93	0.93

Calculated 'true' numbers:

	Cases	Controls	
Exposed	209	82	
Unexposed	291	418	
Total	500	500	Odds ratio = 3.66

Differential misclassification: sensitivity and/or specificity different in cases and controls

	Cases	Controls
Sensitivity	0.86	0.70
Specificity	0.93	0.98

Calculated 'true' numbers:

	Cases	Controls	
Exposed	209	132	
Unexposed	291	368	
Total	500	500	Odds ratio = 2.00

odds ratio is calculated from these data. So, Table 6.7 shows hypothetical data for a case–control study, showing an odds ratio of 2.67. If the sensitivity and specificity of the assessment method used for the exposure are known (from further studies comparing the assessment method used in this study with the true values), then, in each of the case and the control groups, the 'true' numbers of exposed and unexposed subjects can be calculated, as shown. With sensitivity of 0.86 and specificity of 0.93, in both cases and controls, the odds ratio based on the calculated 'true' data is 3.66; showing the expected increase in association seen where non-differential misclassification is removed.

The extent of the reduction towards the null of the observed odds ratio depends on the sensitivity and specificity values, and also on the prevalence of exposure. For example, if sensitivity and specificity are both 90 per cent, which would be regarded as quite good in most circumstances, and the prevalence of exposure in the control group is 20 per cent, a true association with an odds ratio of 5.0 would relate to an observed odds ratio of only 3.4. Non-differential misclassification will dilute the true effect, that is, move the observed odds ratio closer to the null value, as long as the sum of sensitivity and specificity is greater than one. If it is less, reversal of the true effect may occur.

Differential misclassification

If we have data on sensitivity and specificity separately for the case and the control groups, we can adjust for differential misclassification. So in Table 6.7, applying sensitivity figures of 0.86 in cases and 0.70 in controls, and specificities of 0.93 in cases and 0.98 in controls, gives the odds ratio in the 'true' situation as 2.00. With this true odds ratio, the study result of 2.67 shows an over-estimate of the association, produced by differential misclassification.

Table 6.8 Observed odds ratios in a case–control study with non-differential classification, for given true odds ratio, sensitivity and specificity of exposure assessment, and prevalence of exposure in the control group.

Prevalence of exposure in controls	Sensitivity	Specificity	True odds ratio			
			2.0	3.0	5.0	10.0
0.2	0.9	0.9	1.7	2.3	3.4	5.8
		0.8	1.5	1.9	2.8	4.5
		0.6	1.3	1.6	2.1	3.1
	0.8	0.9	1.6	2.1	3.0	4.8
		0.8	1.4	1.8	2.4	3.6
		0.6	1.2	1.4	1.8	2.4
	0.6	0.9	1.5	1.8	2.4	3.4
		0.8	1.3	1.5	1.9	2.4
		0.6	1.1	1.2	1.3	1.5
0.5	0.9	0.9	1.7	2.3	3.3	4.8
		0.8	1.6	2.2	3.0	4.2
		0.6	1.5	1.9	2.4	3.2
	0.8	0.9	1.6	2.0	2.6	3.4
		0.8	1.5	1.9	2.3	2.9
		0.6	1.3.	1.6	1.8	2.2
	0.6	0.9	1.4	1.7	2.0	2.3
		0.8	1.3	1.5	1.7	1.9
		0.6	1.1	1.2	1.3	1.4

Limitations

It is, however, not often that such adjustments can be made reliably. Information on sensitivity and specificity is limited, and may be taken from small studies of questionable applicability. The estimates of sensitivity and specificity have sampling errors dependent on the numbers of observations used to produce them. So although it is possible to use tables such as Table 6.8 or calculations to estimate the odds ratio from an observed odds ratio, such estimates must be treated as approximate. Mathematical adjustment of the observed results of a study is usually used only as a discussion point for interpretation.

Table 6.9 Results based on two data sources: results for the association between breast cancer and use of prescribed drugs in the previous 2 years based on self-report and on pharmacy records that are regarded as move valid. From Boudreau *et al.* [35]

Antidepressants in last 2 years

Breast cancer cases				Controls			
	Pharmacy record				**Pharmacy record**		
	Yes	**No**	**Total**		**Yes**	**No**	**Total**
Self-report: yes	24	2	26	Self-report: yes	17	5	22
Self-report: no	19	145	164	Self-report: no	14	129	143
Total	43	147	190	Total	31	134	165
Prevalence of use, self-report			13.7%	Prevalence of use, self-report			13.3%
Prevalence of use, pharmacy			22.6%	Prevalence of use, pharmacy			18.8%
		Sensitivity	0.56			Sensitivity	0.58
		Specificity	0.99			Specificity	0.97
		Odds ratio using self-report data		1.03			
		Odds ratio using pharmacy records		1.26			

Statins in last 2 years

Cases				Controls			
	Pharmacy record				**Pharmacy record**		
	Yes	**No**	**Total**		**Yes**	**No**	**Total**
Self-report: yes	18	2	20	Self-report: yes	12	2	14
Self-report: no	6	164	170	Self-report: no	2	149	151
	24	166	190		14	151	165
Prevalence of use, self-report			10.5%	Prevalence of use, self-report			8.5%
Prevalence of use, pharmacy			12.6%	Prevalence of use, pharmacy			8.5%
		Sensitivity	0.75			Sensitivity	0.86
		Specificity	0.99			Specificity	0.99
		Odds ratio using self-report data		1.27			
		Odds ratio using pharmacy records		1.56			

Example with sensitivity and specificity data

In a case–control study in the US state of Washington, associations between breast cancer and prescribed drugs were assessed in members of a health plan with its own pharmacies [35]. The primary source of information on the use of medical drugs was interviews, but the interview data could be checked against pharmacy records, which were accepted as a gold standard. As shown in Table 6.9, for antidepressants, 13.7 per cent of breast cancer patients reported use in the last 2 years in the interview, compared to 22.6 per cent reported by pharmacy records, giving an odds ratio of 1.03. Compared to pharmacy records, the sensitivity of self-report was 56 per cent in cases and 58 per cent in controls, and the specificity was 99 per cent in cases and 97 per cent in controls. The 'true' odds ratio based on pharmacy records is 1.26; compared to this, the odds ratio based on self-report (1.03) is reduced towards the null value, as the misclassification is mainly non-differential.

   For statins, the accuracy of the information looks to be better. The use in cases based on self-report was 10.5 per cent, compared to 12.6 per cent based on pharmacy records, and in the control group was 8.5 per cent by both sources. The difference between self-report and pharmacy records is considerably smaller than that for antidepressants, but is more differential. The sensitivity of self-report was 75 per cent in cases but 86 per cent in controls, although the specificity was 99 per cent in each group. The self-reported data gives the association between past use of statins and breast cancer as an odds ratio of 1.27, substantially below the odds ratio of 1.56 that is given by the pharmacy records.

Self-test questions

Answers in Appendix 1, p.400.

Q6.1 Which should be considered first in interpretation of a study: chance variation, observation bias, or confounding?

Q6.2 What is the essential distinction between error and bias?

Q6.3 What is the effect of error (non-differential error) on the results of a study?

Q6.4 What is the effect of observation bias on the results of a study?

Q6.5 What do the terms single-blind, double-blind, and triple-blind imply?

Q6.6 What are the main practical methods available to reduce bias and error?

Q6.7 In a study in which a yes/no question was asked on two occasions, 60 per cent of subjects answered 'yes' on each occasion, 20 per cent answered 'no' on each occasion, 10 per cent answered 'yes' on the first test and 'no' on the second, and 10 per cent answered 'no', then 'yes'. Calculate:

  (a) The proportion showing agreement.

  (b) The expected agreement by chance.

  (c) Kappa.

Q6.8 If the study in Q5.7 showed an odds ratio of 1.8 for the association between the factor assessed and outcome, what would the true odds ratio be?

Q6.9 For general purposes, how would kappa values of 0.9, 0.7, 0.5, and 0.2 be interpreted?

Q6.10 A screening test applied to 1000 subjects identified 100 of them as positive. On further investigation, 50 of these were found to have the disease being tested for. In subsequent follow-up, 10 of the subjects who tested negative developed the disease within a reasonably short time. Calculate the sensitivity, specificity, and predictive value positive of the test.

Q6.11 A survey using a simple portable method of measuring haemoglobin level shows an odds ratio of 1.2 for the association of disease with a unit change in haemoglobin level. The correlation between this field measurement and the best laboratory method is 0.9. What is the estimated true odds ratio?

Q6.12 In a case–control study with a dichotomous exposure variable, 50 per cent of cases and 25 per cent of controls are exposed. For the exposure measurement, the sensitivity is 0.80 and specificity 0.95. Assuming non-differential misclassification, what is the true odds ratio?

References

1. **Brenner H, Arndt V, Stegmaier C, Ziegler H, Rothenbacher D**. Is Helicobacter pylori infection a necessary condition for noncardia gastric cancer? *Am J Epidemiol* 2004; **159**:252–258.

2. **Leclerc A, Martinez CM, Gerin M, Luce D, Brugere J**. Sinonasal cancer and wood dust exposure: results from a case-control study. *Am J Epidemiol* 1994; **140**:340–349.

3. **Schull WJ, Cobb S**. The intrafamilial transmission of rheumatoid arthritis-III. The lack of support for a genetic hypothesis. *J Chronic Dis* 1969; **22**:217–222.

4. **Carter CO, David PA, Laurence KM**. A family study of major central nervous system malformations in South Wales. *J Med Genet* 1968; **5**:81–106.

5. **Mandel EM, Rockette HE, Bluestone CD, Paradise JL, Nozza RJ**. Efficacy of amoxicillin with and without decongestant-antihistamine for otitis media with effusion in children. Results of a double-blind, randomized trial. *N Engl J Med* 1987; **316**:432–437.

6. **Cantekin EI, McGuire TW, Griffith TL**. Antimicrobial therapy for otitis media with effusion ('secretory' otitis media). *JAMA* 1991; **266**:3309–3317.

7. **Rennie D**. The Cantekin affair. *JAMA* 1991; **266**:3333–3337.

8. **Silverman WA**. *Where's the Evidence? Debates in Modern Medicine*. Oxford: Oxford University Press; 1998.

9. **Jaeschke R, Sackett DL**. Research methods for obtaining primary evidence. *Int J Technol Assess Health Care* 1989; **5**:503–519.

10. **Seaton ED, Charakida A, Mouser PE, Grace I, Clement RM, Chu AC**. Pulsed-dye laser treatment for inflammatory acne vulgaris: randomised controlled trial. *Lancet* 2003; **362**:1347–1352.

11. **Medical Research Council**. Streptomycin treatment of pulmonary tuberculosis. *BMJ* 1948; **ii**:769–782.

12. **Tucker JS, Hall MH, Howie PW, Reid ME, Barbour RS, Florey CD, et al**. Should obstetricians see women with normal pregnancies? A multicentre randomised controlled trial of routine antenatal care by general practitioners and midwives compared with shared care led by obstetricians. *BMJ* 1996; **312**:554–559.

13. **Hurt L, ten Asbroek A, Amenga-Etego S, Zandoh C, Danso S, Edmond K, et al**. Effect of vitamin A supplementation on cause-specific mortality in women of reproductive age in Ghana: a secondary analysis from the ObaapaVitA trial. *Bull World Health Organ* 2013; **91**:19–27.

14. Burns KE, Chu MW, Novick RJ, Fox SA, Gallo K, Martin CM, et al. Perioperative N-acetylcysteine to prevent renal dysfunction in high-risk patients undergoing CABG surgery: a randomized controlled trial. *JAMA* 2005; **294**:342–350.

15. Schink T, Kreutz G, Busch V, Pigeot I, Ahrens W. Incidence and relative risk of hearing disorders in professional musicians. *Occup Environ Med* 2014; **71**:472–476.

16. Engdahl B. Noise-induced hearing loss: the diagnosis depends on the doctor's belief. *Occup Environ Med* 2015; **72**:234.

17. Royal College of General Practitioners. *Oral Contraceptives and Health: An Interim Report from the Oral Contraception Study of the Royal College of General Practitioners.* New York: Pitman Medical; 1974.

18. Vessey M, Doll R, Peto R, Johnson B, Wiggins P. A long-term follow-up study of women using different methods of contraception-an interim report. *J Biomed Sci* 1976; **8**:373–427.

19. Vessey MP. Some methodological problems in the investigation of rare adverse reactions to oral contraceptives. *Am J Epidemiol* 1971; **94**:202–209.

20. Collaborative Group on Hormonal Factors in Breast Cancer. Breast cancer and abortion: collaborative reanalysis of data from 53 epidemiological studies, including 83 000 women with breast cancer from 16 countries. *Lancet* 2004; **363**:1007–1016.

21. Doll R, Hill AB. A study of the aetiology of carcinoma of the lung. *BMJ* 1952; **2**:1271–1286.

22. Johannes CB, Crawford SL, McKinlay JB. Interviewer effects in a cohort study: results from the Massachusetts Women's Health Study. *Am J Epidemiol* 1997; **146**:429–438.

23. Paul C, Skegg DCG, Spears GFS, Kaldor JM. Oral contraceptives and breast cancer: a national study. *BMJ* 1986; **293**:723–726.

24. Grayson DA, O'Toole BI, Marshall RP, Schureck RJ, Dobson M, French M, et al. Interviewer effects on epidemiologic diagnosis of posttraumatic stress disorder. *Am J Epidemiol* 1996; **144**:589–597.

25. Cohen J. A coefficient of agreement for nominal scales. *Educ Psychol Meas* 1960; **20**:37–46.

26. Westerdahl J, Anderson H, Olsson H, Ingvar C. Reproducibility of a self-administered questionnaire for assessment of melanoma risk. *Int J Epidemiol* 1996; **25**:245–251.

27. Harlow SD, Linet MS. Agreement between questionnaire data and medical records. The evidence for accuracy of recall. *Am J Epidemiol* 1989; **129**:233–248.

28. Brennan P, Silman A. Statistical methods for assessing observer variability in clinical measures. *BMJ* 1992; **304**:1491–1494.

29. Aitken JF, Youl P, Janda M, Elwood JM, Ring I, Lowe J, et al. Validity of self-reported skin screening histories. *Am J Epidemiol* 2004; **159**:1098–1105.

30. Fleiss JL. *Statistical Methods for Rates and Proportions* (2nd edn). New York: John Wiley & Sons; 1981.

31. Armstrong BK, White E, Saracci R. *Principles of Exposure Measurement in Epidemiology.* Oxford: Oxford University Press; 1992.

32. Thompson WD, Walter SD. Variance and dissent. A reappraisal of the kappa coefficient. *J Clin Epidemiol* 1988; **41**:949–958.

33. Wald NJ, Cuckle HS, Boreham J, Brett R, Stirrat GM, Bennett MJ, et al. Antenatal screening in Oxford for fetal neural tube defects. *Br J Obstet Gynaecol* 1979; **86**:91–100.

34. Institute for Clinical Evaluative Sciences. The jargon decoder—interpreting diagnostic tests. If you expect me to be sensitive, then don't ask me to be so specific. *Informed* 1998; **4**:1–2.

35. Boudreau DM, Daling JR, Malone KE, Gardner JS, Blough DK, Heckbert SR. A validation study of patient interview data and pharmacy records for antihypertensive, statin, and antidepressant medication use among older women. *Am J Epidemiol* 2004; **159**:308–317.

Chapter 7

Confounding

Thus it is easy to prove that the wearing of tall hats and the carrying of umbrellas enlarges the chest, prolongs life, and confers comparative immunity from disease; for the statistics shew that the classes which use these articles are bigger, healthier, and live longer than the class which never dreams of possessing such things.

—George Bernard Shaw: Preface to 'The Doctor's Dilemma'; 1906

Introduction

Confounding is the most challenging issue in the interpretation of studies. This chapter is in three parts. In Part 1, we will define confounding and show what effects it can produce. In Part 2, we will deal with how confounding can be controlled. In Part 3, we will consider some further applications of the logic of confounding.

Part 1. The fundamentals of confounding

Definition and concepts

The ideal experiment

A central concept of science in general, and particularly biology, is the tightly controlled experiment. In the classic laboratory experiment, the investigator uses laboratory rats that have been bred under controlled conditions for many generations, are housed in identical physical environments, are fed and handled in the same way, and are then randomly allocated into the required groups. Observations are then made in a standardized manner, with the observer being 'blind' as to the allocation of the animal. The objective is to achieve a situation where the groups of animals differ in terms of only one factor, the exposure factor being tested. Therefore it is easy to accept that a difference in the outcome between the groups of animals is due either to that exposure factor or to chance. The standardized and blind assessment procedure protects against bias in the observations of outcome (as discussed in Chapter 6), and randomization of animals from a common pool protects against there being other factors that differ between the groups (confounding).

Human studies

In observational studies on humans such tight control is not possible, for scientific or more commonly for ethical or logistic reasons. Human subjects will differ from one another much more than the laboratory animals will, and we cannot only attempt to control a few aspects of their environment and activities. The challenge is to conduct studies of free-living human subjects that will still have a high degree of validity.

We have seen already that the results of a study, in terms of the differences between the groups being compared, may be due to any of four mechanisms: bias, confounding, chance, or causation.

Definition of confounding

Confounding is defined as (Figure 7.1) a distortion of an exposure–outcome association brought about by the association of another factor with both outcome and exposure.

Example of concept

To understand confounding, let us consider some situations intuitively. Suppose we need to assess if there is a causal association between smoking and the incidence of breast cancer in women (a topic on which there is still controversy). There are two standard designs: a cohort study comparing smoking with non-smoking women (simplifying it to two groups), and a case–control study comparing subjects with breast cancer with an unaffected comparison group.

The study gives the observed association between smoking and breast cancer. The question is: is that association influenced by other differences between the two groups? Consider first obesity. There is evidence that women who are obese have an increased risk of breast cancer. There is also evidence, in some communities at least, that people who smoke are more obese than others. Now consider the effect of these two associations on the result of this study. Assume the null hypothesis is in fact true; that is, there is no causal association between smoking and breast cancer. In the cohort study, because the smokers are more obese, they will have a higher risk of breast cancer for that reason. In the case–control study, because obesity is a causal factor for breast cancer, the prevalence of obesity will be greater in the breast cancer patients than in the comparison patients; and, because obesity is associated with smoking, then smoking will also be more common in the breast cancer patients.

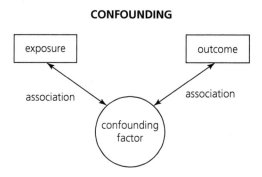

Figure 7.1 Confounding, showing the two associations which are necessary for it to occur.

EXAMPLE OF CONFOUNDING (1)

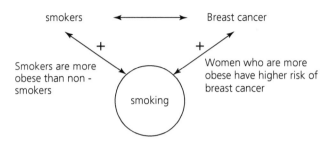

Figure 7.2 An example of confounding; if there is a positive association between smoking and obesity, and a positive association between obesity and breast cancer, the observed association between smoking and breast cancer will overestimate the true association.

Thus both studies will give a result suggesting a positive relationship between smoking and breast cancer, even if there is no true causal relationship (Figure 7.2). If the true situation is that smoking increases the risk of breast cancer, the confounding effect of obesity will mean that the true effect is overestimated. If the true situation is that smoking decreases the risk of breast cancer, the confounding effect will mean that the true protective effect will be underestimated or not detected.

Properties of a confounder

In this situation, obesity is a *confounding factor*. Confounding is produced by the two simultaneous and independent properties: obesity is associated with the outcome in this study, and independently it is associated with the exposure.

The definition of confounding involves a definition of the study hypothesis, because it may be that smoking and obesity are both causal factors for breast cancer. So if we were studying the relationship between obesity and breast cancer in women, we would have to consider smoking as a potential confounding factor.

Direction of effect

The effects of a confounding factor can be in either direction. In the situation given earlier, the exposed group (smoking subjects) has a *higher* prevalence of obesity, and obesity is associated with an *increase* in risk of breast cancer. The net result of this confounding will be to give an apparent *excess* risk of breast cancer in the smoking subjects.

In another situation, consider the relationship of smoking to breast cancer, and the effect of number of children as a confounding factor (Figure 7.3). Suppose that subjects who smoke have had *more* children, and that having had more children gives a *decreased* risk of breast cancer (there is good evidence for this). In this situation, the 'exposed' group who smoke will have had more children, and because of this their risk

EXAMPLE OF CONFOUNDING (2)

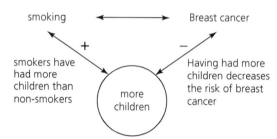

Figure 7.3 Negative confounding: if having had more children decreases the risk of breast cancer, and smokers have had more children than non-smokers, the measure association between smoking and breast cancer will underestimate the true association.

of breast cancer will be *reduced*. If the null hypothesis of no association between smoking and breast cancer is true, the study will give a spurious indication of a protective effect. If there is a real increase in the risk of breast cancer with smoking, the study will underestimate this risk, and may not show it at all, if it fails to take into account the counteracting effect of the difference in numbers of children between the smoking subjects and the non-smokers. This can be called *negative confounding*. The same effect would occur if the exposed group, smokers, had a lower prevalence of a factor that increases breast cancer risk.

How do we know if the two associations critical to confounding exist? The issue is not whether the associations exist in general, for example, whether it is true in general that women who smoke are more obese than non-smokers. That relationship is likely to vary between women of different ages, in different countries, and so on. That is not so important. The crucial issue is, does the association exist within the study population, within the data used in the analysis? Thus, if within the data set given by a particular study it is true that smokers are more obese than non-smokers, and that obese subjects have a higher incidence of breast cancer, then obesity will be a confounding factor in the relationship between smoking and breast cancer. The only other proviso is that the obesity–breast cancer and obesity–smoking associations must be independent; that is, obesity must be associated with smoking use even in women without breast cancer, and obesity must be related to breast cancer even in non-smokers. This may seem difficult logic, but should be clearer after some examples are presented.

Two associations necessary

A factor is therefore a confounding factor only when the *two* associations exist—when *the factor is associated with both the exposure and the outcome* under assessment. Smokers and non-smokers may differ in terms of many other factors; for example, they may differ in the proportion with hypertension. Do we have to consider hypertension as a confounder in assessing the study? The answer is, only if hypertension is itself related to breast cancer. If we have asked data on hypertension in our study, we can assess this by looking at the unexposed women, the non-smokers, and seeing if there is an association between hypertension and breast cancer. If there is not, there is no need to consider hypertension as a confounder: it is associated with the exposure, but not with the outcome. Similarly, the risk of breast cancer is increased in women who have a family history of breast cancer. This will be a confounding factor only if in the study in question the prevalence of a family history of breast cancer differs between smokers and non-smokers.

Confounding in cohort and intervention studies

Because an understanding of confounding is so important, we will look at a number of simple examples, using both hypothetical and real data.

Example of concept

Consider a hypothetical example, Table 7.1. Here are the results of a cohort study in which subjects with low exercise levels are compared to subjects with high exercise levels, the outcome under investigation being the incidence of myocardial infarction in a given follow-up period.

Table A in Table 7.1 shows the simplest form of the results, showing a strong association with low-exercise people having a relative risk of 4.2 compared to high-exercise people. However, let us assume that the subjects vary in obesity, and that obesity and exercise are related; obesity is less common in the high-exercise subjects.

Table 7.1 Confounding: a cohort study assessing the association between the incidence of myocardial infarction and exercise, where obesity is a confounding factor (hypothetical data).

	Myocardial infarctions	Person-years	Incidence/1000
(A) All subjects (n = 8000 person-years)			
Low exercise	105	4000	26.25
High exercise	25	4000	6.25
Relative risk = 26.25/6.25 = 4.2			
(B_1) Obese subjects (n = 4000)			
Low exercise	90	3000	30.0
High exercise	10	1000	10.0
Relative risk = 3.0			
(B_2) Non-obese subjects (n = 4000)			
Low exercise	15	1000	15.0
High exercise	15	3000	5.0
Relative risk = 3.0			

Subtables B_1 and B_2 show the results in an identical format to the first table, separately for obese subjects and non-obese subjects. Subtable B_1 shows that the relative risk for low compared to high exercise in subjects who are obese is 3.0. Subtable B_2 shows that the relative risk for low compared to high exercise in subjects who are not obese is also 3.0. So irrespective of obesity, the best estimate of the effect of exercise is clearly 3.0.

Why then did we get the result of 4.2 in the first table for all subjects? The reason is that obesity is a confounding factor. Obesity is itself a risk factor for myocardial infarction, and this can be seen by comparing the risks for obese subjects for a given level of exercise (subtable B_1) with those for non-obese subjects with the same level of exercise (subtable B_2). For low exercise subjects, the incidence rates per 1000 are 30.0 in obese and 15.0 in non-obese subjects; for high exercise subjects, the corresponding rates are 10.0 and 5.0. Moreover, obesity is related to exercise level, as comparison of the subtables shows that low exercise subjects are much more obese in terms of their distribution by person-years of experience; for the low exercise group, 75 per cent of the person-years apply to obese subjects, while for high exercise the proportion is 25 per cent.

The relationships between these factors, low exercise, obesity, and the outcome of myocardial infarction are shown diagrammatically in Figure 7.4. Low exercise is a risk factor for myocardial infarction, with a true relative risk of 3.0. Obesity is also a risk factor for myocardial infarction, with a relative risk of 2.0, this result being derived from a comparison of subtables B_1 and B_2. However, because low exercise and obesity are positively related to each other, the apparent relative risk of low exercise, based on simply comparing all low-exercise subjects with all high-exercise subjects, is 4.2.

Further, we can add the data in subtables B_1 and B_2 to compare all obese subjects with all non-obese subjects: we obtain the apparent risk ratio of 3.3 for the crude relationship between obesity and myocardial infarction. Thus in this situation there are two independent risk factors for myocardial infarction, low exercise and obesity, which are positively correlated with each other, and therefore each acts as a confounding factor when the relationship of the other to myocardial infarction is assessed.

CONFOUNDING IN A COHORT STUDY (2)

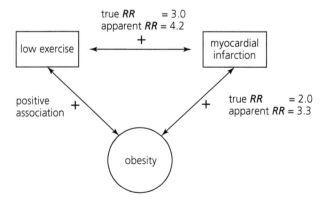

Figure 7.4 Confounding: the associations which exist in Table 7.1. RR = relative risk.

Real example

Consider now a real example of rather simple confounding, shown in Table 7.2. This is derived from a 1986 paper in the *British Medical Journal*, which amongst other comparisons (a third method, lithotripsy, was also assessed) compared the success rate for two different surgical procedures in the treatment of renal calculi [1]. The upper table shows the results as they were described in the summary of the paper. For each surgical technique, open surgery and percutaneous nephrolithotomy, 350 patients were assessed, and the success rates were 78 per cent with open surgery and 83 per cent with percutaneous nephrolithotomy.

In this study, patients were categorized into those who had stones of less than 2 cm in diameter, and those with larger stones. For patients with small stones, the success rate of open surgery was better than that of the other technique, 93 per cent compared to 87 per cent. For patients with larger stones, open surgery also had the higher success rate, 73 per cent compared to 69 per cent. Thus, for either of the two groups of patients, open surgery gave better success rates. An erroneous impression of a lower success rate is created from the pooled data, because open surgery was used much more often on patients with large stones, and those patients had a lower success rate irrespective of the technique used. (As an aside, when this error was pointed out and a more sophisticated analysis suggested, the authors rejected this as '. . . it would only confound the clinicians' [2]. In fact, no complex analysis is needed, just a cross tabulation as in Table 7.2).

Table 7.2 Confounding: a comparison of two surgical methods of treating renal calculi, showing success rates (percentage of patients with no stones at 3 months after treatment). The summary of this paper states 'success was achieved in 273 (78 per cent) of patients after open surgery, 289 (83 per cent) after percutaneous nephrolithotomy . . .'. However, in fact the success rates for open surgery are higher, not lower, than those for the percutaneous technique. The main result of this paper concerns a third method, extracorporeal shock-wave lithotripsy, which was followed by higher success rates than those shown [1].

	Successes	Failures	Total patients	Successes (%)
All stones (n = 700)				
Open surgery	273	77	350	78
Percutaneous nephrolithotomy	289	61	350	83
Stones < 2 cm (n = 357)				
Open surgery	81	6	87	93
Percutaneous nephrolithotomy	234	36	270	87
Stones ≥ 2 cm (n = 343)				
Open surgery	192	71	263	73
Percutaneous nephrolithotomy	55	25	80	69

Source: data from Charig CR et al., 'Comparison of treatment of renal calculi by open surgery, percutaneous nephrolithotomy, and extracorporeal shockwave lithotripsy,' *The British Medical Journal*, Volume 292, Issue 6524, pp. 879–882, © 1989 [1].

Simpson's paradox

In this situation, the confounding factor produced a reversal in the direction of a relationship: while percutaneous nephrolithotomy had in fact the higher success rate, the uncontrolled confounding by size of stone gave results showing a higher success rate with open surgery. While there is nothing fundamentally different in this than in other confounding effects, such a reversal of effect is sometimes called Simpson's paradox, named from the English statistician Edward Simpson who described confounding in a hypothetical clinical example in a 1951 paper [3].

Further example

Often the confounding factor will have more than two categories. A further example of real data (Table 7.3 and Figure 7.5) shows the relationship between physical activity and mortality from coronary heart disease in the prospective study of longshoremen (dock workers) in California, noted in Chapter 4 [4]. Table A in Table 7.3 shows the total data comparing light or moderate exercise level workers with heavy exercise level workers, and shows a relative risk of 3.4 in the light exercise group. However, as one might predict, there was considerable confounding by age in this study. Workers doing the lighter physical work tended to be older than those doing the heavier work. Therefore, their high relative risk could have been because they were older, rather than a direct effect of their lower exercise levels. Thus, in table B the results are sub-divided into four age groups. The relative risks for each age group range from 1.1 to 2.0. We can see that the true effect of exercise averaged over all workers must be some figure between these numbers, and cannot be as high as the observed crude relative risk of 3.4, which is produced partly by the difference in age distribution. It is not intuitively obvious what the best single estimate of the effect of exercise would be; that will be discussed later.

Confounding in case–control studies

The logic of confounding in case–control studies is identical to that in cohort studies, but the arithmetic is slightly different. Table 7.4 shows a hypothetical example of a case–control study comparing patients with skin cancer with controls, the exposure of interest being eye colour, in two categories, blue and brown.

In table A, the results for 500 cases and 500 controls are shown, giving an odds ratio of 1.59 for subjects with blue compared to brown eyes. However, hair colour has been shown to be a risk factor for skin cancer, so subtables B_1 and B_2 show the association between disease and eye colour for subjects with dark or light hair colour separately. For those with dark hair the odds ratio is 1.0, showing no association, and for those with light hair it is also 1.0. Clearly the best estimate of the association of eye colour with skin cancer is an odds ratio of 1.0, showing no association.

We have an apparent association between blue eyes and skin cancer, with the odds ratio of 1.59, although there is no true association. The apparent excess risk in

Table 7.3 Confounding: data from a cohort study of mortality from coronary heart disease and exercise. Confounding by age distorts the association between physical activity and mortality from heart disease. In table A, a comparison of men with light or moderate physical activity with those with heavy activity gives a relative risk of 3.4. Table B shows that (1) mortality rises with age and (2) the proportion of men doing light or moderate work rises with age. Age is a confounding factor, and its effect gives an increase in the observed relative risk between light activity and CHD mortality. This excess is shown as the relative risks within each of four age bands are all much lower than the crude estimate of 3.4 [4]. See also Chapter 4. (page 50–51).

Activity level	Deaths	Man-years	Rate/10 000	Relative risk
(A) All ages				
Light or moderate	532	65 000	81.8	3.4
Heavy	66	27 700	23.8	1.0 (referent)
(B) Age bands				
Age 35–44				
Light or moderate	3	5900	5.1	1.1
Heavy	4	8300	4.8	
Age 45–54				
Light or moderate	62	17 600	35.2	1.9
Heavy	20	11 000	18.2	
Age 55–64				
Light or moderate	183	23 700	77.2	1.7
Heavy	34	7400	45.9	
Age 65–74				
Light or moderate	284	17 800	159.6	2.0
Heavy	8	1000	80.0	

Source: data from Paffenbarger RS and Hale WE, 'Work activity and coronary heart mortality,' *New England Journal of Medicine*, Volume 292, Number 11, pp. 545–550, © 1975 Massachusetts Medical Society. All rights reserved [4].

individuals with blue eyes is because of a positive association between blue eyes and light skin colour. This association can be seen by comparing subtables B_1 and B_2 in terms of the control subjects: the proportion of control subjects with light hair colour who have blue eyes is 67 per cent (100/150); while the proportion of those with dark hair who have blue eyes is only 29 per cent (100/350).

Subtables B_1 and B_2 can also be used to look at the relationship between hair colour and skin cancer. The apparent odds ratio, comparing all light-haired to all dark-haired subjects, is $(300 \times 350) / (200 \times 150) = 3.5$. The true odds ratio is obtained by examining hair colour within the categories of eye colour. For subjects with blue eyes, the odds

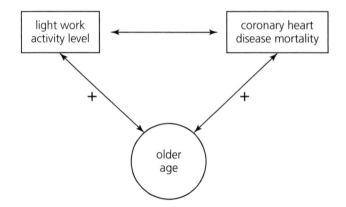

Figure 7.5 Visual representation of confounding data in Table 7.3.

Table 7.4 Confounding in a case–control study: a hypothetical example examining the relationship of eye colour to skin cancer.

	Cases	Controls
(A) All subjects (n = 1000)		
Blue eyes	257	200
Brown eyes	243	300
Total	500	500
Odds ratio = (257 × 300)/(243 × 200) = 1.59		
(B₁) Dark hair colour (n = 550)		
Blue eyes	57	100
Brown eyes	143	250
Total	200	350
Odds ratio = (57 × 250)/(143 × 100) = 1.00		
(B₂) Light hair colour (n = 450)		
Blue eyes	200	100
Brown eyes	100	50
Total	300	150
Odds ratio = (200 × 50)/(100 × 100) = 1.00		

CONFOUNDING IN A CASE CONTROL STUDY (2)

Figure 7.6 Confounding: a diagram showing the relationships present in the data given in Table 7.4.

ratio for the relationship between light hair colour and skin cancer is $(200 \times 100)/(100 \times 57) = 3.5$; for subjects with brown eyes it is $(100 \times 250)/(50 \times 143) = 3.5$. So adjusting for eye colour makes no difference to the association between hair colour and skin cancer; showing that eye colour is not a confounder in the relationship between hair colour and skin cancer. The reason eye colour is not a confounder is that although it is associated with hair colour, it is not itself a risk factor for skin cancer, as shown by its true odds ratio with skin cancer being 1.0.

The associations are shown diagrammatically in Figure 7.6. In fact, the calculation of odds ratio for hair colour within the categories of eye colour was unnecessary. Given that there is no association between eye colour and skin cancer once hair colour was controlled, we can deduce that eye colour cannot be a confounder because it does not fit the definition of a confounder: it is not associated with the outcome under study. Therefore the crude odds ratio relating hair colour to skin cancer will not be affected by controlling for eye colour. A further example of confounding in a case–control study, based on real data, will be shown in the 'Effect modification' section.

Part 2. Methods for the control of confounding

Having understood what confounding is, we can consider the methods available to deal with it. There are only five methods available, as shown in Table 7.5. In the *design* of a study we can *restrict* the participation in the study to certain individuals; we can decide to *match* individuals in the comparison group to individuals in the group of interest; and we may have the option of doing a *randomized* intervention study. Irrespective of what has been done at the design stage, when we come to the *analysis* we may again use *restriction* to certain individuals in the data set; we may divide the data into subgroups by categories of the confounding factor, which is the process known as *stratification*; or we may use *multivariate* mathematical methods to take into account the effect of

Table 7.5 The methods of controlling confounding: one or more may be used.

In the design of the study	Restriction
	Matching
	Randomization
In the analysis of the study	Restriction
	Stratification
	Multivariate methods

more than one confounding factor simultaneously. In practice, a combination of these methods is usually used. We will discuss each of these five methods.

Control of confounding: restriction

Let us go back to our example of a study of smoking and breast cancer, and consider how we could avoid being misled by the effect of obesity or of number of children. One way would be to include in the study only women who were not obese and had not had children. We could do this with either a cohort or a case–control design, and we refer to this method as 'restriction'. It is clearly an effective method, as it removes the confounding, but obviously the disadvantage is that the study then assesses only the association between smoking and breast cancer in women who are not obese and have not had children. We cannot generalize the study results beyond that population.

Suppose instead we do the entire study on women who are obese and have had children. Can there still be confounding? The answer is that there is still potential for confounding. The fact that all the women in the study are obese does not mean they all have the same degree of obesity, and if obesity has a dose–response relationship with breast cancer, and if the degree of obesity is different in smokers and non-smokers, there is still potential for confounding. The same applies to the number of children each woman has had. If, however, we restrict the entire study to women who have a body mass index of between 30 and 40 kg/m^2, and have one or two children, the extra specification in the design will reduce the extent of any confounding. However, such precise restriction would be cumbersome to apply in a practical study.

All studies involve some restriction, if only for practical reasons. The source and eligible populations will be restricted in terms of calendar time, geographical location, and frequently other factors such as age. Restriction should also be considered if there may be small groups of individuals whose results may be appreciably different from those of the main study population; if the study is unlikely to provide much useful information on these subjects, they may be better excluded. For example, a racial or ethnic group which contributes only a small proportion of subjects may have substantially different outcome rates and exposure histories, but there is little value in including such subjects if their total number is likely to be too small for independent consideration.

If information on this group is important, a new study design or a modification to include more of these subjects may be needed.

Randomization

Main advantages

We have dealt with restriction first because some degree of restriction applies to all studies. We deal with randomization next because it has many advantages over the other methods, and therefore there is a major distinction between randomized and non-randomized studies, both in design and evaluation. If a randomized intervention study is feasible, it has many advantages and should be considered first. But it is relevant only for certain situations: prospective intervention studies assessing the effects of an ethical, practical, and acceptable intervention, which is potentially beneficial and not likely to be harmful. Thus while of prime importance in assessing the effectiveness of clinical or public health interventions, randomization is not relevant to most issues regarding the causes of disease, and cannot be applied to retrospective studies.

Methods of randomization

The principle of randomization is that from a pool of study entrants, subjects are randomly assigned to each of the intervention and non-intervention groups. The definition of *random* is that each subject in the study has the same chance of being allocated to any particular group, and that the chance of a particular individual being allocated to one group is not influenced by the allocation of any other individual. It is not simply unsystematic or haphazard assignment. Methods based on an apparently random process, like tossing a coin, will work in principle, but in practice are too open to the possibility of conscious or unconscious manipulation. Randomization is normally done by reference to numbers generated to be completely random, obtained usually from a computer program [5].

The allocation sequence must be random, and the integrity of the process must be protected, and seen to be protected. Each study participant, and the staff working with them, should complete all the study entry requirements before their assignment to an intervention group is made. Subjects should be invited to participate in the study, be confirmed as eligible according to the study protocol, and should give informed consent; and their participation should be recorded. Only then should their allocation to a specific intervention group be given. The assignment and the decision about eligibility should not be changed after the assignment has been revealed. To achieve this, the randomization process is best administered independently from the recruitment of the subjects. The randomization should be done by someone who is not involved in subject recruitment, such as a statistician or pharmacist; in large trials it is often done by staff in an independent central office. There should be a record kept of all subjects assessed and considered eligible for trial entry, showing whether they gave consent to the trial, and then whether they were randomized. All subjects randomized should be considered as trial participants from the time of randomization.

Probabilistic process

The essential logic is that random allocation makes it *likely* that the two groups created will be similar in respect of any particular variable. The essential limitation of randomization is that it is a method based on probability. Therefore its chances of success will be great only if substantial numbers of subjects are used, and we can never be *certain* that randomization will provide equivalent groups. In the extreme, randomization in a study of only two individuals may protect against investigator bias in the assignment, but does not reduce the differences between the two subjects. In a large randomized study, it is highly likely that the groups created by randomization will be comparable with respect to specific factors. If, however, the numbers in each group are relatively small, (a reasonable guideline might be numbers less than 100), then it is quite likely that purely by chance the groups will still vary. If they vary in terms of a factor which is strongly related to the outcome in the study, that factor will be a confounding factor, and we must deal with that in the analysis. The practical message is that randomization is a valuable technique, which with reasonable numbers of subjects should work in most situations; but we should not assume that simply because randomization has been used, the groups being compared cannot differ in terms of any confounding factor [6]. Just as in any other study, data on the factors likely to be the main confounders should be used to compare the groups to make sure they are similar. If they are not, even in a randomized study, other methods of analysis such as stratification or multivariate methods may also be used to take account of any differences of confounding factors.

The value of randomization

Example: iron cooking pots

Table 7.6 shows the value of randomization. In a study previously mentioned in Chapter 3, the provision of iron rather than aluminium cooking pots to families was assessed as a method of reducing anaemia and improving growth in children in Ethiopia [7]. A randomized controlled trial was used, the randomization being by household, with one child per household participating. Without randomization, the families using iron pots and those using aluminium pots could differ in terms of a wide range of characteristics, which could be themselves related to child development. Table 7.6 shows that the groups created by the randomization process are very similar in terms of the age, sex, height, and weight of the children, their recent medical history, characteristics of the mother, and of household access to clean water and sanitation.

We can look at these two groups of subjects and consider whether, if they were subsequently treated in an identical manner, we should expect their outcomes to be the same; there is little in the table that would suggest otherwise. Randomization is the simplest way to achieve such equivalent groups. In principle, we could have a design where the first family seen was allocated an iron pot, and was matched to another family on the features shown in Table 7.6 which would be given an aluminium pot, but such a study would be difficult or impossible to do. The results of this study were that children in households using iron pots had a greater rise in haemoglobin concentration and gained

Table 7.6 The benefits of randomization: in a trial in Ethiopia assessing whether the use of iron pots or aluminium pots affected anaemia and weight gain in children, households were randomly allocated to receive either iron or aluminium pots, and one child per household participated in the study. These data show the similarity of the two groups in regard to characteristics at the time of randomization. SD = standard deviation [7].

	Randomized to iron pots (*n* = 195)	Randomized to aluminium pots (*n* = 212)
Age (months, mean and SD)	31.3 (14.6)	30.5 (15.7)
Male/female (numbers)	99/96	106/106
Weight (kg, mean and SD)	11.6 (2.3)	11.9 (2.3)
Length (cm, mean and SD)	87.2 (8.5)	88.0 (8.7)
Ill in week preceding study	57 (29%)	70 (33%)
Diarrhoea in week preceding study	35 (18%)	40 (19%)
Mother literate	72 (37%)	68 (32%)
Mother ill in last 7 days	50 (26%)	49 (23%)
Access to clean water	148 (76%)	157 (74%)
Adequate sanitation	57 (29%)	72 (34%)

Source: data from Adish AA et al., 'Effect of consumption of food cooked in iron pots on iron status and growth of young children: a randomised trial,' *The Lancet*, Volume 353, Issue 9154, pp. 712–716, © 1999 [7].

more in both weight and height over a 12-month period, so it was concluded that the provision of iron cooking pots may be a useful way to prevent iron deficiency anaemia in similar less developed countries [7].

There is one advantage of randomization that is shared by no other technique. This is that randomization, given reasonably large numbers of subjects, is likely to produce groups that are similar even in respect of variables that we have not anticipated, defined, or measured. Suppose that after the study just described is completed, evidence appears that an infection common in this community is a strong predictor of childhood anaemia. The study would have been better if that infection had been assessed, and if it were shown that the groups were similar in terms of it. But even without those data, as the original study was randomized and had adequate numbers, we can be reasonably sure that the distribution of the two groups in terms of this unmeasured factor would have been similar.

Difficulties with randomized studies

Practical problems

A randomized trial makes heavy demands on participants, health care professionals, and those involved indirectly such as service managers and support staff. Randomization is often difficult to use for reasons of logistics or informed consent. For example, a randomized trial comparing two drugs for the management of heroin withdrawal has been described [8]. The trial required support from a charitable foundation and from the manufacturers of the drugs, logistical support in hospital bed capacity and laboratory services, and the support of hospital staff and the patients themselves. All of these presented difficulties so that the trial could not be completed.

The design of trials has to balance the ideal scientific design with practical considerations. As an example, to evaluate a new method of encouraging smoking cessation in pregnant women, it may be administratively much easier to offer the new programme to all women in a particular clinic and compare them to women in a different clinic, than to allocate women randomly in each clinic. Such a systematic allocation method is weaker than randomization, as there is a greater chance of the groups chosen differing in terms of relevant factors, and analytical methods need to take account of the group allocation (as will be discussed later).

Informed consent

Questions of informed consent may be a critical influence on study design. In a randomized trial in Australian general practice assessing a new method of assessing skin lesions, the choice was between a study design in which individual patients were randomized, and one where general practices were randomized. If patients within each practice were randomized, the general practitioner would need to discuss both the new and the conventional assessment systems, and the randomized design, with each potential participant, and get their written consent. If practices were randomized, the general practitioners would need to give their own consent to being involved in the study, but in their opinion and that of the ethics committees, formal consent from individual patients would not be required, as both management options could be used in ordinary practice. While this ethical distinction is debatable, the result was that a study involving individual randomization was impractical because of the time it would require busy general practitioners to discuss the randomization process with each patient. The trial based on randomization of practices was carried out, with enthusiastic support from practitioners and patients [9].

The limits of randomization; residual confounding

The amount of confounding produced by a factor depends on the strength of its association with the outcome, and the strength of its association with the exposure. Consider a comparison of two treatments for lung cancer. The outcome, mortality, will vary greatly with the extent (stage) of the disease; because this association (stage-outcome) is very strong, stage may have a major confounding effect even if the difference in stage distribution between the treatment groups is small. It is not appropriate to assess confounding by applying a statistical test to compare the stage distribution in the two treatment groups. Stage could be an important confounder even if the difference in stage between the two groups is not statistically significant. Papers describing randomized trials should have a table such as Table 7.6 showing the distribution of relevant factors in the randomized groups, but statistical tests should not be used. This is recommended in the CONSORT statement, which was discussed in Chapter 5 [10].

Remaining differences

Randomization achieves its objectives by a random process. The principle is that it is *likely* that the groups produced by randomization will be equivalent. But some differences between the groups will remain, and on some occasions these differences may be substantial and important.

Example: diabetes trial

Table 7.7 shows a table of baseline characteristics for subjects in a historically important randomized study of the treatment of diabetes, comparing those randomized to receive diet and tolbutamide (an oral glucose-lowering agent) with those randomized to receive diet plus a placebo; the outcome of interest was subsequent deaths, of which many were from cardiovascular disease [11]. Comparing these two groups shows that the patients randomized to receive tolbutamide were older, more frequently had a history of digitalis use or angina, and higher proportions had an electrocardiograph abnormality, high cholesterol levels, high glucose levels, increased relative body weight, and arterial calcification assessed by an X-ray of the lower limb. On the other hand, there was a lower proportion with a history of hypertension. With these data, we cannot be confident that if the two treatments used had identical effects, the two groups would show the same results in terms of subsequent mortality. Several of these factors could have considerable effects on subsequent mortality, and the differences between the groups appear substantial.

Table 7.7 The limits of randomization: this study compared four regimens for the management of diabetes; here the subjects randomized to diet + tolbutamide (an oral glucose-lowering agent) are compared with those randomized to diet + placebo [11].

	Randomized to diet + tolbutamide $n = 204$ (% of subjects)	Randomized to diet + placebo $n = 205$ (% of subjects)
Age > 55	48.0	41.5
Digitalis use	7.6	4.5
Angina	7.0	5.0
ECG abnormality	4.0	3.0
Cholesterol > 300 mg/100 ml	15.1	8.6
Fasting glucose > 110 mg/100 ml	72.1	63.5
Relative body weight > 1.25	58.8	52.7
Arterial calcification	19.7	14.3
Hypertension	30.2	36.8

Source: data from University Group Diabetes Program, 'A study of the effects of hypoglycemic agents on vascular complications in patients with adult-onset diabetes II: Mortality results,' *Diabetes*, Volume 19, Supplement 2, pp. 785–830, © 1970 [11].

'Failure' of randomization

Sometimes this is loosely referred to as a 'failure of randomization', but that is an inappropriate term. The randomization process has been carried out correctly, but being a probabilistic technique it does not guarantee that the groups will be similar in terms of all factors. Statistical tests show that all but one (cholesterol levels) of these differences are not statistically significant at the conventional 5 per cent level, in other words, differences of this or greater magnitude would be expected to occur on more than 5 per cent of occasions. However, that is not the relevant issue; the relevant issue is whether the differences are sufficiently large to influence the subsequent outcome rates in the two groups: a small difference in a factor which is strongly related to outcome will be important. Thus in Table 7.7 we have a randomized study in which there are important differences between the groups being compared. The results of this study showed that total deaths, and particularly deaths from cardiovascular disease, were substantially higher in the group treated with tolbutamide than in the placebo group. The crucial question is whether this difference in mortality can be attributed to the tolbutamide, or whether it is due to the other factors that differ between the two groups. As will be shown later in this chapter, other analytical techniques can be used to address this question.

Pre-stratification

It follows from this that where some major confounding factors can be predicted in advance, it may be better not to rely only on the randomization procedure to produce similar groups [6]. A more reliable procedure is to group the eligible subjects within categories of the strong confounder, and randomize within these categories. Thus in the earlier example we could classify all study entrants by stage of disease, and randomize within each stage, thus ensuring that the stage distribution of the treatment groups will be virtually identical. This is a combination of randomization and stratification, and is sometimes referred to as *randomization within blocks*, or *pre-stratification*. For example, in a trial of perineal pain relief after childbirth, women were randomized within four strata, determined by parity (first birth and later births) and mode of birth (spontaneous and instrumental), as these factors were important in regard to perineal trauma and pain [12]. However, randomized trials are often difficult and time-consuming in practice, and in clinical studies simple designs have great advantages, and pre-stratification should be used cautiously. It is often used to randomize within centres in multicentre studies, ensuring that each centre treats similar numbers of subjects on each of the alternative therapies.

Analysis of randomized trials: intention-to-treat analysis

Not all individuals will complete the treatment to which they have been randomized. Some patients may start the treatment but not complete it; they may decide to discontinue, either for reasons related to the treatment (e.g. side effects) or for other reasons (e.g. change of residence), or their clinical situation may change so that a change in treatment is indicated. Some patients may be randomized but not even commence treatment. Consider Figure 7.7. This represents a clinical trial in which patients are

ANALYSIS OF A RANDOMIZED TRIAL (1)

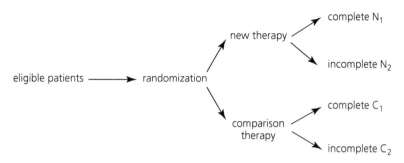

Figure 7.7 Compliance: a randomized trial in which not all subjects complete the treatment course offered. Which groups should be compared?

randomized into two treatment groups, but only some of the patients complete the course of treatment offered. The question is: to assess the effect of the new therapy, which groups of patients should be compared?

One simple answer is to compare patients who received the new therapy with those who did not. The only group who received the new therapy is group N_1; those who were allocated the new treatment and completed it. So we could compare group N_1 with either all other subjects ($C_1 + C_2 + N_2$), all subjects allocated to the comparison treatment ($C_1 + C_2$), or to those allocated to the comparison treatment who completed it (group C_1).

However, if any of these comparisons is used, the value of randomization in controlling confounding is lost, because the comparisons are no longer being made between randomized groups. There may be very considerable differences between the subjects who complete the new treatment (N_1), and those who withdraw or do not receive it (N_2).

Example: lipid-lowering drugs—intention-to-treat analysis

A classic example of this is shown in a randomized double-blind trial comparing lipid-reducing drugs with placebo, carried out in the United States in 1966–69 [13] (Figure 7.8). The outcome was mortality from any cause over the following 5 years. The mortality rate in those patients who were allocated to the lipid-lowering agent clofibrate, and actually consumed over 80 per cent of the allocated dosages, was 15.0 per cent. This rate could be compared to the mortality rate in all patients allocated to the placebo, which was 19.4 per cent, showing a statistically significant difference in favour of clofibrate. However, the patients who were randomized to clofibrate but did not take it had a much higher mortality, 24.6 per cent. This is of course consistent with a beneficial effect of the drug; we would expect patients who did not take the drug adequately to have a higher mortality than those who took it well. But it would be dangerous to ascribe these results to the pharmacological effects of the drug. The point is dramatically illustrated by the mortality experience in relation to compliance

ANALYSIS OF A RANDOMIZED TRIAL (2)

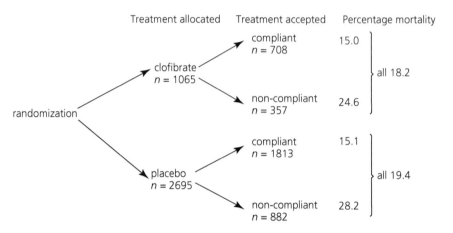

Figure 7.8 Compliance in a randomized trial: the results show the mortality rates from all causes after 5 years of follow-up in patients randomized to either a lipid-lowering agent (clofibrate) or a placebo, in terms of their compliance with the drug regimen. 'Compliant' means taking > 80 per cent of the allocated drug [13].

Source: data from Coronary Drug Project Research Group, 'Influence of adherence to treatment and response of cholesterol on mortality in the Coronary Drug Project,' *New England Journal of Medicine*, Volume 303, Number 18, pp. 1038–1041, © 1980 Massachusetts Medical Society. All rights reserved [13].

with the placebo; those who took more than 80 per cent of the allocated doses of the placebo had a mortality of 15.1 per cent, and those who took less had a mortality rate of 28.2 per cent. The correct analysis of the randomized groups shows that the mortality rate in all those randomized to clofibrate was 18.2 per cent, similar to the rate in all those randomized to placebo, 19.4 per cent. Any other comparison gives an incorrect result because of the confounding effects of factors related to compliance. The results also show that irrespective of what drug is prescribed, subjects who follow the instructions carefully have a lower mortality rate than those who do not. This cannot be ascribed to any pharmacological action, but reflects the influence of factors that are related to compliance, which are confounding factors in the association between the drug allocated and outcome. The correct analysis is referred to as '*intention-to-treat*' analysis; we compare the groups defined by the initial treatment offered.

Example: breast cancer screening

This issue is important both in clinical and in community-based studies. In the first randomized trial of breast cancer screening, women who were members of a health maintenance plan in New York were randomly allocated into two groups [14]. One group continued their normal medical care. Women in the other group were offered an innovative programme of screening for breast cancer, using mammography and clinical examination. About two-thirds of those offered this programme participated. The relevant outcome is death from breast cancer, so the appropriate randomized analysis shows the effect of *offering* a breast cancer screening programme, with a two-thirds acceptance rate, on breast cancer mortality. After some 10 years of follow-up, there was a reduction of around 30 per cent in breast cancer mortality. This randomized trial shows the effect of *offering* a programme of screening. It does not measure the reduction in mortality risk for an individual who agrees to participate, except that this must be higher than the difference shown. Estimates of this can be made, but are uncertain because they depend on how those who participated in the programme differed from those who declined the offered screening in regard to their underlying risk of death from breast cancer.

Management and explanatory trials

In these circumstances, the comparison of randomized groups will be inefficient, as there is a dilution effect as many subjects in the intervention group are not actually receiving the intervention. However, in considering this we have to go back to the question of what the trial is actually for, and how the results will be applied. It is a naive supposition that all patients will follow a doctor's advice, or that everyone will participate in a planned intervention. In many situations, unless the intervention results in an improved outcome, given that a substantial proportion of subjects will not accept it in full, it will not be useful. Trials such as the screening trial address the *management* question: what is the effect of offering an intervention, in a practical situation?

An *explanatory* trial addresses a different question, that is, irrespective of the practical issues involved, what is the effect of the intervention in ideal circumstances, in subjects who do accept it? An explanatory trial comparing two drugs could be done by selecting eligible subjects, obtaining consent, ensuring they all have a high chance of completing the follow-up needed, perhaps by using incentives or requiring they successfully complete a first period of follow-up, and only then randomizing them into groups. Within these precautions, drop-outs and loss to follow-up should be minimal, so that the comparison of randomized groups shows the effects with high participation. Doing such a trial on breast cancer screening, on a large scale, is however, too difficult and has not been done.

Example: iron deficiency

Both types of trial are legitimate: the dangers arise if the results from a study designed or analysed as an explanatory trial are interpreted in management terms. For example, iron deficiency anaemia in adolescence may affect cognitive function, so iron supplementation could protect or improve cognitive function. A randomized trial of iron supplementation carried out on high school girls in the United States assessed this, and showed that the girls who received iron supplementation performed better on tests of verbal learning and memory after 8 weeks than did girls in the control group [15]. However, girls who were clinically anaemic were excluded from the trial, other vitamins or iron supplements were prohibited, many strategies were used to ensure compliance, and the outcome measures used were research tools; and most important, the analysis was based on only the girls who completed treatment rather than being an intention to treat analysis. This was an explanatory study and the results apply under ideal conditions, and therefore show the potential rather than the practical value of iron supplementation [16]. A management study, to directly assess whether iron supplementation in practice would have clinically relevant benefits, would need to use realistic rather than ideal methods of ensuring compliance, use less stringent eligibility criteria, use a more relevant end point and time of assessment, and in particular include in the analysis all subjects randomized.

Pragmatic or practical trials

The terms *pragmatic* or *practical* clinical trials, with meanings similar to management trials, have been used for trials designed to guide clinical or health policy decisions. Trials relevant to policymaking should be based on relevant interventions, and include a diverse population of study participants, recruited from different practice settings, with data collected on a broad range of health outcomes [17].

Example: prostate cancer screening—intention to treat

If a management trial correctly analysed by intention to treat shows no effect that could be because the intervention did not work or because too few subjects accepted it. A controversial example, which also shows the dangers of incorrect analysis, is a randomized trial of prostate cancer screening. Men aged 45–80 years sampled from the electoral rolls in Quebec City, Canada, were randomly allocated in a 2:1 ratio either to receive an invitation to a screening programme using annual measurements of serum prostate-specific antigen (PSA) and digital rectal examination, or to be in a non-invited control group. This is a standard randomized design. The outcome was the death rate from prostate cancer in the 11 years after randomization, reported in two main papers [18,19].

The results based on this randomization (Figure 7.9) show a relative risk of 1.08, an 8 per cent increase in deaths in the group offered screening. However, the published paper shows, in contrast, a relative risk of 0.38, a 62 per cent reduction in mortality, and the authors concluded that their study 'demonstrates, for the first time, that early diagnosis and treatment permits a dramatic decrease in deaths from prostate cancer' [18]. The large mortality reduction is based on a comparison between men who were randomized to screening and were screened, compared to those randomized to no screening who were not screened (groups N_1 and C_1 in the terminology of Figure 7.7, shown earlier). This analysis restricted to compliant subjects is shown in Figure 7.9, and gives the relative risk of 0.38. In the earlier paper, the main comparison was between all the men who were screened, whether they were invited for screening or not, and all other men in the study who were not screened (groups N_1 plus C_2 versus groups N_2 plus C_1 in Figure 7.7); this gave a similar large reduction.

In both these analyses, the benefits of the randomized design have been lost. In the more recent paper, an 'intent to screen' analysis was also made and the lack of effect recognized, but this is given little importance. In this trial, few men invited for screening were actually screened (23 per cent), so that the randomized trial has lost most of its ability to detect an effect of screening because of misclassification (in addition, 7 per cent of the men randomized to the non-invited group were screened, but this is a smaller problem). However, this does not give validity to the non-randomized

ANALYSIS OF A RANDOMIZED TRIAL OF SCREENING

Figure 7.9 Different analyses of a randomized trial of screening: the correct analysis, maintaining the randomized groups, gives a relative risk of 54.4/50.4 = 1.08. Other comparisons lose the advantage of the randomization [19].

Source: data from Labrie F et al., 'Screening decreases prostate cancer mortality: 11-year follow-up of the 1988 Quebec prospective randomized controlled trial,' *Prostate*, Volume 59, Issue 3, pp. 311–318, © 2004 [19].

comparisons, which, presented in papers with the title of a randomized trial, are misleading [20,21].

Stratification

To discuss the next method of controlling confounding, let us go back to the example of studies of smoking and breast cancer, and the problem of confounding by obesity. As we have seen, we could avoid confounding by obesity, by restriction. This could lead to a series of restricted studies, one looking at non-obese women, one at women at a certain level of obesity, and so on. This situation can however be achieved in one study. We could include smokers and non-smokers in a cohort study without any limitations, but with careful recording of each woman's obesity (derived from her height and weight). Then in the analysis, we divide the data, and compare smokers in each category of obesity with non-smokers in the same category, and so on throughout the various levels of obesity. This procedure is '*stratification*', as strata or layers of data are formed. The stratification is done on the basis of the suspected confounding factor. This is the most important and widely used method of controlling confounding. It is used in the majority of studies either on its own or in combination with other methods.

Indeed, we have already used stratification several times. In Table 7.1, we demonstrated the effect of stratification by smoking in a study relating exercise to myocardial infarction. In Table 7.2, we stratified by the size of the renal stone in the study comparing surgical methods in the treatment of renal stones. In Table 7.3, we used four age groups to control confounding by age in a cohort study. In Table 7.4, we used stratification by hair colour in a case–control study relating eye colour to skin cancer. In each of these examples, we went as far as dividing the data into strata, and looking at the measure of association (relative risk or odds ratio) within each stratum of the confounder, and we also made some comments about the range of these results. The extra process, which we will now consider, is how to use the stratified data to produce a *single overall estimate* of effect that has been *adjusted* for the effects of the confounding factor.

Stratification in cohort and intervention studies: Mantel–Haenszel method

The results from the cohort study relating exercise to deaths from heart disease previously shown in Table 7.3, are summarized in Box 7.1, table A, for the four age groups. The total combined data for all ages give a relative risk of 3.44. This is misleading as it is confounded by age; the age-specific relative risks range from 1.06 to 1.99.

A practical difficulty arises when data are divided into a number of strata. The numbers of subjects in one stratum may be small, and therefore the outcome measure, such as the relative risk, for that stratum will be imprecise; so, the relative risk estimates may vary considerably among the strata. There are two issues. First, can we assume that there is a *constant* measure of association, such as relative risk, which can be applied to all strata? At this point we will simply point out that differences based on small numbers are unlikely to be important (such as the youngest age group in Box 7.1), and we should be concerned only about substantial differences between the relative risks in different strata. In Chapter 8 we will present statistical methods to test whether the assumption of a constant relative risk for all the strata is justified. Then, if we assume that the true relative risk is likely to be the same in all strata, we can use the data for all strata to produce a single estimate of relative risk, which is adjusted for the effects of the confounding factor.

This adjusted relative risk will be some type of average of the relative risks in the different strata. There are several methods of producing an overall estimate, which use different methods of averaging. One method indeed would be a simple arithmetic average of the relative risks for each stratum. But this would assume that they are equally precise, and in our example the relative risk for the youngest age group is based only on seven deaths in total, and so we should give it less importance than the relative risks in the other groups.

Calculation of relative risk after adjustment for the confounder

An appropriate method of averaging is to give each stratum an importance related to the amount of information or, in other words, the numbers in the stratum. One widely used method is shown in Box 7.2, and applied in Box 7.1 in table B. The formula for the adjusted relative risk has the same structure as the formula for the relative risk in one stratum. The numerator is the sum of the numerator terms derived from each stratum,

Box 7.1 Stratification in a cohort study: the study shown in Table 7.3 gives, on simple analysis, a misleading result because of confounding by age (table A). Stratification by age avoids this. One method of calculating a summary relative risk measure, adjusting for the stratification, is shown in table B

STRATIFICATION IN A COHORT STUDY: MANTEL–HAENSZEL ANALYSIS

(A) Data stratified by the confounder (age)

Age group	Exposed (light exercise)			Unexposed (heavy exercise)			Relative Risk
	Deaths	Man-years (thousands)	Rate/1000	Deaths	Man-years (thousands)	Rate/1000	
	a_i	N_{1i}	a_i/N_{1i}	c_i	N_{0i}	c_i/N_{0i}	
35–44	3	5.9	0.51	4	8.3	0.48	1.06
45–54	62	17.6	3.52	20	11.0	1.82	1.94
55–64	183	23.7	7.72	34	7.4	4.59	1.68
60–74	284	17.8	15.96	8	1.0	8.00	1.99
All ages	532	65	8.18	66	27.7	2.38	

Crude relative risk (no adjustment for age) = 8.18/2.38 = 3.44

(B) Calculation of summary relative risk, adjusted for the confounder, by the Mantel–Haenszel method

Age group	Total man-years (T_i)	a_iN_{0i}/T_i	c_iN_{1i}/T_i
35–44	14.2	1.75	1.66
45–54	28.6	23.85	12.31
55–64	31.1	43.54	25.91
65–74	18.8	15.11	7.57
Sum		84.25	47.45

Mantel–Haenszel relative risk = (84.25/47.45) = 1.78

and the denominator is a sum of the denominator terms derived from each stratum. The result gives a *weighted average* of the relative risks, in which the weights given to each stratum relate to the amount of information within each stratum. This *adjusted* relative risk is a reasonable summary value of the overall relative risk, adjusting for the confounding effect of the stratification factor, in this case, age. Here this adjusted relative risk is 1.78. This can be seen to be compatible with the four *age-specific* relative risks shown in Box 7.1 table A. This method is derived from a method first developed for use in case–control studies, and is referred to as the Mantel–Haenszel method. (The algebraic notation used in Box 7.1 and Box 7.2 is the same as that used previously in

---

Box 7.2 Stratification: calculation of the Mantel–Haenszel estimate of the summary relative risk in a stratified analysis

---

MANTEL–HAENSZEL ESTIMATION OF RELATIVE RISK

In each subtable i, stratified by the potential confounder:

	Cases	Total subjects or person-years
Exposed	a_i	N_{1i}
Unexposed	c_i	N_{0i}
		T_i = total in the subtable

Relative risk for this subtable = $(a_i/N_{1i})/(c_i/N_{0i}) = a_iN_{0i}/c_iN_{1i}$

The Mantel–Haenszel estimate of relative risk uses the data from all subtables, but gives an estimate of the unconfounded relative risk:

given by $\dfrac{\sum\limits_{i} a_iN_{0i}/T_i}{\sum\limits_{i} c_iN_{1i}/T_i}$

where $\sum\limits_{i}$ indicates summation over all the subtables

---

Chapter 4, except that we indicate the data within one stratum by a subscript $_1$ for the first stratum, $_2$ for the second, etc., which is shown in general terms by the subscript $_i$.)

Example

Stratification can be used in any study design, including randomized trials. We emphasized earlier that while randomization is likely to produce evenly balanced groups, it does not always do so. In Table 7.7, some information from a randomized trial of tolbutamide and placebo in the management of diabetes was given, which suggested substantial differences in the groups being compared. Table 7.8, table A, gives the main results of that study, showing death rates from all causes of 14.7 per cent in the tolbutamide-treated patients and 10.2 per cent in the placebo-treated patients, giving a relative risk of 1.44. We can assess whether these differences are influenced by the differences in the baseline characteristics shown in Table 7.7, by stratified analyses. In Table 7.8, table B, the stratification by arterial calcification is shown. Arterial calcification is a true confounder; it is more common in the tolbutamide-treated group than in the placebo-treated group, and within each treatment group the death rate is higher in the subjects with arterial calcification. However, both within subjects with arterial calcification and in those without arterial calcification, the death rate is higher in the tolbutamide-treated subjects. The best estimate of the relationship between tolbutamide treatment and mortality, adjusted for the differences in prevalence of arterial calcification, is given by the Mantel–Haenszel relative risk calculation, which gives a relative risk of 1.32. We compare this with the original relative risk of 1.44. The conclusion is that the crude increased risk in the tolbutamide group (RR = 1.44) is reduced by stratifying for arterial calcification, but is not abolished and most of the excess risk

Table 7.8 Stratified analysis of a randomized trial: main results of the trial shown in Table 7.7 (table A), and results stratified for arterial calcification (subtables B$_1$ and B$_2$), and adjusted relative risk calculated by the modified Mantel–Haenszel method (Box 7.2) [11]. As often occurs, some data are missing: eight subjects are omitted from the stratified analysis as data on arterial calcification were missing. The crude relative risk for the two subtables combined is 1.42.

(A) Main results (n = 409)

Treatment	Deaths	Survivors	Total	% dead	Relative risk
Tolbutamide	30	174	204	14.7	1.44
Placebo	21	184	205	10.2	1.0(R)

(B$_1$) Stratified: arterial calcification present (n = 68)

Treatment	Deaths	Survivors	Total	% dead	Relative risk
Tolbutamide	13	26	39	33.3	1.93
Placebo	5	24	29	17.2	

(B$_2$) Stratified: arterial calcification absent (n = 333)

Treatment	Deaths	Survivors	Total	% dead	Relative risk
Tolbutamide	16	143	159	10.1	1.09
Placebo	16	158	174	9.2	

Relative risk adjusted for arterial calcification

$$= (13 \times 29/68 + 16 \times 174/333)/(5 \times 39/68 + 16 \times 159/333) = 1.32$$

Source: data from University Group Diabetes Program, 'A study of the effects of hypoglycemic agents on vascular complications in patients with adult-onset diabetes II: Mortality results,' *Diabetes*, Volume 19, Supplement 2, pp. 785–830, © 1970 [11].

is still maintained (RR = 1.32). Analyses of this form can be carried out for each of the variables listed in Table 7.7. However it is clear that this method of analysis is still unsatisfactory, as although it is easy to adjust for each of the variables singly, we are still not answering the more general question which is: does the difference in mortality between tolbutamide and placebo treated patients persist when we take into account the effect of *all* the factors on which we have baseline information? That issue requires more complex analysis that will be shown later in this chapter.

Direct standardization

Another method of taking a weighted average of stratum-specific relative risks is *direct standardization*, which is frequently used in large data sets such as statistical data from whole countries or communities. It is most frequently applied to age, often within the 18 five-year age groups from 0–4 years to 85+ years, or to sex, or ethnic group. It is simply another form of averaging of stratified data, and can be applied to any confounder. For each group being compared, the stratum-specific rates are multiplied by the number of subjects or person-years in that stratum of a '*standard population*'. This standard population may be an intuitively relevant population (such as the whole country in a particular year), or an arbitrary or even artificial population.

The incidence rates for breast cancer in women in 2009 in New Zealand, for the Maori and non-Maori populations, are shown in Table 7.9. In Maori, there were 339 new cases in 332 400 women, giving a crude incidence rate of 102.0 per 100 000 per year. In non-Maori, there were 2420 cases in 1.867 million women, giving a crude rate of 129.6 per 100 000 per year. The rate is 21 per cent *lower* in Maori women, with a risk ratio (Maori: non-Maori) of 0.79. However, the data show that the Maori population is younger, and the rate of breast cancer rises with age, so age is a confounder. To adjust for age, we will use the 'world standard population', an arbitrary population developed by the World Health Organization for this purpose, which approximates the age distribution of the whole world population [22]. For each age group, the observed rate is multiplied by the standard population for that age group, the results are summed, and then divided by the total standard population. The direct age standardized incidence rates produced in this way are 126.2 per 100 000 for Maori, and 89.5 for non-Maori, so the age-standardized rate is 41 per cent *higher* in Maori. The age-standardized incidence ratio is a better description of the relative risk to a woman: thus, on average over the age groups, a Maori women has a 40 per cent higher risk of breast cancer than a non-Maori woman. Of course, other factors—such as the completeness of diagnosis and recording, also have to be considered.

Example: application in a cohort study

Direct standardization can be applied to any stratified data where the stratum-specific rates are known. Table 7.10 shows direct age standardization applied to the study of exercise and heart disease deaths shown earlier. For each exposure group (light or heavy exercise), the death rates for each age group are shown, taken from Table 7.3 Then these are multiplied by the standard population for that age group, to give the 'expected' number of deaths in each age stratum. Here the standard population is the total number of man-years of observation in each age group. Adding these and dividing by the total standard population gives the age-standardized death rate for the low-exercise group (6.99 per 10 000 man-years) and the high-exercise group (3.80 per 10 000 man-years). The ratio of these is the age-standardized relative risk, 1.84. This is not numerically the same as the Mantel–Haenszel relative risk, which as shown in Box 7.1 was 1.78, because a different weighting system has been used. The Mantel–Haenszel estimate is generally preferable, as its weighting system takes into account the different amount of information in each stratum, whereas the age standardization system does not necessarily do this, depending on the standard population chosen. In large data sets, such as routine vital statistics, there is so much data available that this is not really a problem, and that is where direct standardization is most frequently used.

Choice of standard population

A direct age-standardized rate will depend on the standard population used, and that should always be stated when such rates are presented. The World Health Organization

Table 7.9 Age standardization of incidence rates: incidence data for New Zealand women, Maori and non-Maori 2009, using the World Health Organization standard population [22].

Breast cancer incidence, New Zealand, 2009; females

Age	Maori population				Non-Maori population				WHO standard popn
	Cases	Pop. thousands	Rate per 100 000	Rate*std pop	Cases	Pop. thousands	Rate per 100 000	Rate*std pop	
0–	0	41.3	0.0	0.0	0	107.5	0.0	0.0	8.86
5–	0	34.0	0.0	0.0	0	106.5	0.0	0.0	8.69
10–	0	33.5	0.0	0.0	0	111.4	0.0	0.0	8.60
15–	0	33.3	0.0	0.0	0	124.7	0.0	0.0	8.47
20–	0	27.5	0.0	0.0	2	122.2	1.6	13.5	8.22
25–	3	22.4	13.4	106.2	7	120.0	5.8	46.3	7.93
30–	4	22.3	18.0	136.7	34	117.9	28.8	219.5	7.61
35–	12	23.2	51.7	370.0	87	138.3	62.9	449.9	7.15
40–	31	21.1	147.1	969.1	187	141.1	132.5	873.4	6.59
45–	65	20.6	315.1	1903.1	319	145.6	219.1	1323.2	6.04
50–	62	16.1	385.3	2069.2	265	128.7	205.9	1105.5	5.37
55–	54	12.1	445.5	2027.2	292	113.5	257.3	1170.7	4.55
60–	48	8.9	541.8	2015.3	344	103.8	331.4	1232.8	3.72
65–	30	6.3	473.9	1402.8	283	81.4	347.8	1029.6	2.96

(Continued)

Table 7.9 (Continued)

Breast cancer incidence, New Zealand, 2009; females

Age	Maori population				Non-Maori population				WHO standard popn
	Cases	Pop, thousands	Rate per 100 000	Rate*std pop	Cases	Pop, thousands	Rate per 100 000	Rate*std pop	
70–	11	4.5	243.4	537.8	158	63.7	248.2	548.4	2.21
75–	12	2.9	419.6	637.8	154	53.6	287.4	436.9	1.52
80–	5	1.5	328.9	299.3	131	43.9	298.7	271.9	0.91
85+	2	0.9	232.6	147.7	157	43.5	361.3	229.4	0.64
TOTAL	339	332.4		12 622.4	2420	1867.1		8950.9	100.04

Rates	Maori population	Non-Maori population	RR (Maori to non-Maori)
Crude	102.0	129.6	0.79
Standardized	126.2	89.5	1.41

Source: data from Ahmad OB et al., *Age standardization of rates: a new WHO population*, World Health Organization, Geneva, Switzerland, © 2001, available from http://www.who.int/healthinfo/paper31.pdf [22].

Table 7.10 Stratification in a cohort study: direct standardization. The stratified data are the same as in Box 7.1. Here a standard population is chosen as the total man-years at risk in each age group, and to this is applied the age-specific death rates in each of the exposure groups, to give the numbers of deaths expected in each exposure group if each had had the same age distribution. The ratio of these expected numbers is the standardized relative risk.

Age group	Standard population	Exposed (light exercise)		Unexposed (heavy exercise)	
		Observed death rate	Expected deaths in std. pop.	Observed death rate	Expected deaths in std. pop.
	S_i	r_{ei}	$S_i r_{ei}$	r_{ui}	$S_i r_{ui}$
35–44	14.2	0.51	7.2	0.48	6.8
45–54	28.6	3.52	100.7	1.82	52.1
55–64	31.1	7.72	240.1	4.59	142.7
65–74	18.8	15.96	300.0	8.00	150.4
Sum	92.7		648.1		352.0

Age-standardized incidence rate =
(sum expected deaths)/(sum standard population) = 6.99 (exposed); 3.80 (unexposed)
Age standardized relative risk = 6.99/3.80 = 1.84

standard population was introduced to encourage countries to report data using a common standard, so that the rates can be compared. Standardized rates based on different standard populations cannot be compared directly. Further, comparisons will depend on the standard used, as that determines the weight put on each category: for example, if differences are greater in younger people, a standard population with a higher proportion (greater weight) in the younger age groups will show a bigger difference.

Indirect standardization

Another method of standardization is indirect standardization, which gives results often referred to as a standardized mortality ratio or standardized incidence ratio (SMR or SIR). This method is frequently used to compare one smaller group with a larger group that includes it, for example, to compare rates in one occupational group with those of the whole country. Table 7.11 shows an example where 12 deaths from lung cancer occurred in an occupational group, male cooks, over 4 years in New Zealand. To assess this, we calculate the 'expected' number of lung cancers; that is, the number that would arise if the death rates for the standard population (here, all employed men) applied to the cooks. For each age group, we multiply the age-specific rate in the standard population by the numbers of person-years in each age group for the cooks (basically the number of cooks, obtained from census data, multiplied by 4 years) to give an expected number of deaths in that age group. We then add the expected numbers; here, giving 7.1 'expected' deaths. The ratio of the observed number of deaths to this expected number of deaths shows how the actual mortality experience varies from that

Table 7.11 Calculation of a standardized mortality ratio: the data needed are the total number of events in the 'special' population. Here the special population is male 'cooks and related workers' aged 25–64 in New Zealand, 1983–1986. The expected number is calculated by applying the age-specific rates for a 'standard' population, here all employed males in New Zealand, 1983–1986, to the age-specific population at risk for the special occupational group.

Total observed number of events (deaths from lung cancer) = 12			
Expected number of deaths if stratum-specific rates were same as the standard population is calculated as follows:			
Strata of confounder (age group)	Number of person-years P_i	Mortality rate in standard population per 100 000 R_i	Expected number of deaths = $R_i \times P_i$
25–34	7557	0.8	0.06
35–44	4023	4.8	0.19
45–54	2961	47.9	1.42
55–64	2043	265.8	5.43
Total expected number = sum of expected numbers = 7.10			
Standardized mortality ratio = observed/expected = 1.69			

expected, adjusted for age. This is often expressed as a percentage, so that a value above 100 shows a higher mortality rate in the study population than in the standard population. In our example, the age-SMR is 1.69, or 169 per cent.

For this calculation, the only required data for the cooks is the number of cooks (or person-years) in each age group and the total number of deaths. It is not necessary to know the number of deaths within each age group, which is needed for direct standardization or a Mantel–Haenszel analysis; this is fact is the main advantage of the indirect standardization method. If all the data needed is available, the direct standardization or the Mantel–Haenszel method are usually preferable. With indirect standardization the SMR of one specific group cannot be directly compared with that of another group.

Stratification in case–control studies

To apply stratified analysis in a case–control study, we follow the same principle: we divide the data into strata defined by levels of the confounding factor, and calculate the measure of association, usually the odds ratio, for each stratum. As the same issues of small numbers and consequent instability of estimates apply in case–control studies as in cohort studies, we need a method of producing a summary measure of association. The most widely used method is the Mantel–Haenszel estimate of odds ratio, described in a now classic paper [23]. This is a weighted average of the stratum specific odds ratios, the weights being dependent on the numbers of observations in each stratum, as shown in Box 7.3.

Box 7.3 Stratification: calculation of the Mantel–Haenszel estimate of the summary odds ratio in a stratified analysis

MANTEL–HAENSZEL ESTIMATION OF ODDS RATIO

In each subtable *i*, stratified by the potential confounder:

	Cases	Controls
Exposed	a_i	b_i
Unexposed	c_i	d_i

T_i = total in the subtable

Odds ratio for this subtable = $a_i d_i / b_i c_i$

The Mantel–Haenszel estimate of odds ratio uses the data from all subtables, but gives an estimate of the unconfounded odds ratio:

given by $\sum_i (a_i d_i / T_i) / \sum_i (b_i c_i / T_i)$

where $\sum_i$ indicates summation over all the subtables

Example: malignant melanoma

Table 7.12 shows some simplified, but real, data from a case–control study comparing patients with malignant melanoma (a skin cancer) with community-based controls [24]. Table A shows a positive association of melanoma with a history of severe sunburn, giving an odds ratio of 1.40. This association could be due to the trauma of the sunburn, to the sun exposure involved, or to the individual's susceptibility to sunburn. In the subtables B_1 and B_2, we control for susceptibility to sunburn by stratifying the data into two levels of susceptibility (in the actual study, four levels were used). Both in subjects who burn easily and in those who do not, the odds ratio for the association between sunburn history and melanoma is lower than that in the crude analysis; the Mantel–Haenszel estimate gives 1.19 as the unconfounded odds ratio. Thus the crude odds ratio of 1.40 is produced partially by confounding by tendency to sunburn, which is also related to melanoma. Statistical tests on these data will be shown in Chapter 8 (Box 8.4).

Effect modification

In the example in Table 7.12, the odds ratios in individual strata are so similar that there is no obvious utility in the summary estimate. However with many subtables with small numbers of observations in each, the stratum specific odds ratios will be unstable, but the summary estimate provides a stable measure of the overall odds ratio, which has been adjusted for confounding by the factor which has been stratified. Of course, if the odds ratios in the different strata are very different from each other, it may be misleading to use a summary estimate.

Table 7.12 Stratified analysis of a case–control study comparing patients with malignant melanoma with community controls with regard to history of sunburn, and adjusting for tendency to sunburn [24].

	Cases	Controls
(A) All subjects (n = 924)		
Exposed: severe sunburn	136	98
Unexposed: mild sunburn	343	347
Total	479	445
Odds ratio = (136 × 347)/(98 × 343) = 1.40		
(B₁) Subjects who sunburn easily (n = 595)		
Severe sunburn	119	76
Mild sunburn	227	173
Total	346	249
Odds ratio = (119 × 173)/(76 × 227) = 1.19		
(B₂) Subjects who do not sunburn easily (n = 329)		
Severe sunburn	17	22
Mild sunburn	116	174
Total	133	196
Odds ratio = (17 × 174)/(22 × 116) = 1.16		
Mantel–Haenszel estimate of odds ratio		

$$= \frac{119 \times 173 / 595 + 17 \times 174 / 329}{76 \times 227 / 595 + 22 \times 116 / 329}$$
$$= 1.19$$

Source: data from Elwood JM et al., 'Sunburn, suntan and the risk of cutaneous malignant melanoma: the Western Canada Melanoma Study,' *British Journal Cancer*, Volume 51, Issue 4, pp. 543–549, © 1985 [24].

Example

In a case–control study of carcinoma of the uterine cervix, for smoking the overall data show an odds ratio of 6.6 [25] (Table 7.13). When the data are subdivided by age, the odds ratios show great variation, from 27.9 at age 20–29, to 5.9 at age 30–39, and 2.8 at ages over 40. This demonstrates *effect modification*; the association with smoking is *modified* by age. Effect modification can occur with or without confounding. To assess confounding by age, we can use the Mantel–Haenszel odds ratio, calculated as shown in Box 7.3, which gives the odds ratio after age adjustment of 6.3. This is close to the crude odds ratio of 6.6, and shows that there is very little confounding by age in these data.

Table 7.13 Effect modification: in this case–control study relating smoking to cancer of the cervix in women, the crude odds ratio (table A) is 6.6, and the Mantel–Haenszel odds ratio, adjusted for age, is 6.3; there is little confounding by age. However, age modifies the effect; the odds ratios for smoking in the different age groups are very different [25].

(A) All ages

		Cases	Controls	Odds ratio
All ages:	Smokers	130	45	
	Non-smokers	87	198	6.6

(B) Data stratified by age

		Cases	Controls	Odds ratio
Age 20–29	Smokers	41	6	
	Non-smokers	13	53	27.9
Age 30–39	Smokers	66	25	
	Non-smokers	37	83	5.9
Age 40+	Smokers	23	14	
	Non-smokers	37	62	2.8

Mantel–Haenszel odds ratio, adjusted for age = 6.3

Source: data from Lyon JL et al., 'Smoking and carcinoma in situ of the uterine cervix,' *American Journal Public Health*, Volume 73, Issue 4, pp. 558–562, © 1983 [25].

This example illustrates the difference between confounding and effect modification. If a factor is acting only as a confounding factor, it will bias the overall association between exposure and outcome, but the associations in the different strata will be similar. Thus, in Table 7.12, the odds ratio between melanoma and sunburn history was confounded by tendency to sunburn, but there was no substantial effect modification; the association was virtually the same in subjects who sunburnt easily and in those who did not. In the study of exercise levels and heart disease in Table 7.10, there was also substantial confounding by age, but no substantial effect modification; that is, the relative risks comparing light and heavy exercise workers were similar in the different age groups. In contrast, in the current example in Table 7.13, there is relatively little confounding, but there is very clear effect modification. A similar result was seen in the randomized trial analysis in Table 7.8 where the relative risk between tolbutamide treatment and mortality was 1.44 in the crude form, and 1.32 after adjustment for arterial calcification, showing only a small degree of confounding. However, the relative risk for subjects with arterial calcification ($RR = 1.93$) was substantially higher than for the subjects without such calcification ($RR = 1.09$), showing effect modification. The statistical assessment of effect modification in this example of cervical cancer and smoking is shown in Chapter 8, Box 8.5.

Example of both confounding and effect modification

Table 7.14 shows results from a cohort analysis of the case fatality rate from SARS (severe acute respiratory syndrome) in Hong Kong [26]. The fatality rate was, overall, considerably greater in men as compared to women, with a crude relative risk of 1.66. Stratification by age gives a Mantel–Haenszel relative risk, adjusted for age, of 1.35, lower than the crude relative risk, showing confounding by age. This confounding is due to the older age distribution of the men, allied to the increasing death rate with increasing age. The stratum-specific relative risks show that there is also effect modification, with the higher death rate in men being highest in the youngest age group (RR 2.27), and there being no substantial difference between the death rates in men and women at ages 75 years and over (RR 1.02).

Thus in an exposure–outcome relationship, a third factor may act as a confounding factor, may act as effect modifier, may have both effects, or may have neither effect.

Table 7.14 Combined confounding and effect modification: comparison of male and female case fatality rates from SARS in Hong Kong. The death rates are higher in males, particularly at younger ages (effect modification by age), and the overall crude relative risk of 1.66 is partially due to confounding by age, shown by the adjusted relative risk being only 1.35 [26].

Fatality rate in SARS (severe acute respiratory syndrome), comparing males with females, in Hong Kong

(A) All ages

		Cases	Deaths	Survivors	Fatality rate (%)	Male: female relative risk
	Males	776	170	606	21.9	1.66
	Females	979	129	850	13.2	
	Total	1755	299	1456	17.0	

(B) Data stratified by age

		Cases	Deaths	Survivors	Fatality rate (%)	Male: female relative risk
Age 0–44	Males	425	27	398	6.4	2.27
	Females	607	17	590	2.8	
Age 45–74	Males	249	77	172	30.9	1.45
	Females	295	63	232	21.4	
Age ≥ 75	Males	102	66	36	64.7	1.02
	Females	77	49	28	63.6	

Mantel–Haenszel relative risk, adjusted for age = 1.35

Source: data from Karlberg J et al., 'Do men have a higher case fatality rate of severe acute respiratory syndrome than women do?,' *American Journal of Epidemiology*, Volume 159, Issue 3, pp. 229–231, © 2004 [26].

Matching

Concept

Another method of avoiding confounding is to choose the comparison subjects for a study so that they are similar to the case or exposed subjects in regard to pre-specified confounding factors, and then analyse the study appropriately. For example, in a co-hort study assessing high alcohol consumption and the risk of heart disease, factors such as sex, age, and cigarette smoking may be important confounders. For each sub-ject with high alcohol use entering the study, we could select a comparison subject with low alcohol use, with the same sex, age, and smoking history. We thus create two groups of subjects who are similar in terms of these three factors. Within our study therefore there will be no association between sex, age, or smoking status and alcohol consumption, and so these factors will not be confounding. This process is referred to as matching.

Purposes

Matching is a much more complex technique than it appears, and it can be misused. Matching can have three different purposes; it can be used to increase the *efficiency* of the study, to *control confounding*, or to improve the *comparability* of the information collected.

Frequency matching to increase efficiency

Efficiency is the amount of information gained in relation to the size of the study. Sup-pose we want to study health effects of oral contraceptive use; the exposed group will be women, and most will be between 16 and 45 years old. There is no value in enrolling as comparison subjects women who are over 60 years old, or even more obviously, no value in enrolling men in the study. Ideally the ratio of comparison subjects to exposed subjects in each age range should be reasonably constant. An age group in which there are many oral contraceptive users and very few non-users, or vice versa, will give un-reliable information because of the small numbers in one category (in the extreme, a group with no exposed or no comparison subjects gives no information). Thus to increase efficiency, matching can ensure that the groups of subjects being compared are similar in terms of the most important potential confounding factors in the study. This can be achieved by '*frequency matching*': the study is designed so that the distribu-tion of the groups of subjects being compared is similar in terms of major confounding factors. This is an easily applied, useful, and widely used technique, particularly for such characteristics as age and sex. Frequency matching is only a method of ensuring reasonable efficiency, and is not in itself a method of controlling confounding. The confounding factors, both those on which frequency matching has been done and oth-ers, need to be controlled by stratification or multivariate analysis. The analysis is done in the same way as in unmatched studies. The advantage of frequency matching is simply to increase the efficiency of stratification and multivariate methods to control confounding.

Individual matching to control confounding

The second form of matching, 'individual matching', is a precise technique. Rather than simply ensuring broad comparability between the groups being compared, comparison subjects are chosen to match particular index subjects in regard to one or more specified confounding factors. The purpose is not only to improve efficiency, but also to control for the confounding effects of these factors.

In cohort and intervention studies

There is an important distinction in the use of individual matching in cohort or intervention studies and in case–control studies. In cohort and intervention studies, precise matching by important confounding factors will control for the effects of those factors. The analysis is done in the same way as in an unmatched cohort study, and will give estimates of relative and attributable risks which can normally be regarded as free of the confounding effects of the variables on which matching has been done. A caution applies as during the time course of the study, subjects may withdraw or be lost to follow-up, so the initial matched situation will be compromised. This can be dealt with by stratifying or using multivariate methods to deal with any confounding, or in some studies it may be necessary to censor the whole matched set of subjects at the same time.

In case–control studies

In a case–control study, controls are selected by matching them to the cases on specified factors. This will give an efficient study, but to control confounding it is necessary to analyse the study by special methods that keep the data in matched form, in other words, consider each matched group of cases and controls as a unit. As long as this is correctly done, the combination of matching and using a matched analysis should control confounding by the matching factors. The analysis is basically a stratified analysis in which each matched case–control set forms one stratum, or the equivalent 'conditional' multivariate analysis. This is necessary because matching can in fact introduce confounding by the matching factors, and this confounding needs to be controlled. If a matched case–control study is not analysed correctly, the result may be invalid.

Example

The simplest form of analysis is given by a fixed one-to-one matching ratio, where one matched control is chosen for each case, as shown in Box 7.4. Note the format of the table: it shows the *numbers of pairs* classified by exposure and by outcome. The odds ratio is simply the ratio of the number of discordant pairs where only the case is exposed, to the number of discordant pairs where only the control is exposed; here the odds ratio is 4.3 [27]. On the null hypothesis, these numbers will be equal. The *incorrect* unmatched table in the familiar two by two format uses exactly the same data, but the value of the matching is lost. If the matching factors, as in this example, have a strong

Box 7.4 One-to-one matching in a case–control study: this yields a simple analysis. Here 120 male patients with nasal or nasal sinus cancer (a very rare cancer), seen in one clinic over a 38-year period, were matched to male controls with a range of other non-smoking related cancers by age and year of diagnosis. Table A shows a matched analysis; the odds ratio is based only on the pairs with different exposures. Table B shows the unmatched analysis of the same data; this analysis is incorrect as it loses the value of the matched pair comparison, and produces a substantially different odds ratio [27]

ONE-TO-ONE MATCHING IN A CASE–CONTROL STUDY

(A) Distribution of 120 case–control pairs by smoking history

		Controls	
		Smokers	**Non-smokers**
Cases	Smokers	31	30
	Non-smokers	7	52

Matched odds ratio = 30/7 = 4.3

(B) An incorrect unmatched analysis of the same 240 individuals

	Cases	**Controls**
Smokers	61	38
Non-smokers	59	82
	120	120

Unmatched odds ratio = (61 × 82)/(59 × 38) = 2.2

Source: data from Elwood JM, 'Wood exposure and smoking: association with cancer of the nasal cavity and paranasal sinuses in British Columbia,' *Canadian Medical Association Journal*, Volume 124, Issue 12, pp. 1573–1577, © 1981 [27].

confounding effect, the odds ratio based on an unmatched analysis is confounded and is substantially different from the matched, unconfounded, odds ratio. It will be biased towards the null, as shown here. This example, with statistics, is shown in Appendix 2, Table A2.5.

Where another fixed ratio of controls to cases (such as 3:1) is used, the analysis is also relatively simple, but where the matching ratio is variable it becomes complex. Analyses of a fixed ratio matched study are shown in Appendix 2, Table A2.6. Matched analyses also become complex if it is necessary to adjust for further confounding factors after the matched design is set up. Normal stratification procedures are difficult to use, as the matched groups must be kept intact. However, 'conditional' multivariate statistical techniques will allow a matched design to be handled in an analysis that controls other confounding factors; this will be discussed later in this chapter.

Matching to increase comparability of data

A further use of matching is to ensure comparability in terms of the information collected. In a case–control study where some case subjects are interviewed in a hospital and others in their own homes, it is logical to ensure that the comparison subjects are matched for method of interview, and ideally the interviews are conducted on a single-blind basis. This was done in a case–control study of venous embolism and hormone replacement therapy, where most interviews took place in hospital, but 23 per cent were done after discharge [28]. Similar considerations arise if several investigators or centres are involved. The 'type of interview' factor is considered as a potential confounding or effect modifying factor, so stratification or multivariate methods may be used, aided by frequency matching; or individual matching and appropriate analysis may be used.

Potential value of matching

What then are the advantages of matching? There are three main ways in which matching may be useful, but these advantages always have to be considered against the disadvantages of matching when designing a study.

Complex confounding factors

Matching has particular value where there is an important confounding variable that cannot be easily measured or easily defined. Examples include complex social factors, medical care factors, environmental exposures, or circumstances in childhood; these might be controlled by matching with neighbours, other patients, co-workers, or siblings respectively. For example, to assess associations with emotional and behavioural problems, girls with anorexia nervosa were compared with their unaffected siblings, giving control for a range of family and childhood factors [29]. Similarly, to assess the relationship of smoking to Parkinson's disease, using sibling controls may control for other environmental exposures [30].

Thus, studies comparing individuals who are twins with their co-twins, where they differ on the exposure or outcome of interest, can be a very powerful design. Many countries have registries of twins to facilitate such research. Thus, an international case–control study compared women with breast cancer at ages under 50 with their unaffected twin sisters, and showed associations with childhood weight, height, and time of breast development [31]. In a prospective cohort study, twins with moderate alcohol consumption showed a lower incidence of type 2 diabetes than their same-sex co-twins, despite the similarity in genetic and early life factors [32]. Comparisons between monozygotic (identical) and dizygotic (non-identical) twins are a fundamental technique in assessing the contribution of genetic and environmental factors. Using a twin registry in Sweden, respiratory symptoms were compared in smokers and in non-smoking co-twins; from 9319 pairs of twins, 1924 pairs who differed in their smoking were found; the prevalence of cough and of bronchitis was higher in the smoking twins, and the prevalence ratio was similar for non-identical and for identical twin pairs, showing that the association with smoking could not be explained by a genetic confounding factor [33].

Increasing efficiency

Matching is useful where the study has a fixed and limited number of cases, and therefore maximizing efficiency is critical. This may apply to a particularly rare exposure or a particularly rare outcome. For example, in the 1960s some eight cases of vaginal adenocarcinoma were diagnosed in young women in Boston, Massachusetts, United States. Vaginal cancer was previously virtually unknown in young women, and this particular disease was of an unusual pathological type. To study possible causes and increase efficiency, for each patient with vaginal adenocarcinoma, four comparison subjects were individually matched on sex, date of birth (within 5 days), hospital of birth, and ward or private type of service [34].

The same consideration of maximizing efficiency applies if collecting data from the study subjects is expensive, so that the number of subjects needs to be kept a small as possible. For example, if there is a set of subjects with stored blood or tissue samples, careful matching can be done so that fewer samples need to be used for expensive chemical or genetic tests. Thus to assess the relationships of breast cancer with plasma levels of carotenoids and other indicators, stored blood samples collected up to 10 years before diagnosis from over 70 000 subjects in three cohort studies in Sweden were used. For each of 624 breast cancer cases, two controls matched for age, date of blood sample and sampling centre were selected, and biochemical analyses were done only on these samples [35].

Disadvantages of matching

Logistic difficulties

Individual matching involves both practical and conceptual difficulties, and has several disadvantages compared to other methods of controlling confounding. To get matched comparison subjects, many potential comparison subjects may have to be approached, consent obtained, and initial information gathered, making the study more expensive and difficult to set up. If the subjects can be selected from an existing data bank with information already available on the matching factors, this is not a problem, and matching is more often used in those circumstances. The matched design is prone to loss of data; if one member of a matched set does not participate in or complete the study, the whole matched group usually has to be excluded. A further disadvantage has been referred to, that the analysis becomes complex if other factors have to be considered or if the matching ratio is variable.

Matched factor cannot be assessed

The most important disadvantage of matching is that the matching factor cannot itself be assessed in the analysis in terms of its relationship to the outcome. Therefore matching should be used only for factors that are known to be important risk factors and therefore important confounders, and should not be used if it is necessary to assess the relationship between the matched factor and the outcome in the study. Matching is therefore inappropriate for an exploratory study to answer a general question as to what are the causes of the outcome in question.

The further disadvantages of matching are in its inappropriate use resulting in overmatching, which will now be discussed.

Unnecessary matching: 'overmatching'

If the study involves matching on a factor which is not a true confounder, this is often referred to as 'overmatching', although 'unnecessary matching' is a clearer description. It may occur in two situations. Suppose in a case–control study the subjects are matched on a factor which is associated with the exposure, but which is not itself associated with the outcome; it is therefore not a confounding factor, and it is unnecessary to control its effects. Because the matching factor is associated with exposure, the controls are being chosen in a way that will make them more similar to the cases in terms of exposure. The differences in exposure between potential case and control subjects in the source population will be reduced in the study subjects, and an (incorrect) unmatched analysis will lead to an underestimate of the true outcome–exposure association. If a correct analysis is done, stratifying for the matching variable, using multivariate methods, or using an analysis on matched sets, the result of the unnecessary matching will be to increase the proportion of all case–control sets that are concordant for exposure. As these sets do not contribute to the estimate of odds ratio, the study results will not be biased; but the study will be less efficient as fewer sets of observations are contributing to the results. In the extreme, if the matching factor is very closely associated with the exposure, the study will have no ability to assess the exposure. In a cohort study, unnecessary matching also leads to inefficiency, but the study results will still be valid as specific analytic methods are not needed.

Factors not confounding

Consider a case–control study of lung cancer, assessing passive exposure to tobacco smoke. Should lung cancer subjects and controls be matched on their personal smoking experience? As this is a major risk factor and is associated with passive smoking, it needs to be controlled, and matching with a correct analysis would give a powerful study. Should subjects be matched for the size of their family, or for the number of fellow workers they have? These factors are not themselves risk factors for lung cancer, but may be associated with passive smoking: matching would be detrimental. If we wish to guard against the possibility of family size being a risk factor, perhaps by being an indicator of other exposures, it is better to deal with it by stratification or multivariate analysis. Then we have freedom to assess if it is a risk factor, or a confounding factor; if we match on family size we do not have flexibility. The error here is it is in matching for a factor, which is associated with the exposure, but is not an independent risk factor for the outcome and so is not a confounder. Matching for this factor however can make it a confounding factor, which then has to be controlled in the analysis.

Factor in causal pathway

Unnecessary matching will also occur if the matching factor is not a confounding factor because it is part of a causal pathway linking exposure and outcome. In this situation, different methods of analysis may not help, as the study is fundamentally flawed. Consider a case–control study to assess the causes of bladder cancer in a workforce where records of both a chemical exposure and previous bladder cytology are available for the employees. To assess the association between the chemical exposure and bladder cancer, should subjects be matched on prior cytology findings? If they are, and the true causal chain is

chemical exposure $\rightarrow$ abnormal cytology $\rightarrow$ bladder cancer

then a matched study will likely show no difference in chemical exposure. In such situations, the study design used tests a different hypothesis: is chemical exposure related to bladder cancer irrespective of prior cytology findings? This may be a question worth asking, although probably only in specific subgroups; for example, if chemical exposure increases the risk of bladder cancer in subjects with previous abnormal cytology, it may indicate a tumour promotion effect increasing the risk of progression from abnormal cytology to invasive cancer. In these situations the interpretation cannot be made solely on the data: it requires assumptions regarding the causal model and is dependent on whether the third factor is a confounding factor or not. If subjects are chosen without matching, and information on the third factor collected, analyses can be done with and without control for that factor, and its associations with exposure and outcome can be assessed. If matching has been used, this flexibility is lost. The risks of unnecessary matching show again that matching should be used only after careful consideration including of knowledge about the confounding factors relevant to a given situation.

Factor affected by exposure or outcome

Another situation of overmatching arises where the factor which is affected by either the exposure or outcome in the study. This includes symptoms and signs produced either by the exposure or the outcome, including early indications of disease. The issue again is that these factors are not true confounders. For example, in a cohort study of smokers, if smokers and non-smokers are matched in terms of a history of cough, the effect of smoking on the subsequent incidence of lung cancer would be underestimated.

Confounding by indication

This situation particularly applies to studies of the effects of drugs, where the dominant confounder is the underlying disease for which the drugs are prescribed. This is referred to as *confounding by indication*. A strong association between a drug and a disease may arise if the drugs are prescribed for clinical signs or symptoms which are associated with the early stages of the disease, so-called *protopathic bias*. For example, in the assessment of the association between aspirin use and Reye's syndrome (an encephalitis-like illness mainly affecting children, usually after a viral illness), such an association could arise because aspirin was prescribed to children who had symptoms which were early manifestations of Reye's syndrome; this is *reverse causation*—the putative outcome (disease) causes the exposure. A further case–control study concluded that the association was not explicable by such a mechanism, and strengthened the case for aspirin use being causal [36].

Summary of matching

In summary, there are two major types of matching. Frequency matching is used to produce approximately similar distributions of key confounding factors in the groups being compared. It should be considered simply as a method of improving study efficiency, and the matching factors and other confounders should be dealt with in the analysis by stratification and multivariate methods. Specific individual matching is of particular value for complex confounders which cannot otherwise be dealt with, and situations where maximum efficiency is a priority. Such matching should only be carried out for factors which are true confounders. There should be good evidence that the matching factor is a strong risk factor for the outcome, with in addition an association with the exposure. Overmatching is produced if matching is carried out on a factor which is not a true confounder. Matching for a factor associated only with exposure will decrease efficiency, and if not appropriately analysed, will damage validity. Is it important to avoid matching on a factor which is a component in the causal chain linking exposure and outcome, or on a factor which is affected by the exposure or the outcome, such as symptoms or signs.

Multivariate methods

The final method of controlling confounding is to analyse the data using a mathematical model that has the outcome as the dependent variable, and includes both the postulated causal factor and confounding factors in the equation. Multivariate analysis is a major subject in itself, and the purpose of this section is to present the key principles which are important in interpreting the results of these analyses.

Linear regression

While linear regression is not widely used in these studies, it is the simplest model from which the others are derived. It is appropriate for continuous variables. For example, say we want to assess if the birth weight of the baby is related to the mother's pre-pregnancy weight, taking account of any confounding by the mother's height. A linear regression model can be used, with the dependent variable being birth weight, and including two independent (or 'predictor') variables: maternal pre-pregnancy weight, and maternal height. Standard multiple regression methods give a coefficient for the maternal weight variable which shows the relationship between it and birth weight, independent of the confounding effect of height.

The mathematical expression is

$$y = a + b_1 x_1 + b_2 x_2$$

where

y is the outcome, birth weight, and is the dependent variable in the equation

x_1 is the mother's pre-pregnancy weight

x_2 is the mother's height

a is a constant with no intuitive meaning (it is the birth weight if x_1 and x_2 are both zero), and

b_1 and b_2 are the regression coefficients. These coefficients are calculated to be the values that give the best fit of the equation set out above to the observed data. (Terminology varies: y can also be called the outcome variable or regressand; the x variables can be called predictor variables, covariates, or regressors.)

This simple mathematical equation makes several assumptions. It assumes, for example, that the change in birth weight with the change in the mothers' pre-pregnancy weight is linear, and therefore the numerical value b_1 represents the amount of change in birth weight associated with a change in the mother's pre-pregnancy weight of one unit. A similar linear assumption holds for b_2. The equation also assumes that the change in birth weight with pre-pregnancy weight is the same irrespective of the value of the mothers' height, in other words that the effects of maternal height and weight are *independent* and there is no *interaction* between these two variables. These are assumptions inherent in the mathematical form of the equation. The coefficient b_1 with this linear model show the *difference* in the outcome (birth weight) associated with a one unit change in x_1; and independence of the effects of several variables means independence on a linear scale: that is, the risk differences associated with each variable are additive. There are usually other assumptions involved in the ways in which the coefficients are calculated; for example, the usual method of calculation will make the assumption that the variable y has a normal distribution.

Log-linear models: Poisson regression

In many health situations the main variables are not continuous, or even if continuous, such as an incidence rate, they have limits: a rate cannot be negative. Outcomes are often dichotomous (binary): diseased or not diseased, cured or not cured. Exposures may be continuous, dichotomous, or have several categories (e.g. age, sex, stage of disease), so standard linear regression will not be appropriate. Many other models have been developed and applied to these situations.

One model is to take the natural logarithm of the outcome variable, shown by 'ln y', and use the same equation as with linear regression but with ln y

$$\ln y = a + b_1 x_1 + b_2 x_2$$

This transformation means that y cannot be negative, as negative numbers do not have logarithms (ln 0 = 1). This is a log-linear model: the right-hand side is linear, the dependent variable has a logarithmic transformation. It is equivalent to an exponential model

$$y = \exp(a + b_1 x_1 + b_2 x_2)$$

This model is widely used in the analysis of epidemiological cohort studies. The distribution of the dependent variable y determines the best method of fitting the model to the data. In epidemiological cohort studies, where the frequency of positive outcomes is low, a model using a Poisson distribution is often suitable, the method being called *Poisson regression*. The interpretation of the results of any log-linear model is the same.

As these models use a logarithmic, or exponential, model, the interpretation of the coefficients is different from a linear model. Consider a simple model with only one independent variable on the right-hand side, x_1. The coefficient b_1, for variable x_1, estimates the change in ln y for a one unit change in x_1. If $x_1 = 1$ means the subject is exposed, and $x_1 = 0$ means they are unexposed, then the change in outcome associated with x_1 is given by the following.

Let y_e equal the risk in the exposed group, y_u the risk in the unexposed.
If $x_1 = 0$ (unexposed), $\ln y_u = a$ (as $x_1 = 0$, $b_1 x_1 = 0$).
If $x_1 = 1$ (exposed), $\ln y_e = a + b_1$.
So the difference in the equations is b_1, which must equal $\ln y_e - \ln y_u$, and this equals $\ln (y_e/y_u)$. Hence,

$$b_1 = \ln\left(y_e / y_u\right)$$

and, exponential $(b_1) = y_e/y_u =$ risk in exposed / risk in unexposed
= the relative risk associated with exposure.

Thus, in a log-linear model with a binary exposure variable, the exponential of a coefficient equals the *risk ratio* (*relative risk*) associated with that exposure. For a continuous exposure variable, the exponential of a coefficient represents the risk ratio associated with a one unit change in the exposure factor. This is in contrast to the linear model described earlier, where the coefficient showed the risk difference associated with the factor. It follows that where we have two or more independent variables in a log-linear model, the definition of independent effects is that the risk ratio for each factor is constant, so the joint effect of two 'independent' factors is additivity if regard to the log of disease risk, which is *multiplicity* in the effect on the absolute disease risk.

Logistic regression

A further slightly different model is the most appropriate for case–control studies, but it can be used in any study design. It uses a further transformation of y. In the *logistic model* the logarithm of the odds, called the *logit* of disease risk, is used as the dependent variable in a linear regression equation. Where P is the proportion of subjects in the study who have the outcome, or equivalently the probability that a randomly selected subject has the outcome, the *logit* of P is defined: as

$$\log it\, P = \ln\left[P/(1-P)\right]$$

where ln means the natural logarithm (to base e).

The logistic regression equation has the form

$$\ln\left(\frac{P}{1-P}\right) = a + b_1 x_1 + b_2 x_2 + b_3 x_3 \ldots..$$

where as before, the x variables represent exposure factors and confounders, and the b terms are their coefficients. If an x variable is a numerical value (e.g. height), the b coefficient gives the change in logit of P associated with a change of one unit of x, with the assumption of a linear relationship between the two.

Derivation of odds ratio

If x is binary, with the values of 0 or 1, the equation yields the odds ratio associated with x. For example, for sex we might define a variable so that $x_1 = 1$ for males and $x_1 = 0$ for females. For females, $x_1 = 0$, so $b_1 x_1$ is zero. For males, $x_1 = 1$, so the equation for males differs from that for females by having the extra term $b_1 x_1$, which is equal to b_1.

The rest of the equation is the same. So, the difference in the logit of P between males and females will be b_1

$$\ln\left(\frac{P_m}{1-P_m}\right) - \ln\left(\frac{P_f}{1-P_f}\right) = b_1$$

where P_m = the risk for males, and P_f = the risk for females.
  With two numbers r and s, $\ln(r) - \ln(s) = \ln(r/s)$, so

$$\ln\left[\frac{P_m}{1-P_m} \middle/ \frac{P_f}{1-P_f}\right] = b_1$$

where $P_m/(1 - P_m)$ is the odds of the outcome in males; $P_f/(1 - P_f)$ is the odds in females. The quantity in the brackets is the *odds ratio* comparing male to female subjects:

$$\ln(OR) = b_1$$

and

$$OR = \text{exponential}(b_1)$$

Thus with the logistic regression model, the exponential of a coefficient b equals the odds ratio associated with the variable x, if this is a binary variable coded as 0 or 1. If x is continuous, b gives the odds ratio associated with a change in x of one unit.

Example

A simple example is given by the comparison between tolbutamide and placebo, using the data shown in Table 7.8. We will apply a logistic model, as was done in the original analysis.

$$\ln[P/(1-P)] = a + b_1 x_1$$

Where P is the probability of death, and x_1 is 1 for tolbutamide and 0 for placebo.
  For the placebo group $P_p = 21/205 = 0.1024$ (from Table 7.8, table A)
  so

$$\text{logit}\, P_p = \ln(0.1024/0.8976) = -2.171 = a$$

For the tolbutamide group $P_t = 30/204 = 0.1471$
  so

$$\text{logit}\, P_t = \ln(0.1471/0.8529) = -1.758 = a + b_1$$

thus

$$b_1 = -1.758 - (-2.171) = 0.413$$

and

$$\exp(b_1) = \exp(0.413) = 1.511$$

So, the odds ratio is 1.511. We can also calculate the odds ratio from Table 7.8, table A, by the usual method, with the same result: odds ratio = $(30 \times 184) / (21 \times 174) = 1.511$. (Note, in Table 7.8, the relative risk of 1.44 is shown, not the odds ratio).

To account for other factors, the model becomes

$$\ln[P/(1-P)] = a + b_1 x_1 + b_2 x_2 + b_3 x_3 \dots etc.$$

where the other x variables represent other factors. The value of multivariate analysis is that many other factors can be included in the equation. In the analysis of this study, a logistic model was used with 15 other factors (the nine factors shown in Table 7.7, plus sex, race, systolic blood pressure, diastolic blood pressure, visual acuity, and creatinine level). With all these other factors included, the value of b_1 in the presence of these other factors was 0.40, giving an odds ratio of 1.49 for tolbutamide compared to placebo, adjusted for these 15 factors. Thus although there were some considerable differences between the tolbutamide and placebo groups, as shown in Table 7.7, these did not in aggregate produce any great difference in the main result, the odds ratio changing only from 1.51 to 1.49. The results can also be expressed as the difference in mortality rates, as was done in the original paper [11].

Use of dummy variables

Frequently factors with several categories are relevant, and these are often best handled by using a number of 'dummy' binary variables to represent all the categories.

Example

Box 7.5 shows data from a case–control study comparing 83 patients with malignant melanoma with 83 controls chosen from the general population [37], and shows the results for just two factors, the number of palpable moles (naevi) on the upper arm assessed by an interviewer (three categories) and the response to a question on whether the subject had ever had a severe sunburn (two categories). The results from cross-tabulations showed strong associations both with the number of moles and with a history of sunburn. However there were several other factors associated with these two features and also related to melanoma, which therefore are confounding factors. These included the severity of skin freckling (three categories), the usual reaction to sun exposure (four categories), and hair colour (three categories). To control for each of these confounders singly can be done fairly easily by cross-tabulations. However to assess the relationship between moles and melanoma, with control for freckles, sun reaction, hair colour, and sunburn simultaneously by cross-tabulations would mean that $3 \times 4 \times 3 \times 2 = 72$ separate tables showing the case–control distribution by numbers of moles would have to be generated, and in this small study many of these tables would have few or no observations.

It is therefore more useful to include these five factors in a logistic regression equation, expressing each factor as a number of dummy variables, the number being one less than the number of categories. Thus for the number of moles, one binary variable was used with the value 1 for subjects who had one to two moles on the upper arm, and

---

Box 7.5 Multivariate analysis: results from a case–control study comparing 83 patients with malignant melanoma with 83 controls from the general population. Results are shown for two factors, number of moles on the upper arm and history of severe sunburn, derived by (A) cross-tabulation, (B) a logistic regression fitting only the one factor, and (C) a logistic regression fitting five factors, represented by 10 binary variables [37]; fuller results are given in that paper

---

MULTIVARIATE ANALYSIS

(A) Cross tabulations

	No. of moles on upper arm			History of sunburn	
	0	**1–2**	**3+**	**No**	**Yes**
Cases, number	32	16	35	34	49
Controls, number	62	17	4	57	26
Odds ratio	1.0 (R)	1.82	16.95	1.0 (R)	3.16

(B) Logistic regression with one factor only

Coefficient *b*		0.6008	2.830		1.150
Exp(*b*) = odds ratio		1.82	16.95		3.16

(C) Logistic regression with both factors, plus quantity of freckles (3 categories), reaction to sun exposure (4 categories), and hair colour (3 categories)

Coefficient *b*		0.3011	2.587		0.4276
Exp(*b*) = odds ratio		1.35	13.29		1.53

Source: data from Elwood JM et al., 'Malignant melanoma in relation to moles, pigmentation, and exposure to fluorescent and other lighting sources,' *British Journal of Cancer*, Volume 53, Issue 1, pp. 65–74, © 1986 [37].

---

0 otherwise; and another with the value 1 for subjects with three or more moles, and 0 otherwise. Where both these factors are 0 the equation gives the risk in the referent category, subjects with no moles.

If a logistic regression is fitted with just one *x* variable, the result will be identical to a simple cross-tabulation, and the exponential of the coefficient *b* will be equal to the crude odds ratio obtained by the usual calculation on the simple table. These results are shown in table B of Box 7.5, derived from fitting the logistic equation three times, each with only one *x* variable.

Then a model is fitted which includes ten *x* variables, representing the categories of all five factors (moles, sunburn, freckles, reaction to sun, hair colour). The coefficient *b* for each variable gives the odds ratio for that variable, controlled for the effects of all the other variables in the equation. Table C of Box 7.5 shows that with these coefficients, the odds ratios for number of moles are still high, whereas the odds ratio for history of sunburn is 1.53, considerably lower than the crude odds ratio of 3.16. This shows that most of the association with sunburn seen in the simple analysis is not causal, but produced by confounding by one or more of the other factors included in the equation. To determine which factor, analyses can be done fitting each confounding factor singly and seeing how the odds ratio for sunburn changes. The program used will assess the statistical significance of these adjusted coefficients, as shown in Chapter 8 Table 8.3.

Analysis of matched studies: conditional regression

Multivariate analysis for individually matched studies uses methods that take account of the matching, that is, they consider matched sets of cases and controls as sets. These methods are referred to as 'conditional' models. The results are presented in the same way as has been shown, with the same interpretation of the coefficients. They allow a matched analysis that can also include other confounding factors.

Example

In a case–control study within a cohort, the predictive values of various immune and inflammation markers in serum were assessed by comparing 301 patients with non-Hodgkin lymphoma to 301 control subjects [38]. All the subjects were participants in a large US cancer screening trial and had given blood samples at least 5 years earlier. The controls were individually matched to the cases on a 1:1 ratio on age at baseline (55–59, 60–64, 65–69, or 70–74 years), sex, race (white, African American or other), study centre, and time (AM, PM) and date (3-month categories) of baseline blood draw. The analysis used conditional logistic regression, thus taking account of the matching and permitting other factors to be also included.

Outcome and exposure risk scores: propensity scores

Where an analysis has a large number of potential confounding variables, especially when the number of subjects is limited, these factors can be combined to obtain a composite confounding factor [39]. A *propensity score* is derived from a multivariate model with the exposure as the dependent, fitting the potential confounders, so it is summarizing the probability of exposure on the basis of the potential confounders. This is often used in treatment questions, as controlling for the propensity score allows adjustment for a range of factors related to the treatment [40]. An outcome risk score (or 'disease risk' score) is derived from fitting a multivariate model such as a logistic model using the outcome data and the potential confounders, excluding the exposure; thus the model predicts the risk of the outcome on the basis of the joint effects of the confounders. Either of these scores can be considered as a composite confounder, and the exposure–outcome association adjusted for it, by matching, stratification, or multivariate analysis. Adjustment by stratification is useful as then effect modification by the composite confounder can be assessed by stratification or multivariate methods.

Examples

In a study noted in a major review [40], from routine data, patients receiving an antibiotic (azithromycin) were compared to those receiving any of three other antibiotics, or none, matching for a propensity score based on 153 variables [41]. The results showed an increased risk of death, attributed to cardiac effects, and led to regulatory actions.

In a study of the management of patients with significant bleeding following trauma, involving over 20 000 patients in 40 countries, an outcome risk score was developed to predict the risk of death from several factors: age, heart rate, systolic blood pressure, time since injury, type of injury, geographical region, and the patient's condition rated on a coma scale [42]. This led to patients being categorized into four groups by predicted risk of death. The association between transfusion and outcome (death) was then assessed by stratification, showing that transfusion was associated with a reduction in mortality (odds ratio 0.59) in subjects with a high risk of death, and an increase in mortality in those in the lowest risk category (odds ratio 4.87); indeed, data using ten deciles of the risk score showed a fairly regular trend.

Appropriate use of multivariate analysis

To use such models the confounding factors must be recognized in advance, and quantitative information on them must be collected. Considerable care is necessary to use such models properly. Factors to be included in a multivariate model should be examined first by stratification, and issues considered such as the distribution of the observations, the need for transformations, and the appropriateness of assumptions such as a linear relationship to risk. Multivariate analysis is best regarded as a powerful but complex and demanding type of analysis, appropriate to the final stages of analysis of a study, rather than as a magical black box to provide a short cut to a result.

Multivariate analysis can deal with only a limited number of factors. Its scope is constrained by the number of study subjects, which should be much greater than the number of variables included; a minimum of 10 or 15 subjects per variable has been suggested. Factors can be used in different ways: for example, a factor like age can be entered as one continuous variable or represented by a number of categories, each with a corresponding variable. If interactions are to be examined, further interaction terms can be used. Thus for studies which include data on many factors, the most relevant must be selected before a multivariate model is applied. The next section on the use of the principles of confounding in analysis will be helpful in this regard.

Part 3. Further applications of confounding

Application of the definition of confounding to study design

Consideration of the definition of confounding can assist greatly in the design of studies. It provides an answer to the problem of feeling that because there are so many possible confounding factors, no satisfactory study can be designed.

In designing any study, we should make a list of the factors that are likely to be associated with the *exposure* under study, and another list of factors that are likely to be associated with the *outcome*. To do this, we may need to review the literature and consult reference works and people with specialized knowledge. Any factor that appears on both of these lists is a potential confounding factor, and we need to plan how to deal with it. Factors that appear on only one list but which are likely to have a very strong association with either outcome or exposure, may be prudently included as potential confounding factors, as even a small difference in their distribution between the groups being compared may be sufficient to introduce confounding. The use of this approach will often reduce an apparently infinite number of potential confounders to a finite, and often fairly small, list of specific factors.

The options available for confounder control (Table 7.5) can then be considered. In practice, many potential confounders will not in fact be confounding, in that their associations with outcome and exposure in the study data are often weak and unimportant: but this will be known only if data on the confounders are collected. The most commonly used approach in non-randomized studies is to apply some restriction, and to collect data on the potential confounders to allow stratification or multivariate methods to be used in the analysis. Frequency matching can ensure cases or exposed subjects and comparison subjects are similarly distributed in terms of major confounders, such as age and sex, which will be controlled by stratification or multivariate methods. Individual matching should be used only when there are specific advantages to it, and the factors to be matched on are likely to be important confounders.

In randomized studies only one list, of factors likely to be related to the outcome, is needed, and data on these should be collected where possible to assess if the groups are in fact comparable on these factors. In large-scale randomized studies, for example, of population interventions, representative samples of the groups may be selected for this purpose.

Application of the definition of confounding to analysis

Similarly in the analysis there are often a large number of potential confounding factors. Confounding is demonstrated if a stratified or multivariate analysis is performed and the unconfounded relative risk or odds ratio estimate is substantially different from the crude estimate. A practical approach to the analysis of a large data set is therefore to first produce the basic table comparing exposure with outcome, and calculate the crude odds ratio or relative risk. Then each potential confounder is considered in a reasonable number of categories (five are usually sufficient), and stratified or multivariate analyses performed including the potential confounders, calculating the adjusted odds ratio or relative risk. If this adjusted ratio is similar to the crude ratio, there is no substantial confounding by that variable. There are two main approaches to assess if factors are in fact confounding: multivariate methods or stratification. With either, it is the size of the difference between the crude and adjusted risk ratio or odds ratio, not its statistical significance, which indicates confounding.

Multivariate analysis

With logistic regression, the coefficient and therefore the odds ratio estimate for the exposure–outcome association will change when the confounding factors are added into the equation. Sets of potential confounding factors can easily be used, and factors shown to have a confounding effect can be kept in the model while other factors are tested. Concentrating on the change in the coefficient and odds ratio is quite different from using multivariate models to get the best fit to the data, for classification or prognostic purposes, and so methods of selecting factors in multivariate models that are based on statistical significance, such as forward and backward selection methods, are not relevant here. In a large study with many variables, a strategy of setting a maximum acceptable change in the odds ratio or relative risk, such as 10 or 5 per cent, can be applied to potential confounders individually or in groups [43]. In published studies, a statement is sometimes given that many specified potential confounders were assessed, but that none of them changed the risk ratio estimate by more than a given percentage, and so they were not included in the final analysis. Models can be fitted including potential confounders cumulatively, or including all potential confounders and then excluding some; the critical change being the odds ratio for the main association being studied. Thus a large number of potential confounders can be reduced to a small number of actual confounders. Two or more potential confounders considered together may have a confounding effect, even if singly they do not; this is easily assessed using multivariate models. A reasonable approach is therefore to proceed further with a reduced data set, keeping factors that have shown a confounding effect on simpler analysis, plus those of major predetermined importance. This data set should then present a less forbidding challenge.

The use of multivariate models to deal with confounding requires a close attention to the meaning of the various factors in regard to the causal hypothesis that is being assessed.

Stratification

In stratified analysis, the Mantel–Haenszel odds ratio or relative risk is usually used as the adjusted (unconfounded) estimate, and the same logic applies, assessing whether this risk estimate differs from the crude association when the potential confounding factor is controlled by stratification. Stratification will be cumbersome if there are many confounders, but if there are only one or two, stratified analysis allows a more detailed assessment of the data and can show how the confounding effect has come about. Cross-tabulations between each of the factors and outcome, and between each of the factors and exposure, will show these relationships, and a diagram similar to Figures 7.5 and 7.6 can be produced. Strictly, the association between the potential confounding factor and the outcome should be examined within the non-exposed group, and the association between the potential confounding factor and exposure should be examined within the group without the outcome under consideration. Again, it is the strength of these associations, measured by an odds ratio or other measure, that matters, not their statistical significance.

The limits of confounder control and the issue of uncontrolled confounding

A central issue in the interpretation of observational studies is whether the methods of control for confounding can ever be good enough to give complete assurance that confounding has been controlled. On the one hand, studies such as the case–control studies and subsequently the prospective cohort studies of cigarette smoking and lung cancer have provided strong and consistent evidence demonstrating a causal relationship, and explaining it in quantitative terms, so that the strength of the available knowledge on that topic can be regarded as equivalent to the strength of evidence produced by randomized controlled trials in other contexts. Indeed, the aim of those carrying out epidemiological studies using observational methods is often stated in these terms, to come to a similar level of confidence in the results as can be achieved by the randomized trial method. The counter-argument is that no observational study can control for a confounder that is not specifically included in the study, and there may always be other factors that have not be controlled; further, even for those factors included, misclassification errors limit the ability to control their confounding effects.

The key advantage of the randomized trial method is its ability to reasonably exclude confounding, not only by factors that have been measured and assessed, but also by other factors. The real weakness of observational studies is that they provide no protection against the confounding effects of other factors that have not been measured, and may not be recognized or known. The methods described in this chapter can deal with confounding by factors that can be identified and measured, although even for these, confounding may not be completely controlled because of observational errors, limitations in how confounding factors are defined and measured, and statistical issues.

Example: beta-carotene

There are situations where after extensive observational studies produced consistent results, large-scale randomized trials gave quite different results. An influential example is the work on the potential protective effect of beta-carotene, contained in many vegetables. Extensive observational studies, both case–control studies and long-term prospective cohort studies, using the best available methods of dietary assessment and carried out by some of the world's leading research groups, produced generally consistent evidence that subjects with higher serum retinol or beta-carotene levels or with higher beta-carotene intake had substantially reduced cancer risks. This was supported by laboratory evidence that beta-carotene and its metabolites had an anti-carcinogenic action in animals. This evidence grew over many years and a consensus formed that it was strong and consistent enough to justify intervention studies, using beta-carotene dietary supplements to actively prevent many cancers [44]. Although the evidence for benefit was substantial, as Peto and colleagues [44] stated: 'Preventive measures, especially those which may be relevant over a long period to many million people, deserve particularly rigorous evaluation.' So several large randomized trials were set up. However, in contrast to the previous evidence, these trials either showed no beneficial effect, or showed higher cancer rates in those receiving the beta carotene supplements, and such trials had to be stopped promptly [45,46]. 'The cancer prevention community was stunned' by these results [47].

Example: hormones

Another example relates to a reduction in the risk of coronary heart disease in women using oestrogen and/or progesterone hormones. Several observational studies showed that hormone users had a substantially reduced risk of coronary heart disease, with either no change in the risk of stroke or a slight reduction [48]. Therefore hormone therapies became widely recommended to protect against heart disease in women. A randomized trial involving over 16 000 post-menopausal women at 40 centres in the United States was set up to validate this, the Women's Health Initiative (WHI) trial, but it showed an *increased* rate of heart disease and stroke in women randomized to hormone therapy (combined oestrogen-progesterone [49]). As a result, this arm of the WHI trial was terminated early. Similar results were shown in other randomized trials. These clinical trials changed practice and destroyed the case for the benefits of hormone therapy that had been built up through observational studies. It has been pointed out that the confounding effects of socioeconomic status had been inadequately dealt with in the observational studies, and also that an analysis of observational studies taking account of the changes over time in the exposure, hormone use, changed the results, and these two influences together could explain the discrepancies between the observational studies and the clinical trials [50]; this commentary concluded by stating 'however, observational studies are not a substitute for clinical trials no matter how sophisticated the statistical adjustments may seem'.

Example: vitamin C

Antioxidant vitamins such as vitamin C have shown protective effects against cardiovascular disease, cancer, and total mortality in many observational studies, but well-conducted randomized controlled trials of supplements with antioxidants do not show any beneficial effects. The largest observational study shows protective effects of high vitamin C plasma levels on coronary heart disease mortality, with odds ratios of 0.70 in men and 0.63 in women. This study controlled for age, systolic blood pressure, cholesterol, body mass index, smoking, diabetes, and vitamin supplement use. However, the largest randomized trial set up to verify this association showed a small increase in risk associated with vitamin C supplementation, with relative risk of 1.06 [51]. This situation must be due to the influence of unmeasured confounding factors in the observational studies.

Counter example: folic acid

The challenge is the conflict between avoiding premature action on the basis of apparently strong observational studies, and the reality that requiring a randomized trial may delay action for many years, or in some circumstances a randomized trial may never be done. For example, the definitive randomized trial of the preventive action of folic acid on birth defects was described in Chapter 3 [52]. In this situation, an observational study completed 10 years before the randomized trial was completed in fact gave the correct answer [53], and we can now see, in retrospect, that public health action at that time would have prevented many birth defects which otherwise occurred. Would the risk of proceeding on the observation data alone have been justified? Had folic acid or multivitamin supplementation be widely adopted earlier, it is very unlikely that a randomized trial would have been done.

Examples of unresolved situations

The current situation with screening by routine skin examinations with the aim of reducing deaths from melanoma, a dangerous skin cancer, is unsatisfactory. Although authorities generally agree that a screening programme should only be instituted on the basis of randomized trial evidence, no randomized trial of skin screening has been done anywhere in the world, despite a successful pilot study [54] and none may ever be done because of the cost, the numbers of subjects, and the time required. The lack of definite evidence has resulted in many, probably most, doctors in high-risk areas like Australia using and promoting skin screening, while at the same time health authorities and evidence-based reports do not support it, so it is being done, but not funded or organized and evaluated as a cancer screening programme.

There is continued controversy about whether the use of mobile phones (cell phones) causes brain cancers, and whether exposure to power lines causes leukaemia in children. There are many case–control and cohort studies, with mixed results. The main question is whether in the studies that show increased risks, these increases are due to uncontrolled confounding [55].

Self-test questions

Answers in Appendix 1, p.402.

Q7.1 Suppose an as yet unidentified dietary constituent (X) greatly reduces the risk of cancer. It is distributed in foodstuffs in a similar way to an easily measured dietary constituent (D) which itself has no effect on cancer incidence. In a prospective cohort study, dietary intakes of D are measured, and subsequent cancer incidence recorded. What will be the result?

Q7.2 In the same situation as in Q7.1, an intervention trial using pure compound D is carried out. What will the result be?

Q7.3 An innovative pre-school reading programme is launched by asking teachers to volunteer to trial the programme, and the children in the programme are then compared with other children in the same school systems. What are the results likely to show?

Q7.4 Table 7.7 compares the characteristics of two groups in a randomized trial. Why are tests of the significance of the differences between the two groups not presented?

Q7.5 The experience of treating a disease, which can present either early or late, is compared between two hospitals. In hospital A, the success rates are 40 per cent for early disease and 25 per cent for late disease, based on 500 and

100 patients in each category; in hospital B, the success rates are 60 per cent for early disease and 40 per cent for late disease, based on 100 and 200 patients, respectively. How does the performance of hospital B compare with hospital A for each stage of disease; and how does this compare with the crude comparison based on all patients treated in each hospital?

Q7.6 Calculate the Mantel–Haenszel measure of relative risk for the data given in Q7.5.

Q7.7 Again using the example given in Q7.5, assume that over the whole country 25 per cent of patients with this condition are early at presentation. Using a standard population of 25 per cent early and 75 per cent late disease, calculate the direct standardized success rates for each of hospitals A and B. What is the ratio of these direct standardized rates?

Q7.8 In a case–control study, the role of previous injury in producing arthritis of the knee is assessed. In men, 300 of 900 men with arthritis of the knee reported previous injury, compared with 100 of 400 male controls. For women, four of 44 female cases reported previous injury, compared with 50 of 450 female controls. Calculate the overall crude odds ratio, the sex-specific odds ratios, and the Mantel–Haenszel odds ratio.

Q7.9 In an individually pair-matched case–control study, 200 pairs are concordant for exposure and 100 pairs are concordant for lack of exposure; for 200 pairs, the case is exposed and the control is not; for 50 pairs, the control is exposed and the case is not. What is the odds ratio? What would the odds ratio be if an analysis ignoring the matching was performed?

Q7.10 In a multivariate analysis, a binary variable represents oral contraceptive use, being coded 1 for ever use and zero for never use, in a prospective study assessing cardiovascular disease. On fitting ever use of oral contraceptives, plus age, the coefficient is 0.45. When the subject's weight is added to the equation, this coefficient changes to become –0.08. What is the odds ratio for the association with ever use of oral contraceptives, and what is the confounding effect of weight?

References

1. **Charig CR, Webb DR, Payne SR, Wickham JEA**. Comparison of treatment of renal calculi by open surgery, percutaneous nephrolithotomy, and extracorporeal shockwave lithotripsy. *BMJ* 1986; **292**(6524):879–882.

2. **Charig CR**. Confounding and Simpson's paradox—multiple regression would confound the clinicians. *BMJ* 1995; **310**(6975):329.

3. **Simpson EH**. The interpretation of interaction in contingency tables. *J R Statist Soc* 1951; **2**:238–241.

4. **Paffenbarger RS, Hale WE**. Work activity and coronary heart mortality. *N Engl J Med* 1975; **292**(11):545–550.

5. **Altman DG, Bland JM**. How to randomise. *BMJ* 1999; **319**(7211):703–704.

6. **Berger VW**. A review of methods for ensuring the comparability of comparison groups in randomized clinical trials. *Rev Recent Clin Trials* 2006; **1**(1):81–86.

7. **Adish AA, Esrey SA, Gyorkos TW, Jean-Baptiste J, Rojhani A**. Effect of consumption of food cooked in iron pots on iron status and growth of young children: a randomised trial. *Lancet* 1999; **353**(9154):712–716.

8. **Cook CC, Scannell TD, Lipsedge MS**. Another trial that failed. *Lancet* 1988; **331**(8584):524–525.

9. **English DR, Burton RC, Del Mar CB, Donovan RJ, Ireland PD, Emery G**. Evaluation of aid to diagnosis of pigmented skin lesions in general practice: controlled trial randomised by practice. *BMJ* 2003; **327**(7411):375–380.

10. **Altman DG, Schulz KF, Moher D, Egger M, Davidoff F, Elbourne D, et al**. The revised CONSORT statement for reporting randomized trials: explanation and elaboration. *Ann Intern Med* 2001; **134**(8):663–694.

11. **University Group Diabetes Program**. A study of the effects of hypoglycemic agents on vascular complications in patients with adult-onset diabetes. II: mortality results. *Diabetes* 1970; **19**(Suppl 2):785–830.

12. **Dodd JM, Hedayati H, Pearce E, Hotham N, Crowther CA**. Rectal analgesia for the relief of perineal pain after childbirth: a randomised controlled trial of diclofenac suppositories. *BJOG* 2004; **111**(10):1059–1064.

13. **Coronary Drug Project Research Group**. Influence of adherence to treatment and response of cholesterol on mortality in the Coronary Drug Project. *N Engl J Med* 1980; **303**(18):1038–1041.

14. **Shapiro S, Venet W, Strax P, Venet L, Roeser R**. Ten- to fourteen- year effect of screening on breast cancer mortality. *J Natl Cancer Inst* 1982; **69**:349–355.

15. **Bruner AB, Joffe A, Duggan AK, Casella JF, Brandt J**. Randomised study of cognitive effects of iron supplementation in non-anaemic iron-deficient adolescent girls. *Lancet* 1996; **348**(9033):992–996.

16. **Ashby D**. Can iron supplementation improve cognitive functioning? *Lancet* 1996; **348**(9033):973.

17. **Tunis SR, Stryer DB, Clancy CM**. Practical clinical trials: increasing the value of clinical research for decision making in clinical and health policy. *JAMA* 2003; **290**(12): 1624–1632.

18. **Labrie F, Candas B, DuPont A, Cusan L, Gomez JL, Suburu RE, et al**. Screening decreases prostate cancer death: first analysis of the 1988 Quebec prospective randomized controlled trial. *Prostate* 1999; **38**(2):83–91.

19. **Labrie F, Candas B, Cusan L, Gomez JL, Belanger A, Brousseau G, et al**. Screening decreases prostate cancer mortality: 11-year follow-up of the 1988 Quebec prospective randomized controlled trial. *Prostate* 2004; **59**(3):311–318.

20. **Boer R, Schroder FH**. Quebec randomized controlled trial on prostate cancer screening shows no evidence for mortality reduction. *Prostate* 1999; **40**(2):130–131.

21. **Elwood M**. A misleading paper on prostate cancer screening. *Prostate* 2004; **61**(4):372.

22. **Ahmad OB, Boschi-Pinto C, Lopez AD, Murray CJL, Lozano R, Inoue M**. *Age Standardization of Rates: A New WHO Population*. World Health Organization; 2001. Available from: http://www.who.int/healthinfo/paper31.pdf

23. **Mantel N, Haenszel W**. Statistical aspects of the analysis of data from retrospective studies of disease. *J Natl Cancer Inst* 1959; **22**:719–748.

24. **Elwood JM, Gallagher RP, Davison J, Hill GB**. Sunburn, suntan and the risk of cutaneous malignant melanoma: the Western Canada Melanoma Study. *Br J Cancer* 1985; **51**(4):543–549.

25. **Lyon JL, Gardner JW, West DW, Stanish WM, Hebertson RM.** Smoking and carcinoma *in situ* of the uterine cervix. *Am J Public Health* 1983; **73**(5):558–562.

26. **Karlberg J, Chong DS, Lai WY.** Do men have a higher case fatality rate of severe acute respiratory syndrome than women do? *Am J Epidemiol* 2004; **159**(3):229–231.

27. **Elwood JM.** Wood exposure and smoking: association with cancer of the nasal cavity and paranasal sinuses in British Columbia. *Can Med Assoc J* 1981; **124**(12):1573–1577.

28. **Daly E, Vessey MP, Hawkins MM, Carson JL, Gough P, Marsh S.** Risk of venous thromboembolism in users of hormone replacement therapy. *Lancet* 1996; **348**:977–980.

29. **Halvorsen I, Andersen A, Heyerdahl S.** Girls with anorexia nervosa as young adults. Self-reported and parent-reported emotional and behavioural problems compared with siblings. *Eur Child Adolesc Psychiatry* 2005; **14**(7):397–406.

30. **Scott WK, Zhang F, Stajich JM, Scott BL, Stacy MA, Vance JM.** Family-based case-control study of cigarette smoking and Parkinson disease. *Neurology* 2005; **64**(3):442–447.

31. **Swerdlow AJ, De Stavola BL, Floderus B, Holm NV, Kaprio J, Verkasalo PK, et al.** Risk factors for breast cancer at young ages in twins: an international population-based study. *J Natl Cancer Inst* 2002; **94**(16):1238–1246.

32. **Carlsson S, Hammar N, Grill V, Kaprio J.** Alcohol consumption and the incidence of type 2 diabetes: a 20-year follow-up of the Finnish twin cohort study. *Diabetes Care* 2003; **26**(10):2785–2790.

33. **Cederlöf R, Friberg L, Jonsson E, Kaij L.** Respiratory symptoms and 'angina pectoris' in twins with reference to smoking habits: an epidemiological study with mailed questionnaire. *Arch Environ Health* 1966; **13**:726–737.

34. **Herbst AL, Ulfelder H, Poskanzer DC.** Adenocarcinoma of the vagina: association of maternal stilbestrol therapy with tumor appearance in young women. *N Engl J Med* 1971; **284**(16):878–881.

35. **Hulten K, Van Kappel AL, Winkvist A, Kaaks R, Hallmans G, Lenner P, et al.** Carotenoids, alpha-tocopherols, and retinol in plasma and breast cancer risk in northern Sweden. *Cancer Causes Control* 2001; **12**(6):529–537.

36. **Forsyth BW, Horwitz RI, Acampora D, Shapiro ED, Viscoli CM, Feinstein AR, et al.** New epidemiologic evidence confirming that bias does not explain the aspirin/Reye's syndrome association. *JAMA* 1989; **261**(17):2517–2524.

37. **Elwood JM, Williamson C, Stapleton PJ.** Malignant melanoma in relation to moles, pigmentation, and exposure to fluorescent and other lighting sources. *Br J Cancer* 1986; **53**:65–74.

38. **Purdue MP, Hofmann JN, Kemp TJ, Chaturvedi AK, Lan Q, Park JH, et al.** A prospective study of 67 serum immune and inflammation markers and risk of non-Hodgkin lymphoma. *Blood* 2013; **122**(6):951–957.

39. **Deeks JJ, Dinnes J, D'Amico R, Sowden AJ, Sakarovitch C, Song F, et al.** Evaluating non-randomised intervention studies. *Health Technol Assess* 2003; **7**(27):iii–x, 1–173.

40. **Borah BJ, Moriarty JP, Crown WH, Doshi JA.** Applications of propensity score methods in observational comparative effectiveness and safety research: where have we come and where should we go? *J Comp Eff Res* 2014; **3**(1):63–78.

41. **Ray WA, Murray KT, Hall K, Arbogast PG, Stein CM.** Azithromycin and the risk of cardiovascular death. *N Engl J Med* 2012; **366**(20):1881–1890.

42. **Perel P, Clayton T, Altman DG, Croft P, Douglas I, Hemingway H, et al.** Red blood cell transfusion and mortality in trauma patients: risk-stratified analysis of an observational study. *PLoS Med* 2014; **11**(6):e1001664.

43. Maldonado G, Greenland S. Simulation study of confounder-selection strategies. *Am J Epidemiol* 1993; **138**(11):923–936.

44. Peto R, Doll R, Buckley JD, Sporn MB. Can dietary beta-carotene materially reduce human cancer rates? *Nature* 1981; **290**(5803):201–208.

45. The Alpha-Tocopherol Beta Carotene Cancer Prevention Study Group. The effect of vitamin E and beta carotene on the incidence of lung cancer and other cancers in male smokers. *N Engl J Med* 1994; **330**(15):1029–1035.

46. Omenn GS, Goodman GE, Thornquist MD, Balmes J, Cullen MR, Glass A, et al. Effects of a combination of beta carotene and vitamin A on lung cancer and cardiovascular disease. *N Engl J Med* 1996; **334**(18):1150–1155.

47. Duffield-Lillico AJ, Begg CB. Reflections on the landmark studies of beta-carotene supplementation. *J Natl Cancer Inst* 2004; **96**(23):1729–1731.

48. Stampfer MJ, Colditz GA. Estrogen replacement therapy and coronary heart disease: a quantitative assessment of the epidemiologic evidence. *Prev Med* 1991; **20**:47–63.

49. Rossouw JE, Anderson GL, Prentice RL, LaCroix AZ, Kooperberg C, Stefanick ML, et al. Risks and benefits of estrogen plus progestin in healthy postmenopausal women: principal results from the Women's Health Initiative randomized controlled trial. *JAMA* 2002; **288**(3):321–333.

50. Petitti DB, Freedman DA. Invited commentary: how far can epidemiologists get with statistical adjustment? *Am J Epidemiol* 2005; **162**(5):415–418.

51. Lawlor DA, Davey SG, Kundu D, Bruckdorfer KR, Ebrahim S. Those confounded vitamins: what can we learn from the differences between observational versus randomised trial evidence? *Lancet* 2004; **363**(9422):1724–1727.

52. MRC (Medical Research Council) Vitamin Study Group. Prevention of neural tube defects: results of the Medical Research Council Vitamin Study. *Lancet* 1991; **338**(8760):131–137.

53. Smithells RW, Sheppard S, Schorah CJ, Seller MJ, Nevin NC, Harris R, et al. Apparent prevention of neural tube defects by periconceptional vitamin supplementation. *Arch Dis Child* 1981; **56**(12):911–918.

54. Aitken JF, Elwood JM, Lowe JB, Firman DW, Balanda KP, Ring IT. A randomised trial of population screening for melanoma. *J Med Screen* 2002; **9**(1):33–37.

55. Elwood JM. Mobile phones, brain tumors, and the limits of science. *Bioelectromagnetics* 2014; **35**(5):379–383.

Chapter 8

Chance variation

Although men flatter themselves with their great actions, they are not so often the result of a great design as of chance.

—La Rochefoucauld: *Maxims*; 1665

Introduction

In this chapter, we will discuss the effects of chance variation that can be assessed by applying statistical tests. The chapter falls into three parts: Part 1—the application of statistical tests and confidence limits to a simple 2×2 table; Part 2—applications to stratified and matched studies, and to multivariate analysis; Part 3—life-table methods for the consideration of the timing of outcome events in a cohort study or intervention study. Summaries of the statistical methods, with worked examples, are given in Appendix 2. Table A2.15 shows the relationships between the value of a statistic and the probability or *P*-value, and related Excel formulae are listed in Table A2.16.

Part 1. Statistical tests and confidence limits in a simple table

The third non-causal explanation, for an association, after observation bias and confounding, is that it is due to chance variation, or random number variation, the fall of the dice, luck, or whatever synonym you prefer. Statistics is concerned with measuring the likelihood (or probability) that a given set of results has been produced by this mechanism. We will discuss the statistical techniques used most in epidemiological studies and in clinical trials. The principles of interpretation can be appreciated using simple examples, but also apply to results which use much more complex statistics. Many papers will use more complex statistical methods, but working through the widely used statistical methods can clarify most of the general principles of interpretation of statistical tests.

The appropriate place of statistical testing

So far in this text we have discussed the measurement of the association between an exposure and an outcome, in terms of the relative risk, odds ratio, or attributable risk. We have discussed how to judge whether the estimate of association is acceptable, as being reasonably free of bias and confounding. The order of consideration of non-causal explanations, observation bias, confounding, and chance, is important. If there is substantial observation bias, there is no point in adding a statistical analysis to a biased result. The assessment of bias depends on consideration of the design and conduct of the study. Some analysis methods may help to deal with bias, for example, by restricting the study to certain subgroups, using a particular comparison group, and so on. Once observation bias has been dealt with, it is appropriate to consider confounding. We may have a situation in which there could be severe confounding by a factor not included in the study design, in which case further data manipulation is not helpful. More frequently, there may be confounding which can be dealt with by stratification or multivariate analysis, or has been dealt with by randomization, matching, or restriction in the study design. These steps reviewed so far take us to the point of having an estimate of the association, which is, in our best judgement, not compromised by bias and is adjusted as far as possible for confounding. It is this estimate of the association on which we now concentrate and to which we can now apply statistical tests.

Discrete versus continuous measures

We will concentrate on statistical methods applicable to discrete measures of exposure and of outcome, that is, two or a small number of categories. This is for two main reasons. In studies of disease causation and the evaluation of interventions, in most applications, the outcome measures are categorical and often binary (yes/no): the onset of disease, death, recurrence, recovery, return to work, and so on. Even where a quantitative measure can be used, a discrete categorization may be appropriate. For example, in studying ways to control high blood sugar, the change in blood glucose levels in each subject may be assessed, using statistical methods appropriate for this quantitative outcome. However, it may be more relevant clinically to assess the 'success' of treatment by counting subjects who achieve 'well-controlled' levels, defined by preset clinically relevant criteria.

The second reason is that many introductory statistics courses and texts emphasize methods of dealing with continuous data: the normal distribution, t-tests, regression, analysis of variance, and so on. Methods applicable to discrete variables may be less familiar.

The concept of significance

The statistical method the reader is most likely to be familiar with is that of significance testing. The question is: is the difference in outcome between the two groups of subjects larger than we would expect to occur purely by chance? Consider a simple intervention study (Table 8.1).

This study gives the success rate of the new treatment as 20 per cent. Even accepting the study design as being perfect with no bias, we would not interpret this as meaning that for all similar groups of subjects exposed to this intervention, the success rate would be 20 per cent. The 200 subjects chosen are a sample from the uncounted total of all possible subjects who could be given that intervention, and 20 per cent is the

Table 8.1 A simple comparative study: hypothetical data.

Treatment group	Outcome		Total patients	Incidence of success (%)
	Success	**No success**		
New therapy	40	160	200	20
Conventional therapy	20	180	200	10
Total	60	340	400	15

estimate of the success rate in that total group of potential subjects. On the basis of pure chance, we expect that the next sample of 200 subjects would be likely to give a slightly different result. However, 20 per cent is our best estimate of the true success rate. Similarly, in the comparison group, our best estimate is 10 per cent. The significance testing technique tests how likely it is that a difference as large as the one we have seen, or larger, could occur purely by chance, if the true situation is that both the intervention and the comparison groups have the same true success rate. This would occur on the *null hypothesis* that the effect of the new therapy is no different from that of the comparison therapy. This is sometimes referred to as the concept that the two groups of subjects are independent samples drawn from the same population. Therefore statistical tests assess the hypothesis that the true success rate in the two groups is the same, and that the observed differences are produced purely by chance variation around that common value. Our best estimate of the common value of the success rate is based on all the subjects in the study, and therefore is 15 per cent in this example.

Simple statistical tests for a 2 × 2 table

Chi-squared statistic

One commonly used test in this situation is the *chi-squared statistic*, written χ^2, applied to the 2 × 2 table formed from the study results, which gives a value of 7.84 (Box 8.1). To interpret this we need to know the number of *degrees of freedom* of the statistic. The number of 'degrees of freedom' is the number of cells in the body of the table that can vary independently, given the marginal totals (i.e. the totals which appear at the margins of the table). For the table in Box 8.1, if the marginal totals are known, only one number within the table needs to be known—all the rest are then derived from it—and so the table has one degree of freedom (d.f.). An $n \times n$ table has $(n-1) \times (n-1)$ degrees of freedom. Looking up 7.84 in a table of the chi-squared distribution on one degree of freedom (Table A2.15) shows that the probability or *P*-value is between 0.01 and 0.001; alternatively, using an Excel spreadsheet and entering = chidist(7.84,1) gives 0.005 (see Table A2.16). The test shows that, if the true success rate is the same in the two groups, the probability of a difference as large as or larger than the one we have seen occurring purely by chance variation is between 1 in 100 (0.01) and 1 in 1000 (0.001). It is considerably less than 5 per cent (0.05), and so is conventionally accepted as '*statistically significant*'.

Box 8.1 Two appropriate statistical tests applied to a 2 × 2 table: arithmetic examples use the data shown in Table 8.1

STATISTICAL TESTS OF A NULL HYPOTHESIS

Exposure	Outcome		Total no. patients	Success rate (%)
	Positive (success)	Negative		
New treatment	a (40)	b (160)	N_1 (200)	S_1 (20%)
Comparison	c (20)	d (180)	N_0 (200)	S_0 (10%)
Total	M_1 (60)	M_0 (340)	T (400)	S (15%)

Appropriate statistical tests for departures from the null hypothesis:

(a) *Chi-square statistic* $\chi^2 = \dfrac{(ad = bc)^2 T}{N_1 N_0 M_1 M_0} = 7.84$

Equivalently $\chi^2 = \sum \dfrac{(obs - exp)^2}{exp}$ for each of the four cells

$$= \frac{(a - N_1 M_1 / T)^2}{N_1 M_1 / T} + \frac{(b - N_1 M_0 / T)^2}{N_1 M_0 / T} + \frac{(c - N_0 M_1 / T)^2}{N_0 M_1 / T} + \frac{(d - N_0 M_0 / T)^2}{N_0 M_0 / T}$$

$= 7.84$

From the table of the χ^2 distribution on 1 d.f., the probability P of this or a larger value occurring on the null hypothesis lies between 0.01 and 0.001 (from Table A2.15), or using Table A2.16, $P = 0.005$.

(b) *Comparison of two proportions*

$$\text{Standardized normal deviate} = \frac{S_1 - S_0}{\sqrt{\left[S(1 - S) \left(\dfrac{1}{N_1} + \dfrac{1}{N_0} \right) \right]}}$$

$= 2.80$

From a table of the normal distribution (Table A2.15), the two-sided probability corresponding to 2.80 lies between 0.01 and 0.001, or using Table A2.16, $P = 0.005$.

(c) *For a continuity corrected version of the χ^2 statistic, the formulae are:*

$$\chi_c^2 = \frac{\left(|ad - bc| - \dfrac{1}{2} T \right)^2 T}{N_1 N_0 M_1 M_0}$$

and

$$\chi_c^2 = \frac{\left(|a - N_1 M_1 / T| - \dfrac{1}{2} \right)^2}{N_1 M_1 / T} + etc.$$

Hence $\chi_c^2 = 7.08$

From Table A2.15, P is between 0.01 and 0.001, or using Table A2.16, $P = 0.008$.

Difference in proportions

Another commonly used test is a test of difference in proportions, testing whether the 20 per cent success rate in the intervention group is different from the 10 per cent success rate in the control group (Box 8.1(b)). The formula shown assumes each success rate, being a proportion, has a binomial distribution, and yields a *standardized normal deviate* of 2.80. This also corresponds to a two-sided *P*-value of between 0.01 and 0.001 (Table A2.15), or using Excel we can enter = 2*(1-normsdist(2.8)) and this yields 0.005 (Table A2.16).

Comparison of the two tests

We have applied two statistical tests to the same data. They should give the same results. In fact, the chi-squared statistic on one degree of freedom is the square of the normal deviate: $2.8^2 = 7.84$. The cut-off point at 5 per cent significance for χ^2 on one degree of freedom is 3.84, which is the square of 1.96, the cut-off for the normal deviate. As an alternative to calculating the chi-squared statistic from the formula shown in Box 8.1, its square root, the chi statistic, can be calculated and looked up in tables of the normal deviate, which are often more detailed than tables of the chi-squared statistic. This relationship between χ^2 and a standardized normal deviate holds only for the situation where χ^2 has one degree of freedom.

Studies which produce results that can be simplified to the 2×2 format shown here can be dealt with using either of these techniques, and the statistical methods apply to both cohort and case–control designs. The statistic tests the departure of the data from the null hypothesis of no association; therefore it can be regarded as a test of the significance of a risk difference (attributable risk) from the null value of 0, or of the difference of the risk ratio (relative risk or odds ratio) from the null value of 1.

One-sided and two-sided tests

The above-mentioned tests are *two-sided* tests; that is, they estimate the probability that if the null hypothesis were true, a difference would occur which would be as large as or larger than that observed in either direction, that is, the intervention group having either the higher or the lower success rate. A *one-sided test* estimates only the probability of occurrence, on the null hypothesis, of the observed result or results that are more different from the null hypothesis in the same direction. A one-sided test is appropriate in situations where the direction of the effect is established before the data are collected. Thus if Table 8.1 was drawn from a study designed specifically to assess whether the new therapy was better than the conventional treatment, discounting any possibility that it could be worse, a one-sided test could be used. Except with very small numbers, the two-sided probability is simply twice the one-sided probability, and therefore a one-sided test with a probability given as 5 per cent (0.05) is equivalent to a two-sided test with a probability value of 10 per cent (0.1) (see Table A2.15). Chi-squared statistics, because they square the deviations between observed and expected values, directly give two-sided tests, while many tables of the distribution of the standardized normal deviate directly give a one-sided probability value, which is then doubled if a two-sided test is required. In Excel, the command = (1-normsdist(z)) gives the one-sided P-value for a normal deviate z, and = 2*(1-normsdist(z)) gives the two-sided probability.

Small numbers, continuity corrections, and exact tests

The expected value in each cell in a 2×2 table need not be a whole number; it has a continuous distribution. However, the observed values must be whole numbers. In calculating the chi-squared statistic or normal deviate, a '*continuity correction*' which allows for this can be used (see Box 8.1(c)); it is sometimes called a Yates' correction after the statistician Frank Yates who introduced it. Its effect is to reduce the calculated statistic somewhat; this reduction is greater when the number of observations in the table is small. However, its use is controversial; some statisticians argue that the use of a continuity correction gives a more accurate estimation of the P-value, while others disagree [1]. With reasonably large numbers, the continuity correction will make very little difference. For the data in Box 8.1, the continuity corrected χ^2 statistic is 7.08, compared with the uncorrected value of 7.84, corresponding to P-values of 0.0078 and 0.0051, respectively (Table A2.16). The test of comparison of proportions makes an assumption of having reasonable numbers of subjects and gives the square root of the uncorrected χ^2 value.

Thus the issue of whether to use a continuity correction is related to how P-values are interpreted. If we reduce the stress on particular cut-off values of the P-value, such as 0.05, the problem is put into perspective. If the use of a continuity correction changes a result from being less than to being greater than 0.05, this merely shows that the true probability value is very close to 0.05 and should be interpreted accordingly. Also, if the difference is substantial, it means the number of observations is small, and a better solution is to use an *exact probability test*. One of these, the Fisher test for 2×2 tables, is described in Table A2.4, and others are available for other situations; many computer programmes provide exact tests. An approximate rule is that χ^2 statistics become unreliable where any expected numbers in the tables are less than 5. This often occurs if tables with many cells are generated, and the solution may be to combine some categories. The same consideration applies where different results arise from different, but applicable, statistical tests, or even from the same test performed using a different calculator or computer programme. All these serve to emphasize that we should guard against over-interpreting the precise value of the P-value, using it instead as a general measure of probability. We will see later that confidence limits are usually clearer to interpret than statistical tests.

The Mantel–Haenszel test

Although the usual χ^2 tests are appropriate for simple tables, more generally applicable methods that can be extended to deal with stratified data are very useful in epidemiological and clinical studies.

Many statistical tests are derived from the principle that if we calculate the difference between an observed value a and its expected value on the null hypothesis E, square that, and divide it by the variance V of the observed value, the quantity (the statistic) resulting will follow a χ^2 distribution on one degree of freedom (1 d.f.), that is,

$$\chi^2 = (a - E)^2 / V.$$

As we shall see, this general formula can be applied to many different situations, using appropriate calculations to obtain E and V.

The χ^2 distribution on 1 d.f. is simply related to the normal distribution. If a variable χ follows a normal distribution, its square χ^2 will follow a χ^2 distribution on 1 d.f. Thus an equivalent formula to that previously given is

$$\chi = \sqrt{\chi^2} = (a - E) / \sqrt{V}.$$

That is, the difference between the observed value a and its expected value E, divided by the standard deviation of a (the square root of the variance) gives a normal deviate, often referred to as chi, χ, or Z.

The Mantel–Haenszel test for a 2×2 table [2] is shown in Box 8.2 (Nathan Mantel, 1919–2002, and William (Bill) Haenszel, 1910–1998, were both statisticians at the National Cancer Institute in the USA, and this test has been very widely used for over 50 years, both in this form and in other applications). The χ^2 statistic is given by calculating the difference between one observed value in the table and its expected

---

Box 8.2 The Mantel–Haenszel test for a 2×2 table with reasonable numbers. This is applicable to both cohort and case–control data

GENERAL TEST FOR A 2 × 2 TABLE

Table showing fixed marginal totals

	Success	**No success**	**Total**
New treatment	a	b	N_1
Old treatment	c	d	N_0
Total	M_1	M_0	T

General formulae

Observed number of 'exposed cases' $= a$

Expected value of a on null hypothesis $= E = N_1 M_1 / T$

Variance of a under hypergeometric distribution $= V = \left(\dfrac{N_1 N_0 M_0 M_1}{T^2 (T - 1)} \right)$

Chi-squared statistic, 1 degree of freedom $= \dfrac{(a - E)^2}{V} = \dfrac{(a - N_1 M_1 / T)^2}{N_1 N_0 M_0 M_1 / T^2 (T - 1)}$

Normal deviate, $\chi = \sqrt{\chi^2} = \dfrac{(a - E)}{\sqrt{V}}$

Continuity corrected versions: $\chi_c^2 = \dfrac{(|a - E| - 0.5)^2}{V}$ $\chi_c = \dfrac{|a - E| - 0.5}{\sqrt{V}}$

value, squaring that, and dividing by the variance of the observed value. The observed value a is usually taken as the number of exposed cases; the expected number E is derived from the totals in the margins of the table as N_1M_1/T. The variance is calculated from the marginal totals, calculated as shown in Box 8.2. The underlying theory is based on the 'hypergeometric' distribution, and applies to a table where the marginal totals are fixed; this assumption is also made in the Fisher test and the usual χ^2 tests. From this, we can calculate X^2 or X using the formulae given earlier. For a continuity correction, we reduce the absolute value $a - E$ by 0.5, before squaring. For the table in Table 8.1,

> observed value of $a = 40$
> expected value of $a = N_1M_1/T = 200 \times 60/400 = 30$
> variance of $a = N_1N_0M_1M_0/T^2(T-1) = 200 \times 200 \times 60 \times 340/(400 \times 400 \times 399) = 12.78$.

Then

$$\chi^2 = (a - E)^2/V = (40 - 30)^2/12.78 = 7.82$$

and from Table A2.15, P lies between 0.01 and 0.001; and $\chi = 2.80$ and from Table A2.15 or Table A2.16, $P = 0.005$ (two-sided).

These values are almost identical to those given by the tests used in Box 8.1. If a continuity correction is used, $\chi^2 = 7.06$, $P = 0.008$.

The Mantel–Haenszel test, as shown in Box 8.2, was first applied to case–control studies, and is also applicable to cohort studies and surveys using count data. A very similar formula, shown in Box 8.3, is used for cohort data with a person-time denominator. Later in this chapter we will discuss how this basic test, with some variations, can be applied to stratified data, to matched studies, and to cohort studies taking into account follow-up time.

Box 8.3 Person-time data: for cohort data using person-time denominators, formulae very similar to those shown in Box 8.2 are applicable. For a continuity correction, subtract 0.5 from the absolute value of $a - E$

TEST FOR COHORT STUDY WITH PERSON-TIME DATA

	Outcome positive	Person-time
Exposed	a	N_1
Unexposed	b	N_0
Total	M_1	T

Statistical test

Observed no. of 'exposed cases' = a

expected value of a $\qquad E = N_1M_1/T$

variance of a $\qquad V = N_1N_0M_1/T^2$

Chi-squared statistic χ^2, 1 degree of freedom $= \dfrac{(a-E)^2}{V} = \dfrac{(a - N_1M_1/T)^2}{N_1N_0M_1/T^2}$

These formulae are 'asymptotic', that is, they are derived by making assumptions which are valid only where reasonable numbers of observations are available; a guide to 'reasonable' would be that the smallest expected number in the 2×2 table on which the result is based should be greater than five. This limitation does not apply to stratified subtables, which can be smaller if only the summary estimates are to be used. Where numbers of observations are smaller, 'exact' tests can be used, such as Fisher's test for a simple 2×2 table (Table A2.4).

Precision and confidence limits

These tests of significance yield a single value, the P-value. This has quite a long definition: it is the probability of a difference the same as or larger than that observed in the study occurring purely by chance, on the null hypothesis that the outcome is the same in each of the groups being compared. Two studies comparing a new and an old therapy are shown in Table 8.2; in both, the success rate is twice as high with the new therapy. In study A, $P = 0.005$: if there were no true difference, a difference as large as or larger than that seen would have occurred only about once in 200 occasions. In study B, the P-value is 0.14. Using the conventional $P = 0.05$ cut-off, the result in A is *significant*, whereas that in B is *non-significant*.

However, reporting results by using only P-values at best makes poor use of the data, and at worst can be misleading. A superficial review of these two studies might conclude that they are inconsistent, as study A shows a significant benefit while study B shows no significant difference. In fact, the two studies show exactly the same advantage for the new therapy (relative risk of 2.0). It is the precision of the studies, not the estimate of effect, which differs.

A better way to present the results, which uses the information in the study more fully, is to use *confidence limits* for the result rather than the P-value. The concept is as

Table 8.2 Two simple comparative studies: hypothetical data. Statistics calculated without continuity corrections. With a continuity correction they are 7.08 and 1.35, respectively.

	Numbers of subjects		Total	Success rate (%)
	Success	**No success**		
Study A				
New therapy	40	160	200	20
Old therapy	20	180	200	10
Study B				
New therapy	10	26	36	28
Old therapy	5	31	36	14

Study A: relative risk $= 2.0$ $\chi^2 = 7.84$ $P = 0.005$

Study B: relative risk $= 2.0$ $\chi^2 = 2.11$ $P = 0.14$

follows. Any one study provides an estimate of the association, for example, the relative risk shown in the study A (2.0) is an estimate of the true relative risk, which is unknown. This estimate has variability. The variability depends mainly on the size of the study, and the confidence limits show this variability. So for study A, the 95 per cent confidence limits are 1.21–3.30 (the calculation is shown later). So, while we will never know the true value of the relative risk, if our study is free of other biases, we can have 95 per cent confidence that the true value is between 1.21 and 3.30. Of course, the true value could be less than 1.21, or it could be more than 3.30, but that is 'unlikely', meaning it has a probability of less than 5 per cent (1 in 20 times), or less than 2.5 per cent for each of the lower and upper extremes. The value of 1.0 is outside this range, so we can (reasonably) exclude the hypothesis that the new therapy is no better than the old one.

The calculation of confidence limits depends on assuming that, if we did an infinity of similar studies, the results would follow a normal distribution—a bell curve. The curve is centred on the point estimate from our one study. The width of the curve depends on the *standard error* of that estimate: the range of 1.96 standard errors on each side of the point estimate will include 95 per cent of possible values, and so give the confidence limits. For a simple measurement (the mean heights of a sample of adults, for example), the assumption of a normal distribution is reasonable. For ratio measures such as relative risk and odds ratio, this does not apply; but we can assume a normal distribution for the natural logarithm (ln) of the ratio.

Thus, if we know the logarithm of the observed relative risk (ln RR) and its standard error (SE ln RR), we can calculate the 95 per cent confidence limits as follows:

$$95 \text{ percent confidence limits of } \ln RR = \left(\ln RR - 1.96 \times SE \ln RR \right)$$

$$\text{and } \left(\ln RR + 1.96 \times SE \ln RR \right)$$

$$95 \text{ percent confidence limits of } RR = \text{exponential} \left(\ln RR - 1.96 \times SE \ln RR \right)$$

$$\text{and exponential} \left(\ln RR + 1.96 \times SE \ln RR \right).$$

Calculation of confidence limits

For the example in Table 8.2, study A, the RR is 2.0, so the ln RR is 0.6931. The standard error of ln RR, using the notation in Box 8.2, is given by

$$SE \ln RR = \sqrt{\frac{b}{aN_1} + \frac{d}{cN_0}}$$

$$= \sqrt{[(160/(40 \times 200)) + (180/20 \times 200))]} = 0.2550.$$

So the 95 per cent limits of SE ln RR are $(0.6931 - 1.96 \times 0.2550) = 0.1934$, and $(0.6931 + 1.96 \times 0.2550) = 1.1928$. Taking the exponentials of these gives the 95 per cent confidence limits for the risk ratio as 1.21–3.30.

Thus the appropriate way to show the results of study A in Table 8.2 is that the estimated relative risk is 2.0, with 95 per cent confidence limits of 1.21–3.30. The limits exclude the null hypothesis value of 1.0, so the result is 'significant' using a 5 per cent, two-sided, test.

Study B gives the same point estimate, a relative risk of 2.0, with 95 per cent limits of 0.76–5.27. This study is compatible with the true effect being in the range of 0.76 (that is, the new therapy is not as good) up to 5.27 (much better). This presentation of the results of the two studies makes it clear they give similar results, indeed the estimate of RR is the same; they vary in terms of their precision, or power, shown by the smaller study having a larger standard error and therefore wider confidence limits.

Limits other than 95 per cent

Limits other than 95 per cent are calculated using the normal deviate corresponding to that proportion; see Box 8.8 or Table A2.15 or Table A2.16. Thus, for 99 per cent two-sided confidence limits, the normal deviate value is 2.58 instead of 1.96; for 90 per cent it is 1.64. We can use one-sided or two-sided confidence limits. The earlier example is based on two-sided limits.

Why confidence limits should be used

Confidence limits are much more informative than *P*-values. Many leading clinical and epidemiological journals will no longer accept papers using only *P*-values. Confidence limits are particularly useful when the result of the study is non-significant. The presentation of confidence limits may guard against the common fallacy of interpreting studies like study B as showing 'no difference' between the intervention and control group. While the overall result is consistent with the null hypothesis, the confidence limits show that the study is also consistent with a relative risk of 5.0, a considerable effect. A better interpretation of study B is that, while it has demonstrated a relative risk of 2.0, the 95 per cent confidence limits show that the result is consistent with anything from a small detrimental effect of the intervention to a large beneficial effect, and therefore the study is inconclusive rather than demonstrating that the intervention has no effect.

Applications to other designs

The confidence limits of any of the measures of association derived from comparative studies, and also of incidence rates, prevalence, and such measures can all be derived from the general principle that the 95 per cent limits are given by the point estimate plus or minus 1.96 times the standard error. Care is needed to use the right scale: measurements such as incidence and prevalence, and risk difference, require no adjustment, but for ratio measurements such as relative risk and odds ratio, the calculations use the logarithm of the ratio and the standard error of the log transformed ratio. What is needed is a formula for the standard error; that is not always simple to calculate. Formulae for the calculation of standard errors for various study designs are given in Boxes A2.1–A2.3.

Part 2. Statistical methods in more complex situations

Analyses with stratification

The use of stratification to control for a confounding variable was discussed in Chapter 7. The Mantel–Haenszel test is easily applied to stratified data from any type of study, and is a test of the summary relative risk or odds ratio estimate.

The Mantel–Haenszel χ^2 test for a 2×2 table is calculated as (Box 8.2)

$$\chi^2 = (a - E)^2 / V$$

where a is one of the values in the table, such as the number of exposed cases, E is its expected value, and V is its variance. If the data are stratified into several 2×2 tables, a χ^2 test for the association after stratification is given by

$$\chi^2 = \left(\Sigma_i a_i - \Sigma_i E_i\right)^2 / \Sigma_i V^i$$

where $\Sigma_i a_i$ means 'the sum of the values a_i in each table, represented by a_1, a_2, a_3, ... over I tables, where I is the number of tables'. So, the values of a, E, and V are calculated in each stratum and summed, and χ^2 is calculated using the three summations; it still has one degree of freedom irrespective of the number of subtables.

An application to a simple case–control study is shown in Box 8.4; these data were shown previously and relate to the association between melanoma and sunburn history. The single-factor table shows an odds ratio of 1.40, which is statistically significant: $\chi^2 = 4.94$, $P = 0.03$ (Table A2.15). However, part of the association is produced by confounding by tendency to sunburn. Adjustment for this by stratification gives an odds ratio of 1.19, which is not statistically significant; the summary $\chi^2 = 1.16$, $P = 0.3$, indicating that this or a more extreme result would occur in nearly one of three studies of this size if the null hypothesis were true.

Confidence limits can be calculated as shown in Table A2.1; the formula is simple for the crude OR, and more complex for the adjusted OR, but available in many packages such as EpiInfo (http://wwwn.cdc.gov/epiinfo). Here the crude OR has 95 per cent limits of 1.04 to 1.89, and the Mantel–Haenszel adjusted OR is 1.16 with 95 per cent limits of 0.87 to 1.62, based on the standard error of ln OR of 0.02503.

The same formula is applicable to cohort or intervention studies with observations on individuals, as shown in Table A2.2. For person-time data from a cohort study, the values of E_i and V_i are calculated using a formula adapted from that in Box 8.4, which is shown in Table A2.3.

Assumptions in stratification: interaction

The calculation of a summary measure of odds ratio or relative risk implies that this single estimate applies to all the different strata. This is often the most reasonable a priori assumption, but it should be checked by examining the stratum-specific ratios. While substantial variation in stratum-specific odds ratios may be due only to small numbers, a summary estimate may disguise important real variation. With an ordered confounder, such as age, there may be a regular trend in the odds ratio estimates over strata of the confounder.

By comparing the stratum-specific odds ratios (or relative risks) with the summary value, we can test the hypothesis that the summary estimate applies to all strata. A simple test is based on the logic of squaring the difference between an observed value and its expected value, and dividing by the variance, to give a chi-squared statistic. For each stratum, we calculate the difference between the observed ln odds ratio in that stratum (or relative risk) L_i and the summary ln odds ratio L_s (which is its expected value), square that, and divide by the variance (the standard error squared) of the observed stratum-specific ln odds ratio V_i. This gives a measure of the 'goodness of fit' of the model applying the summary odds ratio in each stratum to the observed data. Summing over all subtables gives

Box 8.4 Calculation of the Mantel–Haenszel x^2 statistic from the case–control data shown in Table 7.12

MANTEL–HAENSZEL ANALYSIS OF STRATIFIED DATA

(A) All subjects

	Cases	Controls	Total			
Severe sunburn	136	98	234	$OR = 1.40$		
Mild sunburn	343	347	690	$a = 136$	$E = 121.31$	$V = 43.67$
	479	445	924	$x^2 = 4.94$	$P = 0.03$	

(B$_1$) Subjects who sunburn easily

	Cases	Controls	Total			
Severe sunburn	119	76	195	$OR = 1.19$		
Mild sunburn	227	173	400	$a = 119$	$E = 133.39$	$V = 31.96$
	346	249	595			

(B$_2$) Subjects who do not sunburn easily

	Cases	Controls	Total			
Severe sunburn	17	22	39	$OR = 1.16$		
Mild sunburn	116	174	290	$a = 17$	$E = 15.77$	$V = 8.30$
	133	196	329			

Stratified analysis, adjusting for tendency to sunburn

Summary $OR = 1.19$ (see Table 7.12 for calculation)

$$\text{Summary } \chi^2 = \frac{\left(\sum_i a_i - \sum_i E_i\right)^2}{\sum_i V_i} = \frac{\{(119+17)-(113.39+15.77)\}^2}{(31.96+8.30)}$$

$$= 1.16 \; P = 0.3 \text{ (Table A2.15 or Table A2.16)}$$

Source: data from Elwood JM et al., 'Sunburn, suntan and the risk of cutaneous malignant melanoma: the Western Canada Melanoma Study,' *British Journal of Cancer*, Volume 51, Issue 4, pp. 543–549, © 1985.

$$\chi^2_{(I-1)} = \sum_i \frac{(L_i - L_s)^2}{V_i}$$

where L_i and V_i are the ln odds ratio and its variance for each subtable, and L_s is the ln of the summary odds ratio (e.g. the Mantel–Haenszel odds ratio). Given I subtables, the χ^2 has $I - 1$ degrees of freedom. This is a test of the hypothesis that the odds ratios are homogeneous. Other tests can assess a linear trend in the odds ratios over the strata, which may sometimes be more relevant. However, substantial numbers of observations are required to detect heterogeneity in stratum-specific relative risks. In Box 8.4, the odds ratios in the two strata were very similar (1.19 and 1.16) so a test of heterogeneity is unnecessary (it yields a χ^2 of 0.01).

Box 8.5 shows an example of variation of the odds ratio estimate. In this study, 217 patients with *in situ* carcinoma of the cervix were compared with 243 population-based controls [3]. A significant association between the disease and smoking was seen, with an odds ratio of 6.6 with 95 per cent limits of 4.3–10.0 (table A). After subdivision into three categories by age, the Mantel–Haenszel age-adjusted odds ratio is 6.3, only slightly reduced compared with the crude odds ratio, with 95 per cent limits of 4.1–9.5. Thus age is not a major confounder. However, the odds ratios in each of the three strata of age are considerably different, being 27.9, 5.9, and 2.8 in successively older age groups. The chi-squared statistic testing for heterogeneity of the odds ratio, calculated as above, is 12.1 on 2 d.f., $P < 0.01$, and so there is statistically significant variation in the

---

Box 8.5 An example of interaction defined here as non-homogeneity of the odds ratio in different categories of a third modifying variable. In this case–control study comparing 217 patients with *in situ* carcinoma of the cervix with 243 population-based female controls, a significant association with smoking is seen (Table A); adjustment for confounding by age makes little difference to this result. However, the odds ratios in the three age categories are substantially different, as shown by their confidence limits (C.L.) and by the x^2 test for homogeneity over the three subtables. Calculations shown in Table A2.1. The heterogeneity statistic uses the variance formula in 4A of Table A2.1

INTERACTION IN A STRATIFIED ANALYSIS

(A) Full table

		Cases	Controls	
All ages:	Smokers	130	45	
	Non-smokers	87	198	Odds ratio = 6.6
		217	243	x^2 = 83.1; 95% confidence limits = 4.3, 10.0

(B) Subtables by age

Age 20–29:	Smokers	41	6	*OR* = 27.9
	Non-smokers	13	53	x^2 = 49.7; 95% C.L. = 9.8, 79.6
Age 30–39:	Smokers	66	25	*OR* = 5.9
	Non-smokers	37	83	x^2 = 35.8; 95% C.L = 3.2, 10.8
Age 40 +	Smokers	23	14	*OR* = 2.8;
	Non-smokers	37	62	x^2 = 6.7; 95% C.L. = 1.3, 6.0

Odds ratio after adjustment for age, Mantel–Haenszel method = 6.3

x^2 statistic after adjustment for age, 1 d.f. = 82.3

95 per cent confidence limits of adjusted *OR* = 4.1, 9.5

x^2 for heterogeneity on the three subtables = 12.1 d.f. = 2 $P < 0.01$

Source: data from Lyon JL et al., 'Smoking and carcinoma in situ of the uterine cervix,' *American Journal Public Health*, Volume 73, Issue 4, pp. 558–562, © 1983.

stratum-specific odds ratios. The summary odds ratio of 6.3 is not an adequate description of the relationship of smoking with disease, and so in this study the results for the different age groups should be shown and discussed.

Multiplicative and additive models

This analysis assumes a *multiplicative* model, as discussed in Chapter 4; the relative risk estimates are assumed to be constant. This multiplicative model is assumed in techniques such as the Mantel–Haenszel estimate of odds ratio, and in many multivariate analyses, such as those using the logistic regression model. The attractiveness of this model arises from both its mathematical advantages, as it is a relatively simple model, and the empirical evidence that it appears to apply to a wide range of biomedical applications.

The situations where such a model can be tested are those in which there are two or more strong risk factors, and enough subjects with the various combinations of categories of these risk factors can be identified and their risks assessed directly. Important examples in medicine which have shown that a multiplicative model appears to be an appropriate description include the interplay between several major risk factors for coronary heart disease, as shown in the Framingham Study and other major prospective studies [4,5], and the interactions between factors relating to several cancers, such as smoking and asbestos exposure in relation to lung cancer [6].

There are also examples where this model does not seem to be appropriate. One relatively simple alternative, also described in Chapter 4, is an *additive* model in which the risk of disease in subjects exposed to more than one factor is the sum of the excess risks conferred by each of the factors. With an additive model, the absolute excess risk associated with one factor will be constant in different categories of other factors. This means that the relative risk or odds ratio must vary. For example, in Box 8.5 the odds ratio varies with age. However, the baseline risk of *in situ* carcinoma of the cervix increases with age; therefore it is possible that the decrease in odds ratio with increase in age may reflect a relatively constant attributable risk associated with smoking in different age groups. We cannot directly test this hypothesis from this case–control study alone, although it could be assessed by using information on the absolute risk in different age categories relevant to the same population.

The appropriateness of these different models, and their relevance in both public health and biological terms, has been much discussed. The additive model corresponds to biological independence [1]. With two biologically independent causal factors, the amount of disease (and the absolute increase in disease risk) each causes is not influenced by the action of the other: so there will be additivity of effects on an absolute scale, shown by incidence rates, risk difference, or excess relative risk (relative risk − 1). Biological interaction means that the effect of one factor is modified by the presence of the other factor; for example, the effect of exposure to a virus may be modified by whether the person has been vaccinated, and the effects of sun exposure are modified by skin colour. Evidence that the data support one model better than others will usually require that the risk factors have large effects and the subjects cover a wide range of categories of the joint distribution of the factors involved.

Ordered exposure variables and tests of trend

Often the outcome variable has only two categories, while the exposure or interven-tion variable may have a number of ordered categories. For example, the incidence of lung cancer, a yes/no outcome variable, may be compared in a number of groups of individuals categorized by different levels of smoking; or the survival of a group of patients, a yes/no outcome variable, may be described in terms of a graded measure of the severity of the disease.

To compute relative risks or odds ratios with several exposure categories, an arbitrary category is chosen as the *reference* (or referent) category. This is usually the unexposed or minimally exposed category, although another choice may be made if, for example, that category has very few subjects. The relative risks for each of the other categories of exposure are then calculated by comparing each category with this reference group. If the categories of exposure are logically ordered, there may be a dose–response effect, with increasing (or decreasing) relative risks with increasing levels of exposure. A test for a linear dose–response effect was developed by Mantel [7] as an extension of the Mantel–Haenszel test, which in essence comprises a regression test of the odds ratio against a variable representing the ordered categories of exposure (Table A2.7). Where the exposure categories are defined numerically, such as different amounts of smoking, the categories may be represented by their midpoints, or some variation of it such as its logarithm; otherwise arbitrary values such as 0, 1, 2, etc. can represent ordered catego-ries, such as stage of disease. This test yields a chi-squared statistic on 1 d.f. which tests a linear trend in odds ratio over the ordered categories of the exposure variable, and also a chi-squared statistic on $k - 2$ d.f., where k is the number of exposure categories, which tests the deviation of the data from the linear trend. The sum of these two statis-tics will yield approximately the standard chi-squared statistic for homogeneity, which has $k - 1$ d.f. The linear trend statistic can be significant even if the overall chi-squared statistic is not.

Example

Data from a case–control study assessing risk factors for twin births [8] are shown in Box 8.6. The data show the numbers of cases (twin births) and controls (single births) by maternal parity, in four groups. An ordinary or global chi-squared statistic can be calculated for this 2×4 table; it has 3 d.f. and tests the hypothesis of homogeneity, that is, that the ratio of cases to controls and therefore the odds ratio is the same in each category. The result is $\chi^2 = 91.2$, $P < 0.001$ (Table A2.15 and Table A2.16). This statistic would be the same if the same data were in a different order, for example, if the odds ratios with increasing parity were 1.0, 1.84, 1.36, and 1.17, although such an irregular pattern would make a direct effect of parity less plausible. It is more informative to apply a linear trend test. Using the formula given in Table A2.7, with scores of 0, 1, 2, and 3 for parity, the trend test yields $\chi^2 = 88.0$, d.f. = 1, $P < 0.0001$. The deviation from the linear trend is given by the difference between these, giving $\chi^2 = 3.2$, d.f. = 2, $P = 0.2$; this is non-significant. The interpretation is that there is a positive association between the frequency of twin births and greater parity of the mother, which is consistent with a linear trend.

Box 8.6 Application of a test for trend to an ordered variable. Formulae given in Table A2.7

TEST FOR TREND IN AN ORDERED VARIABLE

	Degree of exposure (parity of mother)			
	0	**1**	**2**	**3+**
Cases (twins)	716	582	454	720
Controls (singletons)	1833	1269	853	1003
Odds ratio	1.0 (R)	1.17	1.36	1.84

Global χ^2 statistic, test for homogeneity $\quad = 91.2$ d.f. $= 3$ P < 0.001

Trend χ^2 statistic, test for linear trend $\quad = 88.0$ d.f. $= 1$ P < 0.001

Residual χ^2 statistic, test for deviations from trend $= 3.2$ d.f. $= 2$ P $= 0.2$

Thus the data are consistent with a linear increase in twinning by parity.

However, this analysis takes no account of confounding.

Source: data from Elwood JM. Maternal and environmental factors affecting twin births in Canadian cities. *Br J Obstet Gynaecol* 1978; **85**:351–358.

The basic data should always be examined. Particularly where there are only a few categories of the exposure variable, a trend can be fitted and may be significant even if inspection of the data shows no regular pattern. The tests are appropriate mainly where there is an a priori hypothesis of an approximately linear relationship between odds ratio or relative risk and the ordered exposure variable. In such circumstances, the test can be more powerful than the standard chi-squared test for homogeneity in an $n \times 2$ table.

The Mantel trend test can deal with stratified data; the Mantel–Haenszel adjusted odds ratios for each category are calculated after stratification, and the test then assesses a linear trend in these adjusted odds ratios. For example, the analysis in Box 8.6 was repeated after stratification for maternal age.

Statistical tests with individual matching

As shown in Chapter 7, in a case–control study, controls can be chosen to be matched to the cases on certain confounding factors, and this technique will control matching if and only if the appropriate matched analysis is used, based on the matched sets of cases and controls. For matched case–control data with one control per case, the resultant analysis is simple, and the appropriate statistical test is McNemar's chi-squared test [9], shown in Box 8.7. This test is a special application of the Mantel–Haenszel test for subtables each representing one matched pair. Note that for the

---

Box 8.7 Statistical test for 1:1 matched case–control studies: note that both the odds ratio and χ^2 depend only on the numbers of discordant pairs

---

MATCHED PAIR ANALYSIS

		Controls	
		Outcome positive	**Outcome negative**
Cases	Outcome positive	31	30 s
	Outcome negative	7 t	52

Odds ratio = s/t = 30/7 = 4.3

χ^2 on 1 d.f. = $\dfrac{(s-t)^2}{s+t} = \dfrac{23^2}{37} = 14.3$ $P < 0.001$

Continuity corrected $\chi^2 = \dfrac{(|s-t|-1)^2}{s+t} = 13.1$ $P < 0.001$

Source: data from Elwood JM, 'Wood exposure and smoking: association with cancer of the nasal cavity and paranasal sinuses in British Columbia,' *Canadian Medical Association Journal*, Volume 124, Issue 12, pp. 1573–1577, © 1981 [27].

---

calculation of both the odds ratio and the statistic, the only contributors are the pairs which are disparate in exposure, that is, the case was exposed but the control was not, or vice versa; on the null hypothesis the numbers of each of these will be the same. For a matched case–control study with a fixed ratio other than one to one, such as two or three controls per case, formulae for the odds ratio estimates and statistical tests are given in Table A2.6.

For matched cohort studies, the measures of association (relative and attributable risk) are calculated in the same way as for an unmatched cohort study. For statistical tests, keeping the matched sets together by stratification or conditional multivariate analysis may increase power and give narrower confidence limits.

Statistical tests in multivariate analysis

The multiple logistic model was described in Chapter 7. In this model, each dependent variable represents an exposure factor. For variables with only two categories, the odds ratio is given by the exponential of the coefficient for that variable. There are two main ways in which statistical tests are applied. First, the computer output will give the each coefficient and its standard error. The coefficient divided by its standard error gives a Z-statistic, or standardized normal deviate, which can be converted to a P-value (see Table A2.15 and Table A2.16). Second, the 'goodness of fit' of an entire model to the data set can be assessed, comparing models by calculating a statistic representing the difference in the log likelihood produced by adding or deleting variables. The log likelihood statistic, or deviance, indicates the deviation of the fitted model from the data, and the better the model fits the data, the smaller it is. If an exposure variable is added to the model, and that exposure is related to the outcome variable, the value of the log likelihood statistic will decrease. The change in log likelihood gives a chi-squared statistic with K degrees of freedom if K variables have been added or subtracted in that change. This method can assess not only if one extra variable is significant, but if a set of variables, representing a number of factors or different categories of a factor, has a significant effect on the fit of the model.

The statistical aspects of the multivariate analysis that was previously presented in Chapter 7 (Box 7.5) are shown in Table 8.3. In this case–control study involving 83 cases and 83 controls [10], the overall model with no independent variables fitted has $n - 1 = 165$ d.f. and a deviance of 230.1. The results of fitting variables singly into the model are equivalent to those from cross-tabulations, shown in Table 7.17. Fitting the two binary variables that together represent the number of moles gives a change in deviance of 38.1 on 2 d.f.; $P < 0.001$. Similarly, for sunburn, coded as one binary variable, the chi-squared statistic is 13.0 on 1 d.f., $P < 0.001$. Therefore both factors show significant associations in single-factor analyses. These chi-squared statistics are the same as those obtained from cross-tabulations (with no continuity correction). The exponential of the coefficient from the model where only one factor is fitted gives the crude odds ratio associated with that variable. Computer programmes give standard errors, which are used to calculate confidence limits.

In this analysis, there were three other relevant factors (number of freckles in three categories, hair colour in three categories, and usual skin reaction to sun exposure in four categories). Therefore the full model fitted had 10 variables representing the number of moles, sunburn history, and the three other factors, and this full model had a deviance of 157.7 with $n - 10 - 1 = 155$ d.f. This full model gives coefficients whose exponentials give the odds ratio of each variable, adjusted for the confounding effects of all the other variables in the model. The overall effect of a factor represented by a number of variables is best judged by comparing the deviance of the full model, with all factors fitted, to that of the model with the variables representing that one factor removed. This change in deviance shows the effect of that factor given that all the other factors are included. Thus, as shown in Table 8.3, the factor of 'number of moles' (two variables) is highly significant in the presence of all other factors, as removing it from the full model gives a significant increase in the deviance. However, if the sunburn is removed from the full model, the increase in deviance is not statistically significant. The interpretation is that the effect of number of moles on melanoma risk is reduced slightly by control for confounding by the other variables included in this analysis, but remains as a strong and statistically significant association, while the association seen with sunburn history in crude data is greatly reduced by controlling for confounding by the other variables, and is no longer statistically significant.

Multivariate analysis for *individually matched studies* uses 'conditional' models which take account of the matching, that is, they consider the cases and controls as matched sets. The results are presented in the same way as has been shown, with the same interpretation of the coefficients. A conditional logistic regression can deal with the matching, and also include other confounders.

Table 8.3 Multivariate analysis: the analysis previously shown in Box 7.5 (p. 179) fitting a multiple logistic model to data from a case–control study of 83 patients with melanoma and 83 controls. Coeff, fitted coefficient; Std error, standard error of coefficient; OR, odds ratio = exponential (coefficient); 95 per cent limits given from exp (coeff ± 1.96 × std error); deviance, log likelihood statistic.

Coefficients and standard errors

Factor	Model with only one factor				Model with 10 variables representing 5 factors			
No. of moles (reference = 0)	Coeff	Std error	OR	95% limits	Coeff	Std error	OR	95% limits
1–2	0.6008	0.4107	1.82	0.82–4.08	0.3011	0.4697	1.35	0.54–3.39
3 +	2.830	0.5705	16.95	5.54–51.84	2.5870	0.6095	13.29	4.02–43.89
Sunburn history (reference = none)								
Yes	1.150	0.3246	3.16	1.67–5.97	0.4276	0.4207	1.53	0.67–3.50

Deviance statistics

Model	Deviance	d.f.	Change in deviance	d.f.
No variables	230.1	165	–	–
Moles only	192.1	163	38.1	2 P < 0.001
Sunburn only	217.1	164	13.0	1 P < 0.001
Full model	157.7	155	–	–
Full model less moles	183.4	157	25.7	2 P < 0.001
Full model less sunburn	158.9	156	1.2	1 P < 0.25

Source: Elwood JM et al., 'Malignant melanoma in relation to moles, pigmentation, and exposure to fluorescent and other lighting sources,' *British Journal of Cancer*, Volume 53, Issue 1, pp. 65–74, © 1986 [37].

Interpretation of statistical results

To interpret any study, we must first assess whether the results reported are free from problems of observation bias and confounding. The statistical significance of the result is in itself no protection against these problems. Indeed, an easy way to produce highly significant results is to use a design which is open to severe observation bias; for example, biased recall between cases and controls in a retrospective study, or an intervention study using a subjective outcome measure made by someone involved in the intervention being assessed. When these issues have been dealt with, the next step is to know whether the statistical methods used are appropriate and correctly applied.

Multiple testing and the Bonferroni correction

Multiple testing is a difficult problem in interpretation. Tests such as those previously described are designed for hypothesis testing, to be applied to one particular result from a study designed to test that association. Where a study produces a large number of associations, such as a study of patient prognosis which assesses 20 factors and uses conventional 5 per cent significance level tests, we expect at least one of these factors to appear as 'statistically significant' if a $P = 0.05$ criterion is used even if none of them in truth is related to the outcome. In some observational studies and in explorations of large data sets, very large numbers of factors can be assessed. For example, studies using death registrations and census data could involve comparisons of perhaps 100 categories of causes of death with several hundred possible occupations. Genetic and proteonomic studies may assess large numbers of subjects, or apply very large banks of biomarkers, and so produce many associations by chance alone. Special statistical methods, some of which are quite complex, have been developed for these situations. In intervention trials, repeated testing may be planned, as discussed later.

If we use one statistical test, with a $P = 0.05$ cut off (referred to as the α level), we are accepting that on 5 per cent of occasions where the null hypothesis is true, we will get a false-positive result. If we use two tests, on independent outcomes, the false-positive rate rises to 10 per cent. So one suggestion is to change the level to α/n, where we are doing n tests, thus bringing the overall false-positive risk back to 5 per cent. So with four tests, we would set $P = 0.008$ (0.05/4) as the significance level for each test: this is the *Bonferroni correction*. However, with large numbers of tests this seems to set the level very high, so the chance of false-negative results (not detecting true associations) will be too high. Also, the correction assumes the tests done are all independent. There is a more basic objection in that it suggests we cannot interpret any test unless we know how many other tests have been applied. Sometimes simply a higher level such as $P = 0.01$ is used. The simplest solution may be to report the tests in the usual way, but also report how many comparisons have been made. (Carlo Bonferroni was an Italian mathematician and economist, 1892–1960, but the test was developed mainly by Olive Jean Dunn, a prominent American statistician [11].)

Example

In a study comparing 301 patients with non-Hodgkin lymphoma to 301 controls, levels of 67 immune and inflammation markers in blood collected 5 years earlier were tested [12]; where all 67 were assessed, a Bonferroni correction α level of 0.00075 was used (0.05/67). Two markers were significant using this criterion, suggesting they may predict the disease ahead of diagnosis.

Hypothesis testing and hypothesis generation

It is valuable to distinguish between results from hypothesis testing studies that have been specifically set up to test a particular hypothesis, and those from studies in which a large number of associations have been examined and data analysis leads to new findings. The latter studies are best considered as hypothesis generating. They raise a new question that should be tested, and then can be confirmed or refuted. Thus in the study just noted [12], the authors distinguish between results that are robust and supported by other evidence, and new results that need testing in further studies. A further issue in the interpretation of positive results is publication bias, which is discussed in Chapter 9.

Appropriate and inappropriate subgroup analyses

In good clinical trials and observational studies, the studies will be designed with adequate statistical power to test the main comparisons specified in the protocol. However, many other differences may be explored, for example, in subgroups. Table 8.4 shows some results of an important randomized trial which assessed both streptokinase and aspirin in reducing the death rate in patients who had a suspected acute myocardial infarction [13]. Some of the results for aspirin are shown. In the whole trial, over 8500 patients were randomized to receive aspirin starting as soon as possible after the onset of symptoms, and a similar number were randomized to placebo. The overall result shows a benefit, a reduced death rate, in the aspirin group with an odds ratio of 0.77 and 95 per cent confidence limits of 0.70–0.85. These confidence limits are calculated by the methods shown in Table A2.2, and are identical to those reported in the paper. This 23 per cent reduction in deaths is obviously clinically important, and is statistically significant. With these data, relative risks could equally easily be used.

Some subgroup analyses were planned in the protocol to the study, but many others were carried out, comparing groups subdivided by sex, age groups, different levels of blood pressure and heart rate, with or without cardiograph abnormalities, and so on. One result was that no beneficial effect of aspirin was seen in patients who had had a previous myocardial infarction (odds ratio 1.02), and the effect was correspondingly greater in those who had not had a previous infarction (odds ratio 0.71). A statistical test of heterogeneity shows that the difference in effects is highly significant ($P = 0.002$). This is important, as it suggests that aspirin is useful only for patients who have no previous history of myocardial infarction. However, this subgroup analysis was unplanned and was the only one of 26 subgroup analyses to show a statistically significant variation. Thus, despite its statistical significance, this is likely to be a chance finding, and in their discussion the investigators suggest it is implausible, given other knowledge of the effects of aspirin on heart disease. To demonstrate the dangers of unplanned subgroup analyses, the investigators also published the results from a subdivision of patients by astrological birth sign. As shown in Table 8.4, this showed that patients with Gemini or Libra birth signs showed no benefit of aspirin (odds ratio 1.09), and the benefit was confined to those with other birth signs (odds ratio 0.72). This difference is also statistically significant with a similar P-value for heterogeneity as was found in the other subdivision ($P = 0.002$).

Therefore, to be reliable, a subgroup analysis should be defined in advance, before the data are examined, giving a specific hypothesis that can be tested. The subgroup analysis by birth sign is not only one of many analyses that could be done, but also the

Table 8.4 Dangers of subgroup analysis: data from a large randomized trial of aspirin in treatment of a suspected acute myocardial infarction, showing total results, and a subgroup analysis by prior myocardial infarction, one of 26 subgroup analyses done. Also shown is an analysis of astrological birth sign.

		Aspirin			Placebo			Odds ratio	95% confidence limits		MH odds ratio	Heterogeneity test	
		Deaths	Total number	Death rate%	Deaths	Total number	Death rate%					Chi sq	P value
All patients		804	8587	9.36	1016	8600	11.81	0.77	0.70	0.85			
Prior myocardial infarct	Yes	219	1454	15.08	219	1484	14.76	1.02	0.84	1.25			
	No	576	7038	8.18	778	7005	11.11	0.71	0.64	0.80	0.78	9.30	0.0023
Astrological birth sign	Gemini / Libra	150	1357	11.05	147	1442	10.19	1.09	0.86	1.39			
	Other	654	7228	9.05	868	7157	12.13	0.72	0.65	0.80	0.77	9.67	0.0019

Source: data from 'Randomised trial of intravenous streptokinase, oral aspirin, both, or neither among 17,187 cases of suspected acute myocardial infarction: ISIS-2. ISIS-2 (Second International Study of Infarct Survival) Collaborative Group,' *The Lancet*, Volume 332, Issue 8607, pp. 349–360, © 1998 Published by Elsevier Ltd [13].

grouping of the birth signs was only one of many ways, and the choice was influenced by the data. Such analyses have been referred to as post hoc, after the fact, data-driven, or the result of data dredging or fishing.

Repeated testing in trials: stopping rules and data-monitoring groups

In intervention trials, it is useful to monitor the results at regular intervals or continuously, so that the trial can be stopped as soon as a definitive result is obtained, or when it is clear that no significant difference will be seen [14]. This involves multiple testing. As the investigators themselves should not know the ongoing results of the trial, most major trials have an independent data monitoring committee, which will assess interim results and decide if the trial should be continued or stopped earlier than anticipated. This is only one of their functions; they can also assess data quality, monitor recruitment, loss to follow-up, compliance, evidence of adverse effects, and other issues [15]. They may also take account of other relevant research and link with other ongoing trials [16]. The statistical methods used take into account the fact that the data are being examined on many occasions, and can be quite complex; a major review includes an appendix on statistical methods [17].

Examples

Several examples have already been noted. During the randomized trial of clofibrate in the treatment of heart disease [18], referred to in Chapter 7 (Figure 7.8), on three occasions during the monitoring of the trial the death rate was significantly lower in the treatment than in the placebo group, if tested using a 5 per cent cut-off. However, the difference was not significant when assessed by methods appropriate for repeated monitoring, and so the trial was continued; the final results showed no significant difference between the clofibrate and comparison groups. In the randomized trial of prevention of neural tube defects noted in Chapter 3 [19], the results passed the level of significance demanded by a sequential test (used to continuously monitor results) when only about two-thirds of the original planned number of participants had been enrolled, and the trial was terminated early as a clear benefit had been shown. In a large randomized trial to assess the anticipated preventive effects of beta-carotene and retinol (vitamin A) involving 18 000 subjects in the United States who were smokers, ex-smokers, or had worked with asbestos, interim results showed a 28 per cent increase in lung cancer incidence and a 17 per cent increase in total mortality [20]. The trial was terminated 21 months early, and the use of beta-carotene supplementation as one part of a further trial involving female health professionals in the USA was also stopped.

Interpreting non-significant results

The interpretation of the results that are reported as not showing statistical significance also raises several issues. The issues of observation bias and confounding must be considered first, assessing whether there are problems that could make the observed result smaller than the true result; these include non-differential misclassification. Again, we must assess if the statistical methods used are appropriate and correctly applied, although multiple testing is not important here. The main issue is the risk of a false-negative result; a *type 2*, or *beta*, error is made if the result is non-significant when there is a true difference.

Confidence limits are much more useful than the *P*-value, as these show the range of values of the association with which the results are compatible. Where limits are not shown in the original material, approximate limits can be calculated from the relative risk or odds ratio if a *P*-value is given, by converting the *P*-value to a normal deviate *Z* (see Table A2.15 and Table A2.16), and using the following relationship:

$$\ln RR \,/\, SE \ln RR = Z, \text{and so } SE \ln RR = \ln RR \,/\, Z.$$

For example, using the data in Table 8.2 for study B, $\ln RR = 0.693$; $P = 0.14$, so $Z = 1.48$; and $SE \ln RR = (\ln 2.0/1.48) = 0.468$. So for the relative risk of 2.0, approximate 95 per cent limits are 0.80–5.0. The more precise calculation gives 0.76–5.27, as shown earlier.

If the non-significant result is based upon a small study, the confidence limits will be wide, making it clear that we cannot conclude that there is no appreciable difference between the groups being compared.

Statistical power and the size of a study

Go back to Table 8.2 and look again at study B. This result is rather unsatisfactory. There is a higher success rate in the intervention group, but as this is not statistically significant and the confidence limits are wide, we cannot confidently decide whether the intervention is beneficial or not. The basic problem is that the study is too small. It does not provide a definite answer. In technical terms, the study lacks *power*. To avoid doing studies like study B, we should predict the power in advance, and modify the design to give the study adequate power. We will review some fairly simple aspects of this; but readers who wish to avoid these may go on to the section that follows, on consulting with a statistician.

Factors affecting the power of a study

Several factors affect the power of a study (Table 8.5). The first is the *strength of the association*, for example, the difference in outcome rates between the two groups, or the relative risk or odds ratio. The larger the true difference, the easier it will be to detect.

The second is the *frequency of the outcome*. The effective size of a cohort or intervention study is not the total number of subjects in the study, but depends mainly on the number of subjects who experience the outcome events. Similarly, the effective size of a case–control study depends mainly on the number of cases and controls who have the exposure under consideration. Study B in Table 8.2 has 72 subjects, but only 15 have the outcome event. If this number were increased by doing the study on patients with a higher frequency of success, or by extending the follow-up time, the study would have more power even though the same number of patients were entered initially. The maximum power for a fixed total number of subjects and a particular relative risk will be when about half the subjects have the outcome, or in a case–control design where half have the exposure under consideration.

Table 8.5 Factors influencing the necessary size of a comparative study.

Strength of the association	Size decreases as the difference in frequency of outcome or exposure increases; size depends approximately on the square of the difference
Frequency of the outcome (cohort and intervention studies) or of the exposure (case–control studies)	Size minimum when frequency close to 50 per cent
Significance level	Size increases as significance level decreases, i.e. a more stringent test is used; higher for a two-sided than for a one-sided test
Power	Size increases as power increases
Confounding	Size increases if confounder control, by stratification or multivariate methods, is required; may decrease in individually matched study
Error	Size increases if non-differential misclassification of either exposure or outcome

The next factors to be considered are the significance level and the power. The *significance level* is the cut-off point at which the association found is regarded as statistically significant. It is most frequently at the $P = 0.05$ level, using a two-sided test. The significance level, or alpha (α), is the frequency of a false-positive result, where a 'significant' result occurs when in truth there is no difference. This type of error is called an *alpha, α,* or *type 1* error. In setting the significance level, we are saying what we will accept as the risk of a false-positive result. In some circumstances the direction of the effect may be regarded as fixed and tests used which assess only effects in one direction, and a *one-sided test* may be used. If we are to apply a 5 per cent one-sided test rather than a 5 per cent two-sided test, fewer subjects will be required.

The *power* of a study is its ability to demonstrate an association, given that the association exists. The frequency with which we will see no significant difference, if in truth there is a difference (a false-negative result), is the *beta, β,* or *type 2,* error. A more powerful study is one that is less likely to miss a true effect; the power of the study is $1 - \beta$. If a true association is present, our ability to recognize it will be greater with a larger sample, a stronger association, and a higher frequency of outcome. A typical value of power is 80 per cent; the study is designed so that the chance of detecting a true difference is 80 per cent, and we accept that we will miss the true difference in 20 per cent of instances. For an exploratory study we may decide that missing a true difference (i.e. obtaining a false-negative result) is unimportant, and we may be content with a lower power, requiring fewer subjects. If we need to be confident that we will not miss a true effect, we may need a power of 90 per cent or more, which will require many more subjects.

For both significance level (α) and power ($\beta = 1 -$ power), the corresponding normal deviates Z_α and Z_β, go into the formula, usually in a term $(Z_\alpha + Z_\beta)^2$, which we call K for convenience. The deviates for commonly used values of α and β, and the corresponding values of K, are given in Box 8.8.

Other considerations

These four factors are the components of the formulae generally used for sample size determination. Other factors also affect the necessary size. If confounder control by stratification or multivariate methods is to be used, the study size required is increased. An individually matched study, where the analysis will use the matched sets, may need a smaller sample size for the same power. Non-differential misclassification, as described in Chapter 6, will lead to a larger sample size being needed. This effect can be assessed by calculating the observable odds ratio or risk difference after allowing for misclassification, as shown in Chapter 6, and using it for the determination of the size of the study needed. Methods of determining study size with allowance for these

---

Box 8.8 Normal deviates corresponding to frequently used values for significance levels (Z_α) and power (Z_β); and table of K where $K = (Z_\alpha + Z_\beta)^2$. The value of Z_β is the normal deviate corresponding to the one-sided test for (1 – power)

CONSTANTS FOR USE IN SAMPLE SIZE FORMULAE

(A) Table relating normal deviates to power and to significance level

Power (1–β) (%)	Z-value (Normal deviate)	Significance level (α) One-sided	Significance level (α) Two-sided
99.5	2.58	0.005	0.01
99	2.33	0.01	0.02
98	1.96	0.025	0.05
95	1.64	0.05	0.1
90	1.28	0.1	0.2
80	0.84	0.2	0.4
70	0.52	0.3	0.6
50	0.0	0.5	

(B) Values of $K = (Z_\alpha + Z_\beta)^2$, for commonly used values of α and β

Significance level		Power 50%	80%	90%	95%	Significance level	
Two-sided value	0.1	2.7	6.2	8.6	10.8	0.05	One-sided value
	0.05	3.8	7.9	10.5	13.0	0.025	
	0.02	5.4	10.0	13.0	15.8	0.01	
	0.01	6.6	11.7	14.9	17.8	0.005	

various factors are available, which is why the formulae given here should be used only as a guide, and expert advice should be sought for any major study. Perhaps most important, the study size given in the formulae refers to the number of study participants in each group being compared who complete the study and provide full data for analysis. In designing a study, allowance has to be made for non-response and possible incompleteness of data.

Design options

The power of a study is increased by increasing the number of subjects in the study, in the intervention or case group, or in the comparison group, or in both. When a similar effort and cost is needed to add a test or a comparison subject, studies with equal numbers in each group are optimal. As the power depends on the number of subjects with the outcome in a cohort study, or the number with the exposure in a case–control study, modifications of the ratio may be used so that the number of outcome events or exposed subjects in each group is likely to be similar. For example, more than half the patients in a trial may be allocated to the new therapy, on the basis of the anticipated benefit yielding equal numbers of deaths in each group. It may be easier to increase the size of the comparison group than of the intervention or case group because more potential subjects are available, data on them has already been collected, or the number of exposed subjects or cases is fixed. The power of the study is increased by increasing the number of controls, but this is less effective than increasing both groups.

Estimating the size of study which is needed

From the four parameters of the expected frequency of the outcome in the control group, the difference in outcome rates, the significance level, and the power, a calculation of the sample size to satisfy those criteria can be made. Some appropriate formulae are illustrated in Box 8.9. The formulae can obviously be used in other ways. It is often useful to calculate the power of the study from the sample size readily available, to show if a proposed investigation is worthwhile or if more ambitious methods need to be used. The following examples will show the application of these formulae.

1. *For a clinical trial.* Suppose that the success rate over 1 year from conventional therapy is 20 per cent, and a new therapy would be useful if the rate increased to 30 per cent. How many patients do we need? Setting a significance level of 0.05 two-sided, and a power of 80 per cent, yields $K = 7.9$ and $n = 292$, that is, 292 subjects in each group. If we were content to detect a larger difference, such as 40 per cent success with the new therapy, then $n = 79$; note the large change in n for a substantial change in $(p_1 - p_2)$.

2. *For an epidemiological cohort study.* We wish to test whether the breast cancer rate is increased in users of a specific drug, and estimate a 10-year cumulative incidence in unexposed women as 0.01 (1 per cent). We set significance at 0.05 two-sided and power at 90 per cent, and wish to be able to detect a doubling of risk to 0.02; hence $K = 10.5$ and $n = 3098$.

3. *Feasibility.* A colleague hopes that a new therapy will increase the proportion of patients recovering from her current 40 per cent to 60 per cent, and is sure the new therapy will not be worse. She sees 100 patients each year who could enter a trial. Is it worth it? Set significance at 0.05 one-sided. Hence $Z_\alpha = 1.64$; $p_1 = 0.4$, $p_2 = 0.6$, $n = 50$; therefore $Z_\beta = 2.04 - 1.64 = 0.40$. From Box 8.9, the power is less

---

Box 8.9 Formulae for calculating the size of a study: for the meaning and values of Z_α, Z_β and K, see Box 8.8. A formula for 1:1 matched studies is given in Table A2.8

Formulae for sample size estimation

For cohort or trial design, with equal groups

$$n = \frac{(p_1 q_1 + p_2 q_2) \cdot K}{(p_1 - p_2)}$$

n = number of subjects in each group

where p_1 = frequency of outcome in group 1 $q_1 = 1 - p_1$
        p_2 = frequency of outcome in group 2 $q_2 = 1 - p_2$

$K = (Z_\alpha + Z_\beta)^2$ where Z_α and Z_β are normal deviates corresponding to significance level α and power $(1 - \beta)$.

     To calculate power

$$Z_\beta = \frac{(p_1 - p_2) \cdot \sqrt{n}}{\sqrt{(p_1 q_1 + p_2 q_2)}} - Z_\alpha$$

For case–control study
Same formulae, where
     p_1 = frequency of exposure in cases
     p_2 = frequency of exposure in controls
        Use of odds ratio

        Given the proportion of controls exposed, p_2, and the odds ratio predicted, *OR*, the proportion of cases exposed, p_1 is given by:

$$p_1 = \frac{p_2 \cdot OR}{1 + p_2(OR - 1)}$$

Unequal groups
If there are c comparison subjects for each exposed subject or case

$$n = \frac{(1 + 1/c) \cdot \overline{pq} \cdot K}{(p_1 - p_2)^2} \quad \text{where } \overline{p} = \left(\frac{p_1 + p_2}{2}\right) \text{ and } \overline{q} = 1 - \overline{p}$$

$$Z_\beta = \frac{(p_1 - p_2) \cdot \sqrt{n}}{\sqrt{((1 + 1/c)\overline{pq})}} - Z_\alpha$$

where n = number of exposed subjects or cases

than 70 per cent. For more accuracy, use Excel to give the one-sided probability of this value of 0.40 in the normal distribution (Table A2.16). This yields 0.35, that is, a power of $1 - 0.35$ or 65 per cent. Her study would miss a difference of the size given on one occasion out of three, and is too weak. For adequate power (e.g. 80 per cent), she would need 74 patients in each group; for 90 per cent, 103 patients. Thus a 2-year accrual period, or collaboration with colleagues, would be advisable to have adequate numbers.

4. *In a case–control study*, we wish to be able to detect a doubling of risk (odds ratio = 2) associated with a factor which is present in 10 per cent of the normal population from which the control series will be drawn. Hence $p_2 = 0.1$ and p_1 is given by Box 8.9 as 0.182; if power = 80 per cent, and significance level = 0.05 two-sided, $K = 7.9$ and $n = 280$. We need approximately 280 cases and 280 controls. If controls are easily found, we could have, say, three controls per case. Keeping the other parameters the same, $p = 0.14$, $q = 0.86$, and $n = 190$; a study design with 200 cases and 600 controls would give similar power to one with 300 cases and 300 controls.

Use of sample size calculations

The formulae given here are fairly simple. This is a large topic, and more complex sample size calculations are available in standard texts [21–23]. In practice, many quantities are unknown when a study is being designed; not only the likely difference between the outcomes, but the extent of loss of information by drop-outs or missing data and the extent to which stratification or other techniques will have to be used which will reduce the power of the study. The main usefulness of these sample size formulae is to indicate the *minimum* number of subjects necessary, or conversely the approximate power that is achievable with the numbers available. Such calculations may show many more subjects are needed, and the study as envisaged may not be worthwhile, or a different approach is needed, such as moving from to a multi-centre study, or testing the question on a different set of subjects or in a different way. These calculations take only statistical sampling variation into account. There is no allowance for incomplete records, drop-outs, or errors in ascertainment, and no allowance for the requirements of more detailed analysis to adjust for confounding or assess results in subgroups.

It is often helpful to compare the power produced by studies with different numbers of subjects, and to calculate a 'power curve', that is, a graph showing the relationship between sample size and power within the other constraints of the study. This will help to choose the most efficient design, which is the one that gives the most information for least cost in subjects, time, and finances.

The major properties of the formulae are useful guides (Box 8.9). The number of patients required is inversely proportional to the square of the difference in outcome rates; in other words, if the difference to be detected is halved, the number of subjects required will be four times as large. The biological effect of a factor will be expected to give a certain ratio of outcome events; the difference in numbers corresponding to a fixed ratio will be greater if the frequency of the outcome is higher, up to 50 per cent. Given that a new intervention reduces mortality by a third, it is easier to detect a difference between 45 and 30 per cent mortality than between 15 and 10 per cent; often a study design can be made more efficient by selecting subjects who have a high risk of the outcome under investigation. There is little room to manoeuvre in terms of significance levels, and one-sided significance levels should not be used unless these are clearly justified. A study with 80 per cent power requires about twice as many subjects as one with 50 per cent power, and a very powerful study with 95 per cent power requires about 60 per cent more subjects than one of 80 per cent power.

As mentioned, studies with more controls than cases can be used. Box 8.9 shows that the power of a study with n subjects in each group is equalled by one with c controls per test subject, and $n[1 + (1/c)]/2$ test subjects; therefore an alternative to finding 100 cases and 100 controls is to use, say, two controls per case and find 75 cases and 150 controls. Unless data for controls are very easy to obtain, for example, by being available on a computer file, it is rarely worth using ratios greater than 5:1.

Ensuring a proposed study will have sufficient statistical power to give an adequately precise result is an ethical as well as a scientific requirement. Reports of completed studies should describe the initial planned study size and its rationale, particularly if the final study includes fewer or more subjects.

Consulting with a statistician about study design

When designing a major study, statistical help should be sought in regard to sample size. The questions the statistician will ask amount in principle to a prediction of the results of the study. In cohort studies and trials, we need to predict the frequency of the outcome in the control group and the size of the difference between control and exposed groups which we regard as worth detecting. It is worth thinking in operational terms; what improvement in results would be needed to make the new therapy worthwhile, or what increased risk for an environmental exposure would be reasonable to detect? For a case–control design, we need the likely frequency of exposure in the comparison group, which may be obtained from literature or a pilot study, and the size of the association to be detected, best expressed as the odds ratio. The remaining questions are to define the significance level and the desired power of the study. There is rarely a good reason to stray from the convention of the 5 per cent level. The question of one-sided and two-sided tests has been alluded to. As to power, a frequently used starting point is 80 per cent in an exploratory study; in a study to reassess a finding or in other circumstances where it is important not to miss a true association, higher power is desirable.

Part 3. Time-to-event analysis: taking the timing of the outcome events into consideration

So far we have given the results of cohort and intervention studies as the numbers of subjects with and without the outcome ('count data'), or the numbers of subjects experiencing the outcome divided by the total person-years of observation ('person-time data'). These methods are valid if the risk of the outcome is constant over the time course of the study, or if the follow-up time is the same for the different groups of subjects being compared. If these do not apply, methods using data on when the outcome occurs are appropriate.

Time-to-event: survival curves

These methods have been widely used in assessing survival after diagnosis or treatment, and so are often referred to as *survival analyses*. However, the methods can be applied to any non-recurrent outcome event, such as death, recovery, onset of a complication, return to work, or discharge from hospital. The results can be expressed either as the proportion of subjects at different times who have *not* undergone the event, as is seen in a survival curve, or as a proportion of subjects who have undergone the event, which gives a cumulative incidence curve. Figure 8.1 shows a survival curve for a group of patients with breast cancer, showing the proportion of the original group who are still alive at various points from the date of diagnosis; at 3 years after diagnosis, 68 per cent of patients are still alive. The same data could be plotted to show the cumulative incidence of death; at 3 years, 32 per cent have died.

To construct such a curve, we need to know for each individual the *starting date* of the period of observation, the *finishing date* of this period, and the *outcome* for that individual. The starting date in a clinical study may be defined as the date of diagnosis, the date of first treatment, or in a randomized study the date of randomization. In an epidemiological cohort study the starting date may be the date of first exposure, such as working in a particular job or using a drug.

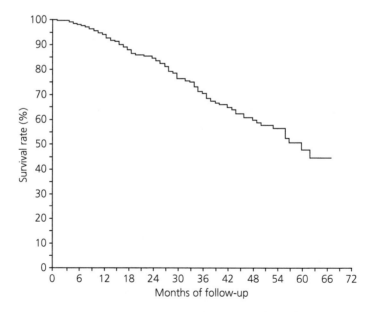

Figure 8.1 Survival of 596 patients with breast cancer from date of confirmed diagnosis, calculated by the product limit method. For this graph, only deaths from breast cancer were counted; the few other deaths were not, the observations being censored at that point.

In a simple example assessing survival in a group of patients, the survival curve is simply the proportion surviving at various points in time. The 'curve' has, in fact, a step-type pattern; if we start with 10 patients the survival rate is 100 per cent until one dies, then it remains at 90 per cent until another dies, and so on. In a larger study, each step will be smaller and the curve appears smoother. Usually we do not know all the dates of death, as some patients will still be alive at the time of analysis and others may have been lost to follow-up, so that their current status will be unknown. The observations on these patients are *censored*. Censoring also occurs if the particular end point under study is precluded by another event; for example, if we wish to count only deaths from a certain cause, other deaths produce censored observations. We shall describe two commonly used methods for constructing a survival curve: the product-limit method (also known as the Kaplan–Meier estimate) and the actuarial or life-table method.

Table 8.6 Hypothetical survival data arranged in order of increasing survival time for a clinical trial with 10 patients in each of two treatment groups. Note: Trials of this size are not recommended; this is for explanation only.

Patient no.	Survival time, (months)*	Treatment group
14	1	A
12	1	A
13	3 +	A
4	4	A
7	6	A
2	9 +	B
9	11 +	A
8	11 +	B
19	12	A
20	13	B
1	15	A
3	16	B
15	22	B
5	22 +	A
10	23	A
6	23	B
16	25 +	B
11	32 +	B
17	32 +	B
18	41	B

*+ indicates a censored observation

The product-limit method

The data in Table 8.6 shows survival times for 20 subjects (at this point ignore the treatment designation). The data show survival time in months, calculated from the date of diagnosis to the date of death, with the subjects arranged in order of increasing survival time. Eight subjects are still alive or have been lost to follow-up. For them, we use the survival time to the date of the last follow-up assessment, and indicate that their survival times are censored. The product-limit method is based on two simple concepts. First, subjects with censored observations are included in the total number of subjects at risk of death only up to the time of their censoring. Second, we use a simple application of probability logic in calculating that the chance of surviving 2 months equals the probability of surviving the first month multiplied by the probability of surviving the second, and so on with subsequent months.

The calculations are shown in Table 8.7. The survival curve changes only when a death occurs; hence a calculation is done only every time a death occurs. Two deaths occurred in the first month, so that the probability of surviving that month was 18/20 or 0.9, and the survival at 1 month (i.e. at the end of the first month) was 0.9. No deaths occurred during the second month and during the third month there was one censored observation but still no deaths, so that the cumulative survival by the end of the third month was $0.9 \times 1 \times 1 = 0.9$; no calculation is needed as no deaths have occurred. During the fourth month one death occurred; at that time there were 17 subjects still under follow-up so the probability of survival was 16/17 or 0.94, and the cumulative

Table 8.7 Calculation of product limit estimate of survival curve from data in Table 8.6. Formula for standard error given in text.

Interval i	Interval between deaths (months)	No. of deaths at end of interval d_i	No. of patients alive immediately prior to end of interval n_i	Probability of surviving interval $P_i = 1 - (d_i - n_i)$	Value of survival curve subsequent to interval $S_i = S_{i-1} \times P_i$	Standard error of survival curve
0	0	–	–	1.0000	1.0000	–
1	0–1	2	20	0.9000	0.9000	0.0671
2	1–4	1	17	0.9412	0.8471	0.0814
3	4–6	1	16	0.9375	0.7941	0.0919
4	6–12	1	12	0.9167	0.7279	0.1054
5	12–13	1	11	0.9091	0.6618	0.1147
6	13–15	1	10	0.9000	0.5956	0.1209
7	15–16	1	9	0.8889	0.5294	0.1242
8	16–22	1	8	0.8750	0.4632	0.1251
9	22–23	2	6	0.6667	0.3088	0.1221
10	23–41	1	1	0.0000	0.0000	

Figure 8.2 Survival curves for the data shown in Table 8.6. The step pattern is the product-limit survival curve calculated in Table 8.7. The dotted line is the actuarial curve calculated in Table 8.8.

survival at the end of the fourth month was 0.94 × 0.9 = 0.85. Therefore each relevant interval ends when one or more deaths occur. The resultant step-type curve is shown in Figure 8.2.

The estimation of survival by this method allows for censoring, and is efficient as in each section of the follow-up period the information available on all subjects observed during that interval is used. The product-limit method gives the survival curve that is the most likely estimate, in statistical terminology the 'maximum likelihood' estimate of the true survival curve.

Bias from loss to follow-up

The adjustment made for censored observations assumes that they are censored randomly, that is, we assume that the subjects whose data are censored at a certain time would have a subsequent course similar to that of the subjects remaining under follow-up. If this is not so, bias will result. For example, if those lost to follow-up do worse than those still being followed, perhaps because very ill subjects no longer attend for treatment, the calculated survival curve will overestimate the actual survival. If those lost to follow-up do better, perhaps as well patients do not return to the hospital, the opposite bias will occur.

Table 8.8 Calculation of actuarial estimate of survival curve from the data in Table 8.6 using 6-month intervals. This example is to show the method; the actuarial method is not advisable with such small numbers, but is useful with large sets of data.

Interval (months)	Patients alive at start r_i	Patients censored c_i	Patients 'at risk' $n_i = r_i - \frac{1}{2}c_i$	Deaths during interval d_i	Probability of surviving interval $P_i = 1-(d_i/n_i)$	Survival curve estimate $S_i = S_{i-1} \times P_i$
0–6	20	1	19.5	4	0.7949	0.7949
7–12	15	3	13.5	1	0.9259	0.7360
13–18	11	0	11.0	3	0.7273	0.5353
19–24	8	1	7.5	3	0.6000	0.3212
25–30	4	1	3.5	0	1.0	0.3212
30–36	3	2	2.0	0	1.0	0.3212
37–42	1	0	1.0	1	0.0	0.0

The actuarial or life-table method

The actuarial or life-table method is often used with large data sets, such as linked incidence and mortality data on populations. It gives an approximation to the product-limit estimate, with the number of calculations being reduced by grouping the data into suitable intervals of follow-up, such as 1 year or 3 months. Calculations for the data used in Table 8.6, with a 6-month interval, are shown in Table 8.8. For each time interval, we calculate the probability of surviving that interval, which is given as 1 minus the probability of dying during that time interval. The probability of dying is given by the number of deaths during the interval divided by the number of subjects under follow-up during that interval. This denominator is estimated as the number of subjects alive at the beginning of the interval minus half the number whose data are censored during the interval. We are making the assumption that if subjects are censored during an interval, their follow-up experience is approximately half that interval. The cumulative probability of survival is calculated, as with the product-limit method, as the product of the probability of survival over each of the intervals up to that point. The resultant survival curve is shown in Figure 8.2.

Presentation

Survival curves are usually shown with an arithmetic horizontal scale, and either an arithmetic or a logarithmic vertical scale. If the risk of death during each section of the follow-up period is the same, a survival curve with an arithmetic vertical scale will show an exponential decreasing curve, while one with a logarithmic scale will show a straight line. Product-limit estimates, being actual calculations of survival rate at every event, are best shown by stepped patterns, while actuarial estimates are an approximation and can be shown as a series of points connected by straight lines. The intervals chosen for actuarial calculation need not be of equal length and are often chosen on a convenient arbitrary basis, such as annual intervals; but they should be short enough to keep the number of censored observations in any interval relatively small.

Confidence limits

The standard error of the survival rate S_i at the end of a given interval is given by

$$SE = S_i\sqrt{\left(\sum_i \frac{1-P_i}{n_i P_i}\right)}$$

using the notation shown in Table 8.7. The summation Σ_i is over all the intervals up to and including the last interval i. This formula is applicable to both product-limit and actuarial calculations and, although approximate, is adequate for most purposes. In the usual way, the 95 per cent two-sided confidence limits are given as the estimate $S_i \pm 1.96 \times$ standard error.

Relative survival ratios and disease-specific survival rates

Analyses of survival for groups of patients are often reported in terms of the *relative survival ratio*. This is observed survival at a point in time divided by the survival expected in a group of similar subjects in the relevant general population. The expected values are derived from *life tables* based on all causes of death, routinely produced from vital statistics data. The life tables may be specified only by age, sex, and year or time period, or in addition may be subdivided by ethnic or racial group, geographical area, or socioeconomic level; the appropriate lifetable to use can be a major issue. This is a way of taking account of the proportion of deaths that will be due to causes other than the disease of interest.

For example, suppose that the survival at 5 years after diagnosis for a group of men in England diagnosed with prostate cancer at age 70 in 2005 is calculated by the product-limit method shown, and is 72 per cent, with 95 per cent confidence limits of 68–76 per cent. From lifetables for men aged 70 in England in 2005, the proportion still alive 5 years later is 83 per cent—that is the 'expected' survival. The relative survival ratio for the group is 0.72/0.83 (i.e. 87 per cent) with confidence limits of 82–92 per cent, obtained by dividing the upper and lower limits of the observed survival by the same factor of 0.83. Similarly, the overall 5-year survival for a group of women with breast cancer diagnosed at age 60 might be 79 per cent, and the expected survival of a group of women of this age is 96 per cent, giving a relative survival of 82 per cent. Although the total survival of the men with prostate cancer was lower than that of the women with breast cancer (72 per cent compared with 79 per cent), their relative survival was higher (87 per cent compared with 82 per cent) as a greater proportion of their total mortality was due to the expected mortality in a group of that age and sex. The relative survival is taken as an indicator of the disease-specific survival, that is, the survival and corresponding mortality specifically due to prostate cancer or breast cancer, respectively.

Alternatively, *disease-specific survival* can be calculated by the methods already shown, counting only deaths from prostate cancer or breast cancer as events, with deaths from any other cause being censoring. The danger with this analysis is that it is open to biases in the allocation of deaths; there is always the suspicion that subjects who have a diagnosis of a severe disease will tend to be certified as dying from that disease, even if their cause of death is in fact independent of it.

In clinical trials and cohort studies with modest numbers of individuals, disease-specific analyses may be appropriate, as attention can be paid to possible biases in outcome assessment and steps taken to ensure that the attribution of the cause of death is not biased by the exposure or intervention of the subject. Thus an independent panel, blind to the treatment allocation in a trial, may review the clinical and pathological information to classify causes of death. Where disease-specific survival is regarded as the prime end point, it is always useful to do an analysis of total survival in addition.

Differences between groups

To compare the survival experiences of two (or more) groups of subjects we could select an arbitrary point in time and compare the survival at that point using a simple 2×2 table of deaths versus survivors at that point, or, rather better, we could compare the actuarial survival rates at that point. The results will depend on the particular time point used. One alternative is to use a mathematical formula which will describe the form of the survival curve adequately and compare the relevant parameters of the formula. These methods are called parametric, as the shape of the curve is assumed; for example, in some situations there may be a simple linear relationship between the logarithm of the survival rate and time. Such methods are clearly dependent on the validity of the parametric model chosen.

To avoid both these difficulties, a non-parametric test is often used. Such a test compares the order in which the outcome events occur in each group of subjects, without reference to the precise timing. Thus the tests evaluate the whole curve, but make no assumptions about its shape.

The log-rank test

Although there are several different non-parametric tests, one method is simple and at the same time powerful and appropriate over a wide range of circumstances [24,25]. This is the log-rank test, and again is an application of the Mantel–Haenszel test. At each point in time at which a death occurs, a 2×2 table showing the number of deaths and the total number of subjects under follow-up is created, as shown in Table 8.9. For each table, the observed deaths in one group, the expected deaths, and the variance of the expected number are calculated in the same way as was shown in Box 8.2. These quantities are summed over all tables, and the Mantel–Haenszel statistic is derived from the summations. The calculation for the data given in Table 8.6 comparing the two treatment groups, is shown in Table 8.10.

Table 8.9 The log-rank statistic: for each time interval, ending when one or more deaths occurs, a 2 × 2 table is created which has usual format (compare Box 8.2). The log-rank statistic is calculated as the stratified Mantel–Haenszel statistic, summing over all time intervals, and yields a χ^2 statistic on one degree of freedom.

For each time interval i:

	Deaths at end of interval i	Subjects still alive at end of interval i	Subjects alive immediately prior to end of interval i
'Exposed'	a_i	b_i	N_{1i}
'Unexposed'	c_i	d_i	N_{0i}
Total	M_{1i}	M_{0i}	T_i

$$\text{Log-rank statistic} = \frac{\left(\sum_i a_i - \sum_i E_i\right)^2}{\sum_i V_i}$$

where $E_i = N_{1i} M_{1i} / T_i$

and $V_i = N_{1i} N_{0i} M_{1i} M_{0i} / T_i^2 (T_i - 1)$

The log-rank test calculations produce the observed to expected ratio for each group, which relates the number of deaths observed during the follow-up period to the number expected on the null hypothesis that the survival curve for that group is the same as that for the combined data. A subgroup of subjects with a mortality rate higher than the whole group will have an observed to expected ratio greater than 1. Therefore, in the data used in Table 8.10, in group A more deaths are observed (7) then expected (3.49). Examination of the survival curves, calculated for each group by the method shown in Table 8.7, shows that there are more early deaths in group A.

Several exposure categories

The log-rank method can be expanded to look at a number of different categories of subjects, which might correspond to graded severities of disease, stages of disease, dose regimens of treatment, and so on. Comparison between the curves can be based on either an overall chi-squared statistic with $(n - 1)$ degrees of freedom, where n is the number of groups compared, which assesses the total variation from the null hypothesis that survival is the same in each group, or by a trend statistic on one degree of freedom which assesses the linear component of a trend in difference in survival experience over the ordered groups.

Thus, Figure 8.3 shows a further analysis of the survival of the breast cancer patients whose overall survival was shown earlier in Figure 8.1. The patients have been divided

Table 8.10 Calculation of log-rank statistic from the data in Table 8.6: the quantities a_i, E_i, and V_i are calculated for each time period i; a time period ends when a death occurs, or two or more deaths occur together. The formula is shown in Table 8.9.

| Interval i | Interval between deaths (months) | No. of deaths at end of interval | | No. of patients alive immediately prior to end of interval | | Expected deaths E_i | Variance V_i |
		Group A a_i	Both groups M_{1i}	Group A N_{1i}	Both groups T_i		
1	0–1	2	2	10	20	1.0000	0.4737
2	1–4	1	1	7	17	0.4118	0.2422
3	4–6	1	1	6	16	0.3750	0.2344
4	6–12	1	1	4	12	0.3333	0.2222
5	12–13	0	1	3	11	0.2727	0.1983
6	13–15	1	1	3	10	0.3000	0.2100
7	15–16	0	1	2	9	0.2222	0.1728
8	16–22	0	1	2	8	0.2500	0.1875
9	22–23	1	2	1	6	0.3333	0.2222
10	23–41	0	1	0	1	0.0000	0.0000
		$\sum a_i = 7$		$\sum E_i = 3.4983$		$\sum_i V_i = 2.16347$	

Log-rank statistic = $(7 - 3.4983)^2/2.1634 = 5.67$

This is a chi-square statistic on 1 d.f., so $P = 0.018$

into four groups in terms of the measurement of oestrogen receptor (ER) concentration in the tumour [26]. The graph shows that survival is better for those with a higher concentration of oestrogen receptors. The log-rank analysis for the four groups gives an overall χ^2 of 60.4 on 3 d.f. ($P < 0.0001$), and the trend statistic, assessing whether survival changes in a linear fashion with a change in receptor concentration, gives a χ^2 of 48.6 on 1 d.f. ($P < 0.0001$).

Control for confounding

Since the log-rank method of analysis is derived from the Mantel–Haenszel statistical method, it can be adjusted for confounding variables. Stratification is used: the comparison between the groups is examined within categories of the confounding factor, by generating survival curves for each group within each subcategory of the confounder. The log-rank statistic allows the data to be summarized over levels of the confounding factor, giving an adjusted observed to expected ratio, and an adjusted

Figure 8.3 Survival curves for 583 breast cancer patients (those shown in Figure 8.1 less 13 with incomplete data) divided into four groups on the quantity of oestrogen receptor (ER) in the breast tumour, measured in femtomoles per milligram.

Reproduced with permission from Godolphin W, Elwood JM, and Spinelli JJ, 'Estrogen receptor quantitation and staging as complementary prognostic indicators in breast cancer; a study of 583 patients,' *International Journal of Cancer*, Volume 28, Issue 6, pp. 667–683, © 1981 Wiley-Liss, Inc., A Wiley Company [26].

chi-squared statistic which assesses the difference between the groups after control for the confounder. For example, the data shown in Figure 8.3 show that survival in breast cancer patients is related to oestrogen receptor concentration. It is important to know whether this effect is independent of the effect of other prognostic factors such as staging. Therefore a stratified analysis was done, assessing differences in survival by oestrogen receptor status within clinical stage categories, and the calculating an adjusted log-rank statistic. This showed that the observed to expected ratios were little changed; the ratio for subjects with the highest receptor concentration was 0.44 before control for clinical stage and 0.45 after such control, and the trend statistic was 48.6 before controlling for stage and 47.3 afterwards. This shows that the prognostic effect of oestrogen receptor quantity is independent of clinical stage.

Multivariate analysis: proportionate hazards model

Multivariate methods can be applied to survival data. Such methods are similar in principle to the logistic regression model described earlier in this chapter. A powerful method with wide applicability is the proportional hazards model developed by Cox [27]. (Sir David Cox is a prominent British statistician.) This model allows the survival curve to take any form, that is, the hazard function, or instantaneous mortality rate, is allowed to vary with the time from the start of follow-up. However, it is assumed that the relative effect of any factor on the hazard function will be constant over time. Thus, if the hazard function at time t in the referent group of subjects is expressed as $\lambda_{0,t}$, the function for subjects with a factor x_1 is given by

$$\lambda_{1,t} = \lambda_{0,t}.\exp(b_1 x_1)$$

or

$$\ln\lambda_{1,t} = \ln\lambda_{0,t} + b_1 x_1$$

where b_1 is the coefficient related to x_1. If x_1 has the values 0 or 1, the exponential of b_1 will be the ratio $\lambda_{1,t}/\lambda_{0,t}$; that is, the ratio of the hazard function, which is a relative risk. With multiple factors, the model becomes

$$\lambda_{k,t} = \lambda_{0,t}.\exp(b_1 x_2 + ...b_k x_k)$$

Of course, methods that can deal with a multivariate analysis and the complexity of censored survival data are complex, and specialist statistical and programming advice is required.

As stated at the beginning of the chapter, this review of key statistical methods emphasizes that statistical methods are one component of the process of assessing causation, along with the consideration of observation bias and confounding. In subsequent chapters, we will consolidate and develop this theme.

Self-test questions

Answers in Appendix 1, p.403

Q8.1 Two studies of the effects of a new treatment on recovery from a disease are available. The first study gives a relative risk of 2.2, with a chi-square statistic on one degree of freedom of 9.6. The second study gives a relative risk of 4.6, with a chi-square statistic of 1.8. How would you interpret these results? (Use Table A2.15 or the Excel functions shown in Table A2.16).

Q8.2 In a study of injury in different work groups, there were 16 injuries in 1 year in a group of 1000 employees working on special processes, while for a larger group of 10,000 workers there were 40 injuries in a year. What is the relative risk of injury and the associated chi-square statistic (use Box 8.3)? What are the 95 per cent two-sided confidence limits for the relative risk? (Use Table A2.2, section 4A).

Q8.3 In a case–control study, 52 of 400 controls are exposed to the agent in question compared with 34 of 100 cases. Calculate the odds ratio, the Mantel–Haenszel chi-square statistic, and the 95 per cent two-sided confidence limits. Use Box 8.2 and Table A2.1.

Q8.4 A cohort study gives a result showing a relative risk of 2.25 with 95 per cent two-sided confidence limits of 0.88–5.75. How do you interpret this?

Q8.5 The background rate of smoking cessation over 1 year is assumed to be 10 per cent. A specific programme is thought worthwhile if it would double this to 20 per cent. It is assumed that the cessation programme could not reduce the cessation rate. You want to design a study which has high confidence (90 per cent) that you can detect an effect of this magnitude. How many subjects do you need? Use Boxes 8.8 and 8.9.

Q8.6 If the answer from the last question suggests a number beyond your resources, how could you design the study to use a smaller number?

Q8.7 You want to set up a case–control study to assess a factor that you expect to be present in 10 per cent of the control sample. You want to be able to detect a relative risk of 2, with 80 per cent power and using a two-sided 0.05 significance level. Cases and controls are equally difficult to recruit. What is the minimum number of subjects you require?

Q8.8 If in the case–control study described in Q8.7, controls are much easier to recruit than cases, how many cases are needed if four controls per case are recruited?

Q8.9 In an individually matched case–control study there are 200 pairs in which the case is exposed and the control is not, and 50 where the control is exposed and the case is not. What is the odds ratio, the chi-square statistic, and the approximate 99 per cent two-sided confidence limits? Use Table 8.4 and Box 8.5.

Q8.10 In a case–control study, 50 of 100 cases and 20 of 100 controls in men have the exposure of interest. In women, 60 of 100 cases and 10 of 100 controls are exposed. What are the results? Are the results different for men and women?

Q8.11 From the data in Figure 8.2, calculate the survival curve for each of groups A and B. What is the survival rate and 95 per cent confidence limits for each group at 18 months? Do these results agree with the log-rank statistic calculated in Table 8.10.

References

1. **Rothman KJ, Greenland S, Lash TL**. *Modern Epidemiology*, 3rd edn. Philadelphia, PA: Walters Kluwer and Lippincott Williams and Wilkins; 2008.
2. **Mantel N, Haenszel W**. Statistical aspects of the analysis of data from retrospective studies of disease. *J Natl Cancer Inst* 1959; **22**:719–748.
3. **Lyon JL, Gardner JW, West DW, Stanish WM, Hebertson RM**. Smoking and carcinoma *in situ* of the uterine cervix. *Am J Public Health* 1983; **73**(5):558–562.
4. **Truett J, Cornfield J, Kannel W**. A multivariate analysis of the risk of coronary heart disease in Framingham. *J Chronic Dis* 1967; **20**(7):511–524.
5. **Pooling Project Research Group**. Relationship of blood pressure, serum cholesterol, smoking habit, relative weight and E.C.G. abnormalities to incidence of major coronary events: final report of the Pooling Project. *J Chronic Dis* 1978; **31**(4):201–306.
6. **Saracci R**. Asbestos and lung cancer: an analysis of the epidemiological evidence on the asbestos-smoking interaction. *Int J Cancer* 1977; **20**:323–331.
7. **Mantel N**. Chi-square tests with one degree of freedom; extensions of the Mantel-Haenszel procedure. *Am Stat Assoc J* 1963; **58**:690–700.

8. **Elwood JM**. Maternal and environmental factors affecting twin births in Canadian cities. *Br J Obstet Gynaecol* 1978; **85**:351–358.

9. **McNemar Q**. Note on the sampling of the difference between corrected proportions or percentages. *Psychometrika* 1947; **12**:153–157.

10. **Elwood JM, Williamson C, Stapleton PJ**. Malignant melanoma in relation to moles, pigmentation, and exposure to fluorescent and other lighting sources. *Br J Cancer* 1986; **53**:65–74.

11. **Dunn OJ**. Multiple comparisons among means. *J Am Statistical Assoc* 1961; **56**:52–64.

12. **Purdue MP, Hofmann JN, Kemp TJ, Chaturvedi AK, Lan Q, Park JH, et al**. A prospective study of 67 serum immune and inflammation markers and risk of non-Hodgkin lymphoma. *Blood* 2013; **122**(6):951–957.

13. **ISIS-2 (Second International Study of Infarct Survival) Collaborative Group)**. Randomised trial of intravenous streptokinase, oral aspirin, both, or neither among 17,187 cases of suspected acute myocardial infarction: ISIS-2. *Lancet* 1988; **332**(8607):349–360.

14. **Workshop on Early Stopping Rules in Cancer Clinical Trials**. Cambridge, United Kingdom, 13–15 April 1993. *Stat Med* 1994; **13**(13–14):1289–1499.

15. **DAMOCLES Study Group**. A proposed charter for clinical trial data monitoring committees: helping them to do their job well. *Lancet* 2005; **365**(9460):711–722.

16. **Chalmers I, Altman DG, McHaffie H, Owens N, Cooke RW**. Data sharing among data monitoring committees and responsibilities to patients and science. *Trials* 2013; **14**:102.

17. **Fernandes RM, van der Lee JH, Offringa M**. A systematic review of the reporting of Data Monitoring Committees roles, interim analysis and early termination in pediatric clinical trials. *BMC Pediatr* 2009; **9**:77.

18. **Coronary Drug Project Research Group**. Influence of adherence to treatment and response of cholesterol on mortality in the Coronary Drug Project. *N Engl J Med* 1980; **303**(18):1038–1041.

19. **MRC (Medical Research Council) Vitamin Study Group**. Prevention of neural tube defects: results of the Medical Research Council Vitamin Study. *Lancet* 1991; **338**(8760):131–137.

20. **Omenn GS, Goodman GE, Thornquist MD, Balmes J, Cullen MR, Glass A, et al**. Effects of a combination of beta carotene and vitamin A on lung cancer and cardiovascular disease. *N Engl J Med* 1996; **334**(18):1150–1155.

21. **Pocock SJ**. *Clinical Trials: A Practical Approach*. Chichester: Wiley; 1983.

22. **Machin D, Day S, Green SB**. *Textbook of Clinical Trials*, 2nd edn. Chichester: John Wiley; 2006.

23. **Fleiss JL, Levin B, Paik MC**. *Statistical Methods for Rates and Proportions*, 3rd edn. New York: John Wiley & Sons; 2003.

24. **Mantel N**. Evaluation of survival data and two new rank order statistics arising in its consideration. *Cancer Chemother Rep* 1966; **50**:163–170.

25. **Peto R, Pike MC, Armitage P, Breslow NE, Cox DR, Howard SV, et al**. Design and analysis of randomized clinical trials requiring prolonged observation of each patient. II. analysis and examples. *Br J Cancer* 1977; **35**(1):1–39.

26. **Godolphin W, Elwood JM, Spinelli JJ**. Estrogen receptor quantitation and staging as complementary prognostic indicators in breast cancer; a study of 583 patients. *Int J Cancer* 1981; **28**:667–683.

27. **Cox DR**. Regression models and life-tables. *J R Statist Soc Series B* 1972; **34**:187–220.

Chapter 9

Combining results from several studies: systematic reviews and meta-analyses

And differing judgements serve but to declare.
That truth lies somewhere, if we knew but where.

—William Cowper: *Hope*; 1782

Introduction

In the first part of this chapter, we will discuss systematic reviews and the role of meta-analysis. In the second part, we will present the most widely used statistical methods for meta-analysis and related issues such as exploring differences between studies.

Part 1. Systematic reviews and meta-analysis

So far in this book, we have concentrated on the assessment of the methods and results of a single study. For most topics there will be many studies available, which need to be assessed, compared, and summarized.

Narrative reviews

Traditionally, reviewing many studies was done by ad hoc methods, now referred to as a *narrative review*. Authors of reviews and textbooks would select the studies they thought most relevant, comment on them in a narrative fashion, and give their conclusions. The criteria used to select and assess studies were not defined, and often not recognized by the author. These criteria might include the type of study, the size of the study, and the reputation of the investigators and the journal publishing the study. Such criteria may have some validity, but the key issue is that the criteria were not explicitly defined. As a result different experts reviewing the same material could come to very different conclusions, and the reasoning behind their conclusions was hidden.

Systematic reviews

In contrast, in a *systematic review* the key feature is that the methods of doing the review are explicitly documented, just as the methods of any other study are described, so that in principle they can be reproduced by others. It is now accepted good practice that the methods by which studies are identified, the criteria determining whether a study is included in the review or excluded, the criteria used to assess the importance and quality of the different studies, and the methods used to consolidate the results and come to conclusions, are all explicitly described. Such systematic reviews are at the centre of developments in *evidence-based medicine* and *evidence-based health care*.

Meta-analysis

Within this overall process of systematic review, *meta-analysis* refers to statistical methods using the data from numerous studies to produce an estimate of an overall association, and explore variations between the studies. A systematic review need not include a meta-analysis, as meta-analysis is only relevant if several studies provide data that can be sensibly combined. Thus only a few years after the first randomized trial of tuberculosis treatment (described in Chapter 2, Figure 2.6), a comparative review of the three studies on the topic then available was published [1]. The first published meta-analysis may be by Goldberg in 1906 from a review of 44 studies of bacteriuria in typhoid [2]. Systematic reviews and meta-analysis have developed very rapidly since the 1980s as a result of the development of good statistical methods for combining study results, the recognition of the importance of using all available information to avoid publication bias, the greater power and accessibility of computer-based systems for retrieving literature, and the development of Cochrane (previously known as the Cochrane Collaboration). All of these influences will be discussed in this chapter.

Examples

Two examples will show the power and relevance of meta-analysis, both in regard to breast cancer. An international effort to combine data from all randomized trials of treatment of early breast cancer started in 1983–84, and is still continuing (http://www.ctsu.ox.ac.uk/research/meta-trials/ebctcg), with results on outcomes up to 20 years after diagnosis [3,4]. Analyses on recurrences and deaths up to 15 years since randomization were based on data on 150 000 women in 200 trials and have influenced treatment practices worldwide [5]. The definitive information on the treatment of breast cancer now comes from these analyses, rather than from a reviewer's choice of the 'best' trial or from the most 'authoritative' textbook.

A similar effort in regard to breast cancer aetiology was set up in 1992, and is also continuing (http://www.ceu.ox.ac.uk/research/29/collaborative-group-on-hormonal-factors-in-breast-cancer). Analyses of the effects of oral contraceptive use, based on 54 case–control and cohort studies, 53 000 women with breast cancer, and 100 000 controls [6] included about 90 per cent of the worldwide information on the question, and produced some new findings, not shown in any of the individual studies, such as a small but important increased risk of breast cancer in current users that decreased after cessation of use. The assessment of the effects of abortion has been mentioned in Chapter 6 [7]. The assessment of the effects of ages at menarche and menopause included data from 117 studies, 119 000 breast cancer cases, and 306 000 controls [8].

Cochrane

In 1992 in Britain, the Cochrane Centre was founded with support from the National Health Service. It is named in honour of Professor Archie Cochrane, a Scottish physician (1909–1988) who in a long career in epidemiology and health care research argued strongly that all health care interventions should be tested for their efficacy, where possible by randomized trials [9]. He wrote a thought-provoking autobiography [10]. This developed into the international Cochrane Collaboration, launched in 1993—the organization is now known as Cochrane. Participants in this international network prepare systematic reviews of health care interventions, using a standard approach and meta-analysis methods. At first restricted to randomized controlled trials, the work also extends to meta-analyses of observational studies. The Cochrane website (http://www.cochrane.org) provides freely accessible information on the extensive databases available, and on methodological issues in systematic reviews and meta-analysis. The *Cochrane Handbook for Systematic Reviews of Interventions* [11] is a valuable reference source discussing methods of accessing literature, formatting systematic reviews, and conducting meta-analyses. The website also provides access to the Review Manager (RevMan) computer software, which supports Cochrane format reviews, and includes meta-analysis [12].

Meta-analyses based on individual subject data, or on results of each study

There are two major types of meta-analysis. A meta-analysis may be based on the results of each study, published or unpublished, or may be a new analysis using the original data for each participant in each of the studies. The use of only the study results is obviously much easier; however, there is little ability to deal with limitations or biases in these results. Terminology varies. We will use *meta-analysis* to refer to all combined analyses, and use the terms *pooled analysis* or *individual patient (or participant) data* (IPD) analysis to refer specifically to analyses using individual subject data [11]. This terminology is used by the Cochrane system and by PRISMA [13].

A meta-analysis with individual participant data can summarize the main results and can also produce new analyses, such as the assessment of effects within sub-groups, the interactions between two or more factors, and the more adequate control of confounding. The meta-analyses of aetiological and treatment issues of breast cancer mentioned previously used individual subject data. Such pooled analyses are particularly valuable where the major limitations of individual studies are not only in sample size, but in the adequacy of confounder control and the limited analysis of sub-groups. Such meta-analyses require the active support of the investigators of each original study, and a great deal of work in editing, perhaps recoding, and checking the original data to produce consistently formatted data for analysis.

The most successful efforts have had substantial funding for these central functions, and support for meetings of investigators who are involved throughout the process. The analysis of these pooled data sets is in principle the same as the analysis of one large study, with the individual studies being treated as strata in the analysis.

However, most meta-analyses are simpler, being based on the results of previous studies, and these too are very valuable. The great majority of systematic reviews in the Cochrane database include only meta-analyses of published results. The methods available for the analyses of the results of many studies, to produce summary estimates of the overall effect, measures of the precision of that summary measure, and to explore issues of variation between studies, will be discussed in the second part of this chapter.

Systematic review and meta-analysis: the process

The term 'systematic review' describes a process with several important steps, one of which is meta-analysis (Box 9.1). These steps are to define the objective and the question; to set the criteria for studies to be included in the review; to identify, retrieve, and review these studies; to abstract the data required for the review and analysis; to perform a meta-analysis when appropriate, to report and interpret the results; and finally to plan for the review of new evidence as it arises.

Defining the question: PICOS

The objectives of any systematic review and any meta-analysis within that review need to be clear and explicit, just as the objectives of any other scientific study should be. So far in this book we have discussed the assessment of the results of a single study in terms of internal and external validity. In systematic reviews and meta-analysis, internal and external validity are assessed in terms of the evidence provided by all the studies included in the review. As with one study, we need to define the key association, and interpret this this in terms of a cause and effect relationship, with attention to both internal and external validity.

Care in defining the question is crucial. The acronym PICOS is suggested [14]: define (P) the patient population or disease that is addressed; (I) the interventions or exposures; (C) the comparators—the groups representing non-intervention or non-exposure; (O) the main outcome assessed; and (S) the study designs included. Many

---

Box 9.1 Steps in a systematic review

Steps in a Systematic Review

1. Define the objective and the question.
2. Define the criteria for inclusion of studies.
3. Find all eligible studies.
4. Review the methods and results of each study.
5. Summarize the results of each study in a standard format.
6. Apply statistical methods to produce a summary result.
7. Assess variation between studies (heterogeneity).
8. Review and interpret findings, and report them.
9. Set up plan for monitoring new evidence and revising the review.

productive meta-analyses have addressed broad questions. The reviews of breast cancer treatment noted earlier assessed major comparisons, for example, comparing patients randomized to treatment with tamoxifen with those not offered it, including trials in which the other treatments received and the selection of the patients varied greatly. One of the values of meta-analysis is that it may indicate variations between studies that show the importance of other factors.

Strengths of a meta-analysis

Increased precision

Within the overall objective of the systematic review, a meta-analysis will have certain objectives, which come from the strengths of this method. The first is to increase statistical power and therefore the precision of the estimate of effect. Meta-analysis was originally designed to counteract the prime weakness of individual randomized trials, which was small size and therefore imprecision of the results. Meta-analysis, by combining data from a number of studies, increases statistical power and increases the precision of the estimate of association. For example, the pooled analysis referred to earlier shows an improvement in 15-year mortality from 60 per cent to 55 per cent in patients with advanced breast cancer with the use of radiotherapy: a clinically important but, in absolute terms, small benefit that would not be apparent in a single study, but is clear and highly significant statistically in the combined analysis [15]. Clearly this objective is only met if the studies combined are compatible, and the overall association based on all studies can be accepted as valid.

Increased detail

Especially using individual patient data, pooled analyses can explore relationships within the data that may lead to conclusions which an individual study cannot assess. Thus the pooled analysis of data from many studies of breast cancer and oral contraceptive use showed a relationship between current use and increased risk, which decreased rapidly after cessation of use. This had not been recognized in any of the separate studies [6].

Testing hypotheses

A meta-analysis may assess hypotheses that have arisen from individual studies. In the same example as earlier, some previous studies of breast cancer and oral contraceptive use had led to specific hypotheses that risk was increased with use at young ages, or use before a first pregnancy, and biological hypotheses had been produced to match these epidemiological associations. Meta-analysis, particularly using pooled individual patient data, can test such hypotheses on the larger set of data; in this example, neither of these specific hypotheses was sustained.

Simplify questions

A further result of many meta-analyses has been to simplify the questions. Many meta-analyses have shown that the results of related but non-identical interventions or exposures have been consistent. Meta-analyses of clinical trials may show that different combinations of drugs or different dosages give similar effects. For example, for effects of blood pressure-lowering agents, meta-analyses have shown differences between classes of drugs, but few important differences between individual drugs or dosages [16]. Similarly, the meta-analysis of oral contraceptive use and breast cancer showed consistent results for studies of women in different countries and ethnic groups and differing risks of breast cancer [6].

Format of reports of systematic reviews: PRISMA

The PRISMA (preferred reporting items for systematic reviews and meta-analyses) statement is a guideline to issues which should be addressed in a systematic review, with a flowchart and 27-item checklist, produced by the international group [13,14] (http://www.prisma-statement.org/). An example is given in Figure 9.1. There is also a guide to producing the protocols for a systematic review [13].

Publication bias and outcome reporting bias

We can only assess the studies we can access. It has been estimated that about half of health-related research studies are never published [17]. If, of all studies done on a topic, we have access to only a subset, and if that subset differs from the others, *publication bias* exists. The bias arises if the results of the study influence whether we know about it or not. This has been explored mainly in the context of randomized trials of therapy. There is good evidence that positive and statistically significant results are generally more likely to lead to publications, for example, from tracing later publications of conference abstracts [18]. This was described back in 1979 as the '*file drawer*' problem by Rosenthal [19], who summarized it by saying that 'journals are filled with the 5 per cent of studies which show type 1 errors, while the file drawers back at the lab are filled with the 95 per cent of the studies that show non-significant results'.

Consequences of publication bias

A conceptual approach to this, considering what may happen in one situation, that of clinical trials of new therapies for cancer, was given by Peto and colleagues [20]. Suppose that over a given period there are 120 large clinical trials with several hundred patients involved in each, and 1200 small clinical trials with maybe 50 subjects involved in each (Table 9.1). These large trials test therapies that have survived preliminary evaluation, and so we will assume that of the 120 new treatments tested, 20 are actually beneficial. If the power of these large trials is 90 per cent, 18 of the 20 will be correctly reported as beneficial. Of the 100 therapies that are not beneficial and are assessed by large trials, five will be expected to show significant results because of the use of a significance level of 5 per cent (type 1 error). Further, because large trials are major undertakings, even those with negative results are likely to be reported. So, the published literature should give a fair representation of the total results from large trials. Now consider the 1200 small trials. As these test treatments for which less previous work has been done, assume that 100 of the interventions tested are in fact beneficial. As the power of a small study to detect these benefits is only 50 per cent, there will be

Figure 9.1 Flowchart using the PRISMA system for a systematic review of studies of body mass index and the outcome in renal transplant recipients [37].

Reproduced from Lafranca JA et al., 'Body mass index and outcome in renal transplant recipients: a systematic review and meta-analysis,' *BMC Medicine*, 13:111, DOI 10.1186/s12916–015–0340–5, © 2015 Lafranca et al.; licensee BioMed Central. This is an Open Access article distributed under the terms of the Creative Commons Attribution License (http://creativecommons.org/licenses/by/4.0), which permits unrestricted use, distribution, and reproduction in any medium, provided the original work is properly credited [37].

50 correct reports of benefit, and 50 false-negative results. Of the 1100 non-beneficial new interventions assessed by small trials, some 55 may have erroneously positive results; so there are 105 positive results from small trials. These may all be published. The 1095 results of small trials that show no significant difference may not be published. The consequence is that about half of the *statistically significant* benefits reported for new therapies on the basis of *small* trials may be incorrect (Table 9.1). So, we should regard a new significant result from a small trial as not definitive, and needing further evidence from other studies. It may be useful to ask whether the study would have been published if it had shown no benefit of the new intervention. The better solution, of course, is to publish all trials, not necessarily individually, but within a systematic review.

Table 9.1 Publication bias: the problem of judging one result in terms of others, and the issue of publication bias, in that small trials with no significant difference will often not be published.

Type of trial	True situation	No. of trials in progress	Numbers with results which show		
			No significant difference	New therapy better	
Large (several hundred patients)	No difference	100	95	5	Significance level 0.05
	New therapy better	20	2	18	Power 90% (optimistic)
Small (several dozen patients)	No difference	1100	1045	55	Significance level 0.05
	New therapy better	100	50	50	Power 50%
Proportion of trial results which are correct (no adjustment for publication bias)	Large trials showing no difference	98%			
	Large trials showing a significant difference	78%			
	Small trials showing no difference	95%			
	Small trials showing a significant difference	48%			

Source: data from Peto R et al., 'Design and analysis of randomized clinical trials requiring prolonged observation of each patient. II. analysis and examples,' *British Journal of Cancer*, Volume 35, Issue 1, pp. 1–39, © 1977 Cancer Research UK [19].

This issue is not restricted to trials of new drugs: the same applies to observational, epidemiological, and genetic studies [21,22].

Reasons for selective publication

Publication bias arises through research studies that produce less 'exciting' results, or those with no commercial or other benefit, not being as accessible [23]. Not all research studies are completed; not all are submitted for publication; not all are accepted, particularly by high-profile journals, where the acceptance rate of submissions may be very low; and not all published papers will be included in computerized databases. The most common reason is that the study is not submitted for publication, this applying to 85 per cent of unpublished studies in a systematic review [24]. The reasons for this given by investigators were most often lack of time or low priority, with many others including unimportant or negative results. Fear of rejection by journals was more common than actual rejection [24]. Several recent studies suggest that selective acceptance by journals is not a major factor, although these studies tend to cover high-quality journals [25]. Publication bias may be inevitable or even desirable, as while researchers and particularly those who conduct meta-analyses want to get access to the complete spectrum of research on each topic, most users of research results rely on scientific journals to filter the information and present them with a selection which is of high quality, relevant, digestible, and even interesting. Scientific journals are commercial enterprises which to stay in business have to be read, whether owned by commercial companies or by professional societies. Papers with non-significant or expected results require much greater effort to make them acceptable for publication.

Types of publication bias

Publication bias can mean that the study is never published in any form, or just that the results are less accessible. There may be *delayed publication*, or publication in less frequently cited or indexed sources—*citation bias*. Studies published in languages other than English are less cited (*language bias*). Most literature searching processes depend on words identified as keywords, or words in the title or the abstract of an article; results only noted in the body of the article will be harder to access. Studies not published in journals, but appearing in book chapters or reports from governments, voluntary organizations, or commercial reports, will be harder to find. The contrast is that studies whose results are of benefit to commercial interests or are otherwise newsworthy may be published in multiple forms and highly publicized.

Outcome reporting bias

Even if a study is published, there may be selection of which outcomes are reported or emphasized in the publications—*outcome reporting bias*. This has similar effects to publication bias, but can be subtle and difficult to detect; a clue may be outcomes described in the methods or, if available, in the protocol, that are not shown in the results. For example, a comparison of protocols and publications for 102 randomized trials approved in 1994–95 showed that many pre-specified outcomes were incompletely reported and 62 per cent of reports had at least one primary outcome changed, introduced, or omitted, compared to the protocol [18].

Deliberate withholding of results

The deliberate suppression or delay in publication of research results by commercial interests is a major scandal [17]. Many trial results, estimated to include 60 per cent of all trial data up to 2011, of the anti-influenza drug oseltamivir (Tamiflu) were not reported, giving a false impression of its efficacy and supporting sales of billions of dollars [26]. Trials showing increased mortality seen with lorcainide, a cardiac antiarrhythmia drug, were not reported leading to many thousands of preventable deaths [27,28]. Non-reporting or delayed and selective reporting of results showing increased heart problems in users of the analgesic and anti-inflammatory drug rofecoxib (Vioxx) may have led to over 100 000 myocardial infarctions [29]. Delays in reporting trials of vitamin

A supplementation, which showed much less benefit than had been assumed, may be attributed to researchers anticipating hostile reviews and extensively re-checking results [30].

Several of these issues have come to light only because results had to be released to regulatory authorities. There have been major efforts to increase transparency, and some of the leaders of these efforts have been praised [31]. The European Medicines Agency, from 2015, now requires publication of trial results for successful applications to the Agency [31].

Finding the relevant studies

Some studies are much easier to locate than others. A search for all available published information on a topic is a major undertaking, may never be complete, and much of the information obtained may be of dubious quality. If unpublished information is to be included, the difficulties are greatly increased. While a complete search is the ideal, more limited searches of published literature identified through major databases will be a considerable improvement on a casual search of a few textbooks and journals.

Studies published in the major medical and scientific literature, which is abstracted on to easily available databases such as Medline, will be the most easily found. But even here, the number of relevant studies found will depend on the search technique and how thoroughly it is applied. Many studies are not included in computerized databases, because they appear as chapters in books, or reports of governments, research institutions, or companies. Such information is much less readily accessible; it is sometimes referred to as 'grey literature' (white literature being easily accessible, and black being kept confidential, such as the internal records of a drug company or government department). Material that is published in languages other than English, in countries with weaker research bases, or in journals which are not indexed by major indexing systems, can all easily be missed. Then of course, some studies may be performed but never published, as discussed earlier.

Electronic databases of scientific literature

The two main electronic databases of scientific literature in health are Medline and Embase, which are the electronic versions respectively of Index Medicus (published by the US National Library of Medicine) and Excerta Medica (published by Elsevier). A search of one major database such as Medline, while simple to do, is unlikely to identify all relevant studies. Medline has the great advantage of being freely available on several sites including PubMed (http://www.ncbi.nlm.nih.gov/pubmed). Embase covers European journals more thoroughly, but access requires a subscription (http://www.embase.com). There are many other systems. Cochrane has given rise to the Cochrane library, comprising several important databases, accessed through the website (http://www.cochrane.org). The *Cochrane Database of Systematic Reviews* comprises the detailed reviews of specific clinical questions, mainly on the effectiveness of interventions, which have been produced and published within the collaboration, plus protocols and editorials. This database extends to public health policy issues (such as the prevention of tooth decay by fluoridation), and a wide variety of other issues related to clinical care. By December 2014, over 8000 reviews had been produced. The *Cochrane Central Register of Controlled Trials* (CENTRAL) is a large database of randomized controlled trials. Another major source of literature is the Centre for Reviews and Dissemination, operated by the British National Health Service and based at the University of York, whose website gives access to DARE (the *Database of Abstracts of Reviews of Effects*) and PROSPERO, an international registry of systematic reviews (http://www.york.ac.uk/crd/). The *Health Technology Assessment Database,* with information on ongoing projects and completed reports from health technology assessment organizations worldwide, and the *NHS Economic Evaluation Database* (NHSEED), which contains structured abstracts of articles describing economic evaluations of healthcare interventions, are accessible through the Cochrane sites.

Optimal search strategies

The Cochrane Handbook [11] gives good advice on search strategies. Studies have identified optimal search strategies for use with Medline and other databases to retrieve various types of studies, such as systematic reviews [32], treatment studies [33], and other topics. These studies were done by applying the logic of screening (described in Chapter 6) to the assessment of the accuracy of specific search strategies. To derive the 'gold standard' for comparison, a substantial team of research staff *hand-searched* each issue of 161 clinical journals for the year 2000. The results of each search strategy were compared to this gold standard in terms of sensitivity, specificity, and overall validity. Using a search strategy with high specificity will yield a relatively small number of articles, most of which will be relevant, which is appropriate for quick searches seeking an immediate answer to a question. Using search strategies with high sensitivity will include almost all relevant material, but also a considerable amount of less relevant material, which will be appropriate for those conducting systematic reviews, for example, for the development of clinical guidelines.

Trials in intensively researched mainstream areas of medicine are usually easier to locate. For example, for a meta-analysis of the effects of beta-blockers in treating hypertension, it was sufficient to search the Cochrane library, which of course includes several databases, and PubMed [34]. However, for a meta-analysis of the effect of sedative hypnotics in older subjects with insomnia the authors used Medline/PubMed, Embase, the Cochrane clinical trials database, Psychlit, bibliographies of published reviews, and contacted the manufacturers of the newer drugs; they identified 24 eligible studies [35]. For a meta-analysis of placebo-controlled trials of homeopathy and allopathy, searches were carried out using 19 electronic databases, reference lists of relevant papers, and contacts with experts [36]. In this analysis, larger beneficial effects were shown in small trials and in trials judged to be of lower quality.

Inclusion criteria

The definition of which studies will be included in a systematic review needs to be set. This can be a complex process. The criteria for the inclusion or exclusion of individual studies from the whole systematic review, or from aspects such as a meta-analysis, should be explicit, well documented, and reproducible. Both studies and publications need counting, as one study can give several publications, and one report can include several studies. Eligibility criteria for the studies will include the PICOS features; criteria for publications may include type of publication (peer-reviewed journals, or other sources as well), language, and start and end dates for the searches done.

All studies that fulfil the stated inclusion criteria should be accessed and assessed. Typically, a large number of studies are identified and assessed quickly, for example, by assessing the title and abstract, and a much smaller group of studies is assessed in more detail. Studies may have major limitations or weaknesses, such as not providing information on the most relevant outcomes, not giving results in sufficient detail for further assessment, presenting results on only a subset of the participants, and so on. The reasons for exclusion of studies from further consideration should be documented, and the process can be described in a flowchart. Figure 9.1 shows the PRISMA flowchart for a systemic review of the effects of body mass index on outcomes of renal transplantation [37], and shows that 5526 publications were identified, 242 assessed in more detail, to yield 56 studies which were included in the systematic review, covering over 209 000 transplant recipients. Of 37 different outcome measurements, 26 were included in meta-analyses.

Each set of data from a study should be counted only once, so multiple publications from the same study can cause difficulties. Only one result from each study should be used in one meta-analysis; if several different outcomes or exposures are to be assessed (e.g. an effect of a drug on mortality, and on incidence of a complication), each should be analysed separately. In observational studies, there are often multiple measures of exposure, for example, different methods of assessing a complex exposure such as exercise or sun exposure.

The process should avoid the use of inappropriate exclusion criteria, which sometimes appear in less scientific processes. For example, the association between passive smoking and lung cancer has been of great importance both scientifically and legally. A meta-analysis of all available studies by the US National Research Council gave an overall relative risk of 1.34; a subsequent meta-analysis derived a lower risk of 1.12 based only on the studies which were conducted in the USA, this being justified on the basis that only studies based on the population to which the policy decisions would apply should be used [38]. A similar restriction was suggested in a US Senate report on breast cancer screening, even though most of the randomized trials have been done outside the United States [39,40].

However, the decision to exclude or place less emphasis on certain studies because of such methodological criteria may itself introduce more bias, as will be discussed later in this chapter.

Extraction of data

Once the studies have been identified, the relevant results have to be abstracted from the reports. This requires definition of the comparisons and outcomes to be assessed, and is often a quite complex process. It is also open to subjective influences, so the extraction of the key data from each study should involve two or more investigators working independently and disagreements and compromises should be documented. Standardized reporting forms and computer entry procedures with error checks are desirable. The abstraction of key data could be blinded, with information on, for example, the title of the paper, the journal, the authors, and other aspects removed before the data is abstracted, but the value of this extra investment is not generally accepted.

Care needs to be taken in defining the exposure or intervention and the outcome for each specific comparison. Different studies of the same topic may use different outcome measures or may report a number of outcomes, and for a meta-analysis the outcome must be relevant and consistent.

Detecting publication bias: funnel plots

If there are a number of good (that is, unbiased) studies of an association, each will give an estimate of the true association, subject to chance variation. The results should centre on the true value of the effect, with the variation being greater in the smaller studies because they have lower precision. So if we plot the estimate given by each study against a measure of the precision of that study, we expect a pattern centred on the true value of the association, with the low precision studies having greater variability, and therefore more spread on the graph, than the high precision studies. A funnel plot is a graph with one point for each study, the horizontal axis showing the estimate of the association in the study (with ratios on a log scale), and the vertical axis showing the variability of the estimate, for example, the inverse of the standard error. If all the studies are unbiased, and we have information on all the studies, there will be a symmetrical pattern with an overall shape of a funnel (an upright or inverted triangle), centred on the true value. Publication bias means (usually) that small, low-precision studies that give positive associations tend to be published, but small, low-precision studies that show null results or a negative association tend to be ignored. If so, the plot will be asymmetric.

Example

Figure 9.2 shows a funnel plot for 17 studies (8 cohort and 9 case–control studies) giving associations between occupational exposure to extremely low-frequency (electric power) electromagnetic fields and the incidence or mortality from amyotrophic lateral sclerosis, a neurodegenerative disease [41]. The logarithm of the relative risk or odds ratio is on the horizontal axis, and its standard error on the vertical axis, so the larger studies with greater precision appear at the top of the graph. The vertical line shows the log of the 'average' risk ratio, 0.255, giving a risk ratio of 1.29 (calculated by methods shown later in this chapter). If there were no publication bias, the results from each study would be symmetrically distributed around this average value. Here there are many more data points to the right, being small studies which show an increased risk (a hazard), and very few data points to the left, corresponding to small studies which show no hazard. The implication is that there are other small studies showing no association or no hazard (relative risks less than one), but these have not been published or identified for the review.

Asymmetry in a funnel plot is not necessarily due to publication bias or selective outcome reporting; some studies may have poor design or analysis, or true variation in the association between different studies could be related to the size of the studies [42]. Statistical tests may be useful if there are at least 10 data points; these are weighted

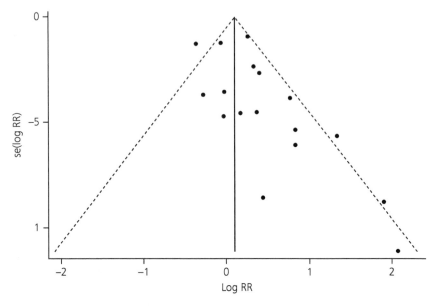

Figure 9.2 Funnel plot from a meta-analysis of 17 cohort and case–control studies of the association between occupational exposure to power frequency electromagnetic fields and the risk (incidence or mortality) of amyotrophic lateral sclerosis [41].

Reproduced from Zhou H et al., 'Association between extremely low-frequency electromagnetic fields occupations and amyotrophic lateral sclerosis: a meta-analysis,' *PLoS ONE*, Volume 7, Issue 11, e48354, © 2012 Zhou et al. This is an open-access article distributed under the terms of the Creative Commons Attribution License, which permits unrestricted use, distribution, and reproduction in any medium, provided the original author and source are credited [41].

regressions of measures of effect size against measures of variability, with variations in detail [43,44]. These are developments of Egger's test [45], which was used for the funnel plot in Figure 9.2; this gave $P = 0.034$, indicating significant asymmetry.

Assessing 'quality' and risk of bias

The abstracted studies can be assessed using various quality criteria. The PRISMA statement [14] recommends the term '*risk of bias*' rather than 'quality', and that this should be assessed several components. The Cochrane risk of bias tool [11] sets components for randomized trials, specifying details of randomization (sequence generation and allocation concealment), blinding, incomplete outcome data, and selective outcome reporting, with all other issues considered as 'other sources of bias'. For studies other than randomized trials, this is inadequate. The appraisal process set out in this book and summarized in Chapter 10 is a 'risk of bias' tool that can be applied to all types of studies. The underlying issue is that of internal validity: can we accept the association reported as a valid measure of the true situation.

Many semi-quantitative systems have been proposed, so that studies can be scored and compared on a simple scale, but these depend on the definition and weighting of each item in the score, and are less useful than describing the assessment of each component, as different aspects will have different impacts depending on the topic. Thus, in a meta-analysis of 17 trials comparing types of heparin for the prevention of deep venous thrombosis, the overall relative risk was significantly greater in trials if the outcome assessment was not blind, although other components did not show differences [46].

The results of quality assessment can be applied in different ways. First, studies that do not fulfil pre-set quality criteria can be excluded from the analysis completely. This is simple with some criteria (such as only including randomized trials) but for less clear issues it is usually unwise to exclude studies completely, because quality criteria are of questionable validity. It may be difficult to ascertain whether a study actually is deficient in a certain area (such as in the checking of validity of information) or whether the relevant information is simply not reported in the papers available. However, the assessment of quality may make a formal meta-analysis inappropriate, or urge caution in its interpretation. Thus, a systematic review of cholinesterase inhibitors for patients with Alzheimer's disease assessed cognitive outcome, and most of the trials assessed showed small but positive benefits. However, the authors noted many methodological limitations including multiple testing without appropriate statistical corrections, and exclusions of patients after randomization, and therefore did not perform a meta-analysis. They concluded that the information was insufficient to support the benefits of these drugs [47].

Second, analyses may be carried out comparing studies which differ in terms of specific components of quality. Thus Schulz and colleagues [48] further reviewed 33 meta-analyses, which had themselves involved 250 controlled trials, and analysed the associations between assessments of methodological quality of the trials and the estimated treatment effects. Amongst several results, they found significant differences in outcome in trials which were not double-blind compared to those that were, and in those where the randomization allocation was inadequately concealed, with the weaker studies reporting larger odds ratios. Moher and colleagues [49] assessed 11 meta-analyses including 127 trials, also finding larger effects in studies with inadequate allocation concealment, but finding no difference in those which were not double-blind. In the meta-analysis of occupational exposures shown in Figure 9.2 [41], significantly increased risks of disease were seen in case–control studies, for exposures based on the job title only, and for incidence; and risks were small and non-significant if based on cohort studies, detailed job-exposure matrices, or on deaths.

Some studies show how the measure of effect changes as studies with decreasing quality scores are cumulatively included in the analysis. If the result changes rapidly, this would suggest that the quality scoring is relevant and justifies putting more emphasis on it. Thus, in a meta-analysis of seven randomized trials assessing mammographic screening in women under the age of 50, Glasziou and colleagues [50] presented the results by cumulatively including studies in the rank order of a quality score. This showed that a beneficial result, although non-significant, was seen in the study they regarded as having the best design characteristics, but inclusion of any further studies changed this risk ratio to a null result.

If the component has many ordered categories or is quantitative, for example, year of publication or an overall quality score, an analysis can be done assessing the relationship between the results and the quality variable, using *meta-regression* methods. These are discussed later in this chapter.

Limitations of meta-analysis

If all the studies have a similar limitation, a meta-analysis will not overcome that limitation. For example, a meta-analysis of observational studies found that women who practised breast self-examination tended to have smaller cancers than those who did not, with the conclusion that self-examination is beneficial [51]. However, all the observational studies included have the same problem, that women who choose to practise self-examination differ from those that do not, not only in regard to measurable factors such as age, but in regard to a complex matrix of factors which relates to their own health care practices and their use of medical resources. None of the studies individually can deal with this confounding, so the meta-analysis does not help with this.

Exploring differences between studies: heterogeneity, effect modification, and meta-regression

One of the main values of meta-analysis is that it can demonstrate differences between study results and lead to explanations of such differences. The interpretation of such results is similar to the situation in a single study where the results differ between subgroups. If the split was anticipated, that is, if it had been predicted for some logical reason or from other results that there should be this type of variation, the results are reasonably robust. If they are unexpected, their interpretation has to be cautious, and should be looked on as generating a new hypothesis.

Such analyses are assessing effect modification, that is, the effects of factors which influence the main association that is being studied. The analysis may be by stratification assessing whether the main effect differs between the strata. Thus, in a meta-analysis of hormone replacement therapy and the incidence of stroke, there was an excess risk of borderline significance shown in the studies published before 1986, but a significant reduction in stroke in studies published after 1986 [52]. A meta-analysis of nine randomized trials and four case–control studies assessing screening mammography in reducing breast cancer mortality showed that the overall benefit, a 26 per cent mortality reduction, did not vary with the number of mammographic views per screen, the time interval between screenings, or the duration of follow-up; but it did vary with the age of the woman, with no benefit being seen in women entering the studies under age 50 [53]. Statistical methods to assess heterogeneity are discussed in the second part of this chapter.

Whether the factor being considered as an effect modifier has ordered categories or is quantitative, stratification can be augmented by regression analyses relating this factor to the main effect. In the context of meta-analysis, this approach to the study of effect modifying factors is referred to as *meta-regression*. For example, in a meta-analysis of studies reporting operative mortality rates for surgical repair of ruptured abdominal aortic aneurisms, examination by time showed a steady reduction in the operative mortality rate over a 40-year period [54]. In a meta-analysis of 10 cohort studies, the percentage reduction in risk of heart disease for the same reduction in serum cholesterol decreased with increasing age of the subjects, from 54 per cent at ages 35–44 to 19 per cent at ages over 75 [55].

Variables commonly assessed by stratification or meta-regression methods in therapeutic trials include age, sex, previous therapy, aspects of the current therapy such as dose, method of administration, and the time at which the therapy was given. The baseline risk of the patients treated, assessed by the severity or extent of the underlying disease, or by co-morbidity and general factors such as clinical performance status, is often of particular interest. The outcome measure used will be relevant. If the therapy has a constant relative risk for different risk categories of patients, that is, a similar proportional reduction in the underlying hazard, the absolute measure of benefit expressed as a risk difference will be larger in those with a higher baseline risk, and the number needed to treat will be smaller. Also in subjects with a lower baseline risk of the disease being targeted, other diseases (competing mortality and morbidity) will be more important, so the effects of the therapy on total mortality or general quality of life may be reduced.

These issues may be explored in a meta-analysis using the results of individual studies, but of course will be limited by the extent of variation in the factors to be assessed in the studies available. Much more powerful and informative analyses can be done in pooled analyses of individual subject data from the various studies.

Meta-analyses of observational studies

Meta-analysis was first developed for application to randomized trials, on the logic that the chief issue to be overcome was that of the small study size of most trials, with the advantage that randomized trials represent a consistent study design, so that the results of different trials can be reasonably combined.

Meta-analytical methods are also used for observational studies, both cohort and case–control studies, as well as being applied to studies of screening and diagnostic testing, economic valuations, and other classes of study. The principles and methods are the same, but the objective may be different.

Observational studies are often weak not primarily because of small study size, but because of a limited ability to account for confounding and susceptibility to observational bias. Meta-analyses can be very valuable in dealing with confounding and observation bias, but considerable care is needed. If all the studies included in a meta-analysis have the same limitation, for example, use the same methods of the assessment or are all inadequate in dealing with confounding factors, a meta-analysis will not necessarily help. As with randomized trials, meta-analyses using individual subject data are particularly powerful in exploring these issues of observation bias and confounder control.

Several important meta-analyses of observational studies have already been mentioned, such as the analyses of aetiological factors in breast cancer. The main advantages of these meta-analyses compared to the individual studies that contribute to them are the reasonably precise measures of association produced and the greatly increased ability to assess confounding and effect modification. For example, the meta-analysis of studies relating previous induced abortions to breast cancer showed that there was no increased risk in studies in which abortions were documented prior to the onset of the breast cancer, and the positive associations came from retrospective case–control studies open to recall bias, as discussed in Chapter 6 [7].

A meta-analysis of observational studies using individual subject data is a complex process. Unless the studies have been designed in common, the methods of assessment of exposures such as diet are often very complex, and it may be difficult or impossible to assess the equivalence of measures used in different studies. For example, there are many studies from different places in the world assessing sun exposure in relationship to skin cancers, but as well as needing to ensure that the questionnaires used in different studies are compatible, there is the issue that 1 hour's sun exposure in Sydney is not the same as 1 hour's exposure in London. Often the data needs to be considerably simplified to make it consistent between studies. Thus in a meta-analysis of case–control studies of childhood leukaemia related to measured electromagnetic fields, the meta-analysis had to use a simplified assessment which could be obtained from all the studies available, and ignore the more sophisticated and perhaps more valid assessment methods used in the most extensive studies [56]. However, the advantage of the meta-analysis is that by having greater numbers of subjects the association between increased risk and different levels of exposure can be assessed quite precisely.

The ideal is to have international collaboration from the study design phase, so that observational studies carried out in different places are designed to be combined in an individual subject data analysis, and use the same questionnaires and methods. This was done in the 'Interphone' studies relating to use of mobile phones and brain cancers, where case–control studies were conducted in several countries using a commonly agreed protocol and data collection methods [57]. The objective was to produce a statistically powerful pooled analysis of all the data, although individual studies were funded from each country and also published as separate studies. Even more ambitious are international prospective studies such as the European Prospective Investigation into Cancer and Nutrition (EPIC) [58], which is continuing (http://epic.iarc.fr/).

Part 2. Statistical methods in meta-analysis

Obtaining a measure of overall effect: fixed effects methods using data from each study

The most widely used statistical methods for meta-analysis are based on a 'fixed effects' model, that is, they derive a summary estimate of effect only from the data given by the studies included in the analysis.

Averages weighted by the inverse of variance

The underlying principle of these methods is straightforward. Each study included in the meta-analysis contributes an outcome measurement: relative risk, odds ratio, risk difference, or another measure. For each outcome measurement, its precision is indicated by its variance; the more precise the measure, the smaller the variance.

A reasonable overall measure of effect based on all studies is the weighted average of the outcome measurements from each study. The weight is the inverse of the variance of the study. In this way, the studies which have the greatest weight and therefore contribute the most to the overall measure of effect are those with the lowest variance and the greatest precision. They will usually be the largest studies.

In mathematical terms, to obtain the weighted average we multiply the measure of effect for each study by its weight, add these terms for all studies, and divide the result by the sum of all the weights. Where the effect measure is a ratio, relative risk or odds ratio, we need to work in logarithms.

Where $\ln OR_i$ is the log odds ratio from each study i, and w_i is the weight for that study (the inverse of the variance of $\ln OR_i$), the summary measure of effect $\ln OR_s$ is given by

$$\ln OR_s = \left(\frac{\sum_i (w_i \times \ln OR_i)}{\sum_i w_i} \right)$$

The most widely used methods of meta-analysis use this approach, the details vary with the measure of effect and the formula for the variance.

In Table 9.2, the results of three randomized trials of the treatment of acute conjunctivitis (eye infection) are shown, comparing the antibiotic chloramphenicol to placebo [59]. The outcome assessed is microbiological remission, assessed by eye swabs taken for culture. The trials were all fairly small, and the result of each trial is shown on one line as the number of successes, that is, remission, and the number of failures, for patients randomized to chloramphenicol (the treated group), and to the placebo control group. The odds ratios range from 2.52 to 11.25. We will show the two most commonly used methods applied to these data. The two methods both use the observed number of successes in the exposed group, the expected number, and the same formula for variance; they use the same statistical test, but different measures of the odds ratios and summary odds ratio.

Mantel–Haenszel method

The Mantel–Haenszel process [60,61] is the same as that used in the analysis of stratified data; here the stratification variable is the individual study. Thus, for each study the quantities ad/T and bc/T are calculated, then these are summed, and the summary odds ratio is calculated as the ratio of these. The summary χ (or χ^2) statistic is calculated using the formula given in Box 8.2 and in Table A2.1 in Appendix 2. The Mantel–Haenszel calculation gives an odds ratio of 4.77, and a χ statistic of 6.62, which has a P-value of much less than 0.0001. Confidence limits for the overall odds ratio are based on the formula given in Table A2.1, 5D, which gives 95 per cent limits of 2.91–7.82.

Peto method

In the Peto method [62], for each trial the number of observed events in the intervention group (O_i) is known, and the number of events expected (E_i) is found as shown; the value $O_i - E_i$ is then calculated. The variance of the expected number (V_i) is calculated

Table 9.2 Application of the Mantel–Haenszel and Peto methods to a meta-analysis of three randomized trials of chloramphenicol (antibiotic), compared with placebo, for acute conjunctivitis, assessing the outcome of microbiological remission after 2–3 days.

Results of each study

Study	Treated group: Success	Treated group: Fail	Control group: Success	Control group: Fail	Total	Odds ratio
	a	*b*	*C*	*d*	*T*	
1	24	10	6	26	66	10.40
2	132	8	22	15	177	11.25
3	53	23	32	35	143	2.52

Mantel–Haenszel method

	a = obs	*E*	*V*	*ad/T*	*bc/T*	Odds ratio	Chi
1	24	15.45	4.15	9.45	0.91	10.40	4.19
2	132	121.81	3.33	11.19	0.99	11.25	5.59
3	53	45.17	8.65	12.97	5.15	2.52	2.66
Sum	209	182.44	16.12	33.61	7.05		

$OR = \text{sum } (ad/T)/\text{sum } (bc/T) =$		4.77	
95% confidence limits for OR		2.91,7.82	
$\text{Chi} = (\text{sum } a - \text{sum } E)/\text{sum } V^{.5} =$		6.62	<0.0001
Heterogeneity chi sq (2 df)		8.09	0.017

Peto method

	a = obs	*E*	*V*	*O–E*	Odds ratio	*Z* deviate
1	24	15.45	4.15	8.55	7.84	4.19
2	132	121.81	3.33	10.19	21.39	5.59
3	53	45.17	8.65	7.83	2.47	2.66
Sum	209	182.44	16.12	26.56		

Summary results: ln OR = sum $(O - E)$/sum $V =$	1.65	
$OR = \exp (\ln OR) =$	5.19	
95% limits for OR	3.19, 8.46	
Normal deviate = sum $(O - E)$/sum $V^{.5} =$	6.62	<0.0001
Heterogeneity chi sq	12.13	0.002

Source: data Sheikh A et al., 'Antibiotics for acute bacterial conjunctivitis,' *Cochrane Database Systematic Reviews*, Volume 2, CD001211, © 2000 The Cochrane Collaboration. Published by John Wiley & Sons, Ltd [59].

by the same method as in the Mantel–Haenszel test (Box 8.2). As a measure of effect, the differences between the observed and expected numbers in each study are summed. The natural logarithm of the summary odds ratio is given by this term divided by the sum of the variances [62]; so

$$OR_s = \text{exponential} \left\{ \frac{\sum_i (O_i - E_i)}{\sum_i V_i} \right\}$$

To assess significance, the summary normal deviate statistic is calculated over i trials as

$$x = \frac{\sum_i (O_i - E_i)}{\sqrt{\sum_i V_i}}$$

This is the same as the Mantel–Haenszel summary statistic shown earlier (Box 8.2).

In this example, the Peto method shows an overall odds ratio of 5.19, and a normal deviate of 6.62 ($P < 0.0001$) showing a highly significant effect. The statistical test is the same in these two analyses. They use different calculations for odds ratio, and in this example the differences in odds ratio are substantial. The variance of the Peto summary odds ratio is 1/(sum of the variances of each study), and the 95 per cent confidence limits are 3.19–8.46.

Comparison of Mantel–Haenszel and Peto methods

These two methods are both justifiable on statistical grounds. The Peto method uses only odds ratios; the Mantel–Haenszel, with minor variations, can use odds ratio, risk ratio, or risk difference. The Peto method has been very widely applied to meta-analyses of randomized trials, and works well even with small numbers or zero cells in some studies. The measure of effect (observed minus expected number) is simple to understand and to report. Where there are considerable differences between the individual studies in the ratios of exposed to unexposed subjects, or of cases to controls, and where effects are large or the outcome is fairly common, the Mantel–Haenszel method is statistically superior, as the Peto method can produce a biased measure of effect [63]. This applies to the data in Table 9.2, where the two methods give quite different results. For this reason, the Mantel–Haenszel method is preferable in the analysis of cohort and case–control studies, where such variation is more likely than in clinical trials. Thus the Peto method was used in the large meta-analysis of the treatment of breast cancer, based on randomized trials using survival data [64], while the Mantel–Haenszel method was used in the meta-analysis of observational studies relating oral contraceptive use to breast cancer incidence [6]. Both methods are used in the Cochrane RevMan software, with the Mantel–Haenszel being the default method.

Both methods, however, have two major disadvantages. The results of each individual study need to be available as a 2 × 2 table. As only these data are used, confounding effects of other variables cannot usually be taken into account (although a simple confounder may be dealt with by using stratified data from each study, e.g. data by sex, if available). So, these methods are of less value where the estimate of effect given by the simple 2 × 2 table is not a good measure of the final result of a study, because of confounding or matching. This applies in the diabetes trial referred to in Chapter 7, where a final result was given by multivariate analysis incorporating confounding variables. In randomized trials, this situation is unusual, so the methods can usually be applied. In observational studies however, it is less likely that a simple 2 × 2 table gives an adequate summary of the overall result, as adjustment for other confounding factors is often essential. Indeed, the results may not be published in a form that allows a 2 × 2 table to be constructed. These limitations are overcome by methods based the final measure of association and its confidence limits.

Choice of outcome measures

Most meta-analyses of treatment effects follow the logic that treatment is designed to reduce the frequency of unwanted events, such as deaths, recurrences, or complications, and therefore a beneficial effect is shown by an odds ratio or risk ratio less than 1 and a risk difference less than 0. However, other clinical outcomes may be positive outcomes, such as the achievement of function, discharge from hospital, and so on. Binary outcomes such as survival can be reported as either the proportion of patients surviving or the proportion of patients dying. If analyses are expressed in terms of deaths as distinct from survival, the odds ratios in the two situations are reciprocals of each other, and risk difference measurements will be the same with a reversed sign. However, with risk ratios, that is the ratio of incidence rates, the ratio itself will be different, and its statistical significance and heterogeneity between studies may be different.

In Table 9.2, we showed the Mantel–Haenszel and Peto methods using odds ratios. The Mantel–Haenszel method can also be applied using relative risks or risk differences (Table A2.2). The relative risks for the three studies shown in Table 9.2, in the order given, are 3.76, 1.59, and 1.46, and the adjusted Mantel–Haenszel relative risk is 1.71, with 95 per cent limits of 1.41 to 2.08. They are substantially different from the odds ratios because the outcome, the success rate, is quite high and varies in the control groups of the studies, being 19 per cent in study 1, but 60 per cent in study 2 and 48 per cent in study 3. The overall Mantel–Haenszel risk difference, using methods shown in Table A2.2, is 33 per cent, with 95 per cent limits of 23–43 per cent. All these can be generated by the Cochrane RevMan software.

Methods based on the result and confidence interval for each study

These methods use the best estimate of effect obtained from each study, and its 95 per cent (usually) confidence limits. Usually the final result in a paper or report is used, after adjustment for confounding. This may be given from the results of a multivariate analysis, a matched analysis, or a stratified analysis after controlling for confounding. The variance of each risk estimate is calculated from its confidence limits, and the overall effect is given by a weighted average of the results for each study, using the inverse of each study's variance as the weight [65,66]. In using this method, care needs to be taken in abstracting the information to ensure that the confidence limits used are correct.

In some studies, confidence limits may not be given but may be calculated from the raw data; if only a *P*-value is given, the variance can be estimated (Chapter 8).

Example

Table 9.3 shows the application of the confidence limits method to a meta-analysis of seven case–control studies that assessed the association between sunburn in childhood and the incidence of melanoma in later life [67]. The result of each study is adjusted for various confounders such as ethnic origin and skin type. From each published study the best estimate of odds ratio, OR_i, after appropriate confounder control, and its 95 per cent upper and lower confidence limits, OR_U and OR_L is abstracted.

The variance is calculated as

$$\text{Variance } OR_i = \left(\frac{ln(OR_U / OR_i)}{1.96} \right)^2$$

$$\text{or, Variance } OR_i = \left(\frac{ln(OR_i / OR_L)}{1.96} \right)^2$$

These two expressions should give the same result, apart from rounding errors; it is a useful to calculate the variance using each of the lower and the upper confidence limits, and use the average. The weight for each study w_i is the inverse of its variance, and then the summary ln odds ratio ln OR_s is given by

$$ln\,OR_s = \frac{\sum_i (w_i \times ln\,OR_i)}{\sum_i w_i}$$

The analysis based on the seven studies shows an overall odds ratio of 1.88. The confidence limits are

$$95\% \text{ limits of } OR_s = exp\left[ln\,OR_s \pm 1.96\sqrt{V_s} \right]$$

$$\text{where } V_s = \text{variance of } ln\,OR_s = \frac{1}{\sum_i w_i}$$

and here the summary odds ratio of 1.88 has 95 per cent limits of 1.56–2.28.

Display of results: the forest plot

The results of a meta-analysis are often displayed as a *forest plot*. The name presumably relates to the forest- or tree branch-like appearance, but the origins are not clear [68]. This method has been adopted by Cochrane and built into the RevMan software. The results of the meta-analysis just discussed are shown as a forest plot in Figure 9.3. The individual studies are each summarized on one line. The graph for each study shows a square indicating the weight assigned to that study, and a horizontal line showing (in this example) the 95 per cent confidence interval for the odds ratio, on a logarithmic scale. The text shows the odds ratio and its confidence limit, and the weight expressed as

Table 9.3 Meta-analysis using the confidence limits method: results of seven case control studies relating a history of sunburn in childhood to the incidence of melanoma.

(A) Meta-analysis of 7 case–control studies

Study i	Odds ratio OR_i	95% CL lower	95% CL upper	Variance	Weight w_i	$w_i \ln OR_i$	Heterog. Q_i
1	1.30	0.90	1.80	0.03	31.86	8.36	4.39
2	1.20	0.60	2.30	0.12	8.50	1.55	1.73
3	3.70	2.30	6.10	0.06	16.14	21.12	7.35
4	2.40	0.80	7.30	0.32	3.14	2.75	0.18
5	6.50	3.40	12.30	0.11	9.29	17.40	14.25
6	1.49	0.97	2.32	0.05	20.20	8.06	1.11
7	1.60	1.00	2.60	0.06	16.83	7.91	0.45
				Summation	105.97	67.14	29.47

summary $\ln OR_S = \dfrac{\sum_i (w_i \times \ln OR_i)}{\sum_i w_i} = \qquad$ 0.63

Summary $OR_S = \exp(\ln OR) = \qquad$ 1.88

95% CI for summary OR_S $\qquad$ lower $\quad$ 1.56

$= \exp\left[\ln OR_S \pm 1.96 / \sum_i w\right] = \qquad$ upper $\quad$ 2.28

(B) Excluding studies 3, 5

Study i	Odds ratio OR_i	95% CL lower	95% CL upper	Variance	Weight w_i	$w_i \ln OR_i$	Heterog. Q_i
1	1.30	0.90	1.80	0.03	31.86	8.36	0.28
2	1.20	0.60	2.30	0.12	8.50	1.55	0.25
4	2.40	0.80	7.30	0.32	3.14	2.75	0.85
6	1.49	0.97	2.32	0.05	20.20	8.06	0.04
7	1.60	1.00	2.60	0.06	16.83	7.91	0.22
				Summation	80.54	28.63	1.64

summary $\ln OR_S = \qquad$ 0.36

summary $OR_S = \exp(\ln OR) = \qquad$ 1.43

95% CI for summary $OR = \qquad$ lower $\quad$ 1.15

$\qquad$ upper $\quad$ 1.78

Source: data from Elwood JM and Jopson J, 'Melanoma and sun exposure: an overview of published studies,' *International Journal of Cancer*, Volume 73, Issue 2, pp. 198–203, © 1997 Wiley-Liss, Inc [67].

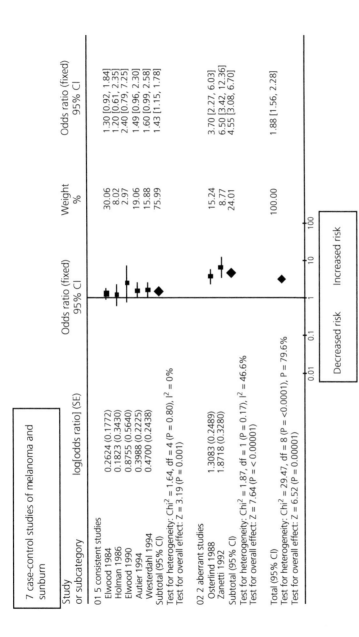

Figure 9.3 Display of meta-analysis of data: data shown in Table 9.3, produced by the Cochrane RevMan software (version 4.2.8, 2005); the graphical display is a forest plot.

Source: data from Elwood JM and Jopson J, 'Melanoma and sun exposure: an overview of published studies,' *International Journal of Cancer*, Volume 73, Issue 2, pp. 198–203, © 1997 Wiley-Liss, Inc [67].

a percentage of total weight of all studies. The combined estimate of effect based on the meta-analysis is shown by a diamond, with its width showing the 95 per cent confidence interval. Other data presented are the statistical test for the significance of the overall effect, and the statistical test for heterogeneity, which will be discussed later. This output can be produced for odds ratios, relative risks, or risk differences (which are shown with an arithmetic scale), and using Peto (odds ratios only), Mantel–Haenszel, or confidence limits calculations, or with the random effects models discussed later in this chapter.

Tests of heterogeneity

An important part of any meta-analysis is testing whether the overall summary estimate is an adequate representation of the set of data. To do this, a *heterogeneity* test is used, comparing each of the individual study results with the summary estimate. The demonstration of heterogeneity will focus attention on why there are differences between studies. If one or two studies stand out from the rest, there may be reasons for this, such as differences in the intervention, the exposure, the study design, or the population studied.

If there is significant heterogeneity between studies, the overall measure of effect cannot be simply interpreted. The studies need to be assessed to see if there is a logical reason for the heterogeneity; if such a reason is found, subdivision of the studies into meaningful groups will be helpful. As well as the overall statistic, the heterogeneity statistics produce a value for each individual study, based on the comparison of that study's result to the summary result. Where there is heterogeneity, it is therefore logical to exclude the studies with the greatest differences from the summary value, and then repeat the analysis, recalculating the summary measure of effect and the heterogeneity statistics compared to this new summary measure. Often the results have to be presented as showing a summary statistic based on a certain number of studies, and pointing out one or more studies with results which are inconsistent with this overall estimate.

Q test

A widely used test of heterogeneity, sometimes called Cochran's Q test, (after William Cochran) is analogous to the test used in stratified analysis, shown in Chapter 8. For each study a term Q_i is calculated, using the w_i terms used in the main meta-analysis

$$\text{where } Q_i = w_i \cdot (\ln OR_i - \ln OR_s)^2$$

so that Q_i depends on the weight w_i, and the squared difference between the odds ratio OR_i for that study and the summary odds ratio OR_s.

Then the sum, $\sum_i Q_i$ is a χ^2 statistic on $(n-1)$ degrees of freedom, where n is the number of studies. For the analysis of the seven studies of sunburn and melanoma (Table 9.3 and Figure 9.3), the overall heterogeneity statistic is 29.5, on six degrees of freedom, which is highly significant ($P < 0.001$). Examination of the heterogeneity statistics for each study shows that the major contributors to this are studies five and three, which have the highest odds ratios. Exclusion of these studies allows the calculation of a summary odds ratio based on the remaining five studies, which is 1.43, and the heterogeneity statistic (recalculated using this revised summary odds ratio) is no longer significant. The next step is to consider why two of the studies give considerably higher odds ratios than the remaining five studies. This may relate to a real difference in the populations studied or to a difference in methods, for example, in the methods used to ascertain sunburn. Heterogeneity does not necessarily mean that the studies which are in the minority are in error; they may be as or more valid than the rest. Heterogeneity statistics for the Mantel–Haenszel and Peto methods are shown in Table A2.12, and for confidence limits methods in Table A2.13 in Appendix 2.

I^2 statistic

The Q test has low power (i.e. limited ability) to detect heterogeneity if there are few studies, and tends to be oversensitive with many studies [69]. The I^2 statistic measures the proportion of total variation attributable to between-study heterogeneity, the remainder being sampling error. The quantity I^2 is calculated as

$$I^2 = 100 \times \left[Q - (k-1) \right] / Q$$

where Q is the sum of all Q_i given previously, and k is the number of studies in the analysis. Confidence limits can be calculated. It is descriptive, with no defined cut-off, but values below 30 per cent are usually regarded as showing no substantial heterogeneity. For Figure 9.3, the I^2 based on all seven studies was 80 per cent, but based on the five consistent studies was 0 per cent.

Random effects models

The methods described so far are all *fixed effects* models, that is, they estimate the overall measure of effect given the studies which have been included in the analysis. A different approach assumes that the studies which have been included are a representative sample of a hypothetical larger population of studies, and therefore uses a different method of estimation, a *random effects* model. Where there is no heterogeneity between studies, these two approaches give the same results. Where there is heterogeneity, the random effects model may give substantially different results [70]. It gives a greater importance (weight) to the smaller studies in the set, and this can be criticized as the smaller studies may be more likely to suffer from methodological limitations or from publication bias (in the presence of publication bias, it is the smaller studies that are a biased sample).

The calculations for the most widely used random effects model, the DerSimonian–Laird method [71], are shown in Table A2.14. The fixed effect models (the Mantel–Haenszel and Peto methods), and the random effects model, the DerSimonian–Laird method, both produce weighted averages of the results from the individual studies. The fixed effect models use as weights the inverse of the within study variance for each study, $1/v_i$. The DerSimonian–Laird method weights the studies by the inverse of a combination of within study variation and between study variation $1/(v_i + D)$; as this variance will be larger, the confidence interval of the summary measure of effect will be wider. The term D depends on the heterogeneity between studies (it includes the sum Q_i mentioned earlier) and is zero if this is small, in which case the results given are the same as for fixed effect models; D cannot be negative. With substantial between-study variance, that is, heterogeneity, the DerSimonian–Laird method gives relatively more importance to the smaller studies within the set. With this difference, the random effects model can be applied to count data and to confidence limits data.

For the data shown in Table 9.3 and Figure 9.3, using all seven studies, the random effects model gives a summary odds ratio of 2.1 with 95 per cent confidence limits of 1.36–3.23; the calculations are shown in Table A2.14 in Appendix 2. The odds ratio is higher than the fixed effects estimate, as some small studies have high odds ratios and they are given more weight in the random effects model; and the confidence interval is wider as between-study variation is incorporated.

An example of heterogeneity and publication bias

The funnel plot shown in Figure 9.4 is from a meta-analysis of 15 randomized controlled trials of magnesium treatment to reduce deaths following myocardial infarction, published between 1964 and 1975 [72]. The forest diagram for these trials is shown in Figure 9.5 with the studies in order of their weight in the analysis (the forest plot has the larger studies at the bottom, the funnel plot has them at the top). Most of these trials were small, with nine of them having less than 100 patients and less than 10 deaths in the treated group. One trial published in 1992 was much larger than the rest, with over 1000 patients in each arm and about 100 deaths, and appears at the top of the plot. The meta-analysis for these 15 studies shows a statistically significant

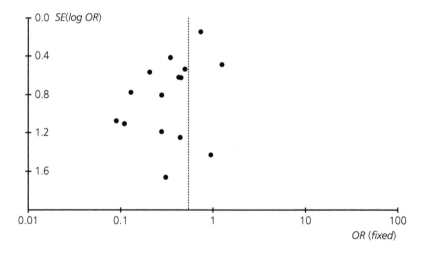

FUNNEL PLOT OF 15 TRIALS

Figure 9.4 Funnel plot: a funnel plot of 15 randomized trials of magnesium in reducing mortality after myocardial infarction. The horizontal axis shows the logarithm of the odds ratio, and the vertical axis shows its standard error; the least precise studies are at the bottom. The asymmetry of the plot suggests publication bias.

Source: data from Sterne JAC and Egger M, 'Funnel plots for detecting bias in meta-analysis: guidelines on choice of axis,' *Journal of Clinical Epidemiology*, Volume 54, Issue 10, pp. 2001; 54(10):1046–1055, © 2001 Elsevier Science Inc. All rights reserved [72].

META-ANALYSIS: RESULTS AND FOREST PLOT (2)

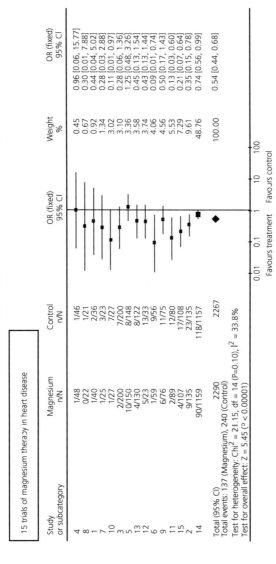

Figure 9.5 Display of meta-analysis of data: forest plot for 15 trials of magnesium therapy in heart disease, also shown in Figure 9.4, produced by the Cochrane RevMan software. Addition of one much larger trial changed the summary odds ratio from 0.54 to 1.01 (see text).

Source: data from Sterne JAC and Egger M, 'Funnel plots for detecting bias in meta-analysis: guidelines on choice of axis,' *Journal of Clinical Epidemiology*, Volume 54, Issue 10, pp. 2001; 54(10):1046–1055, © 2001 Elsevier Science Inc. All rights reserved [72].

benefit of magnesium therapy, with approximately a 50 per cent reduction in deaths, shown by the odds ratio of 0.54, with 95 per cent confidence limits of 0.44–0.68, using the Mantel–Haenszel method. There is, however, moderate heterogeneity (shown by the I^2 of 33.8 per cent). The larger studies have results closer to the null value, and the smaller studies show a pattern of results extending mainly to the left, representing results showing benefits of magnesium therapy. There is a noticeable absence of results on the right-hand side, suggesting publication bias.

Subsequently (published in 1995), a very large randomized trial was performed [73], which involved almost 30 000 patients treated with magnesium and 30 000 controls, with over 2000 deaths in each group. Its statistical weight is sufficient to outweigh all the other trials combined by a large margin. This large study showed no benefit from magnesium therapy, with indeed a slight excess of mortality in the magnesium-treated subjects (Mantel–Haenszel odds ratio 1.06, 95 per cent limits 1.00–1.13). Adding this large trial to the previous meta-analysis changes the combined odds ratio to 1.01 (limits 0.95–1.07), showing no effect of magnesium. The overwhelming results from the large trial shows that the meta-analysis based on the previous 15 studies had given an erroneous conclusion, because of publication bias.

Meta-regression

Meta-regression applies regression models to explore the influence of features of the studies included in a meta-analysis on the overall results. These factors may be categorical grouping of studies (such as comparing cohort with case–control studies) or a quantitative feature, such as year of publication. For example, a meta-regression of the age of the subjects against the relative risk of ischaemic heart disease with lowered cholesterol levels showed that the extent of the risk reduction decreased with increasing age. This was shown by a regression of the relative risk against age, and also by stratification by age [55]. The statistical methods for meta-regression are basically a regression analysis, where the measure of effect such as odds ratio or relative risk (on a log scale) or risk difference is the dependent variable, the other factors such as age are the independent variables, and the analysis assesses the relationships between the measure of effect and the other factors. Single-factor analyses are analogous to regression with one variable, and methods analogous to multivariate regression can be used. However, the appropriate estimation of variances, appropriate weighting, and other statistical issues may be complex.

Self-test questions

Answers in Appendix 1, p.405.

Q9.1 What is publication bias, and what effect is it likely to have on a review of published data?

Q9.2 What are the main arguments for and against including all possible studies in a meta-analysis?

Q9.3 In a review of personal versus group counselling for alcohol-related problems, two randomized trials were found. In one, there were 40 'successes' out of 70 clients given individual therapy compared with 20 successes in 60 clients treated in groups; in the other trial, the success rates were 60/75 for individual intervention compared with 20/35 for group intervention. Use the Peto and Mantel–Haenszel methods to estimate the overall odds ratio and the associated statistical test.

Q9.4 In reviewing studies of environmental smoke and asthma, you find four cohort or case–control studies, with the following results, given as odds ratios and 95 per cent confidence limits: 3.0 (2.2, 4.1); 6.0 (2.6, 13.8); 3.22 (2.78, 3.73); 1.40 (0.34, 5.76). What is the summary odds ratio and its confidence limits? Is there significant heterogeneity?

References

1. **Daniels M, Hill AB**. Chemotherapy of pulmonary tuberculosis in young adults. An analysis of the combined results of three Medical Research Council trials. *BMJ* 1952; **1**(4769):1162–1168.

2. **Winkelstein W**. The first use of meta-analysis? *Am J Epidemiol* 1998; **147**(8):717.

3. **Darby S, Davies C, McGale P**. The Early Breast Cancer Trialists' Collaborative Group: a brief history of results to date. In: Davison AC, Dodge Y, Wermuth N (Eds). *Celebrating Statistics*. Oxford: Oxford University Press; 2005:185–198.

4. **McGale P, Taylor C, Correa C, Cutter D, Duane F, Ewertz M, et al**. Effect of radiotherapy after mastectomy and axillary surgery on 10-year recurrence and 20-year breast cancer mortality: meta-analysis of individual patient data for 8135 women in 22 randomised trials. *Lancet* 2014; **383**(9935):2127–2135.

5. **Early Breast Cancer Trialists' Collaborative Group**. Effects of chemotherapy and hormonal therapy for early breast cancer on recurrence and 15-year survival: an overview of the randomised trials. *Lancet* 2005; **365**(9472):1687–1717.

6. **Collaborative Group on Hormonal Factors in Breast Cancer**. Breast cancer and hormonal contraceptives: collaborative reanalysis of individual data on 53 297 women with breast cancer and 100 239 women without breast cancer from 54 epidemiological studies. *Lancet* 1996; **347**(9017):1713–1727.

7. **Collaborative Group on Hormonal Factors in Breast Cancer**. Breast cancer and abortion: collaborative reanalysis of data from 53 epidemiological studies, including 83 000 women with breast cancer from 16 countries. *Lancet* 2004; **363**:1007–1016.

8. **Collaborative Group on Hormonal Factors in Breast Cancer**. Menarche, menopause, and breast cancer risk: individual participant meta-analysis, including 118 964 women with breast cancer from 117 epidemiological studies. *Lancet Oncol* 2012; **13**(11): 1141–1151.

9. **Cochrane AL**. *Effectiveness and Efficiency: Random Reflections on Health Services*. Oxford: Nuffield Provincial Hospitals Trust; 1972.

10. **Cochran AL, Blythe M**. *One Man's Medicine: An Autobiography of Professor Archie Cochrane*. Cardiff: Cardiff University; 2009.

11. **Higgins JPT, Green S (Eds)**. *Cochrane Handbook for Systematic Reviews of Interventions, Version 5.1.0* [updated March 2011]. 2011. Available from: http://handbook.cochrane.org/

12. **The Cochrane Collaboration**. *RevMan 5.3* [updated June 2014]. 2014. Available from: http://tech.cochrane.org/revman

13. **Moher D, Liberati A, Tetzlaff J, Altman DG**. Preferred reporting items for systematic reviews and meta-analyses: the PRISMA statement. *BMJ* 2009; **339**:b2535.

14. Liberati A, Altman DG, Tetzlaff J, Mulrow C, Gotzsche PC, Ioannidis JP, et al. The PRISMA statement for reporting systematic reviews and meta-analyses of studies that evaluate healthcare interventions: explanation and elaboration. *BMJ* 2009; 339:b2700.

15. Clarke M, Collins R, Darby S, Davies C, Elphinstone P, Evans E, et al. Effects of radiotherapy and of differences in the extent of surgery for early breast cancer on local recurrence and 15-year survival: an overview of the randomised trials. *Lancet* 2005; **366**(9503):2087–2106.

16. Turnbull F, Blood Pressure Lowering Treatment Trialists' Collaboration. Effects of different blood-pressure-lowering regimens on major cardiovascular events: results of prospectively-designed overviews of randomised trials. *Lancet* 2003; **362**(9395):1527–1535.

17. Chan AW, Song F, Vickers A, Jefferson T, Dickersin K, Gotzsche PC, et al. Increasing value and reducing waste: addressing inaccessible research. *Lancet* 2014; **383**(9913):257–266.

18. Chan AW, Hrobjartsson A, Haahr MT, Gotzsche PC, Altman DG. Empirical evidence for selective reporting of outcomes in randomized trials: comparison of protocols to published articles. *JAMA* 2004; **291**(20):2457–2465.

19. Rosenthal R. The file drawer problem and tolerance for null results. *Psychol Bull* 1979; **86**(3):638–641.

20. Peto R, Pike MC, Armitage P, Breslow NE, Cox DR, Howard SV, et al. Design and analysis of randomized clinical trials requiring prolonged observation of each patient. II. analysis and examples. *Br J Cancer* 1977; **35**(1):1–39.

21. Ioannidis JP. Why most published research findings are false. *PLoS Med* 2005; **2**(8):e124.

22. Boffetta P, McLaughlin JK, La VC, Tarone RE, Lipworth L, Blot WJ. False-positive results in cancer epidemiology: a plea for epistemological modesty. *J Natl Cancer Inst* 2008; **100**(14):988–995.

23. Dwan K, Altman DG, Arnaiz JA, Bloom J, Chan AW, Cronin E, et al. Systematic review of the empirical evidence of study publication bias and outcome reporting bias. *PLoS One* 2008; 3(8):e3081.

24. Song F, Loke Y, Hooper L. Why are medical and health-related studies not being published? A systematic review of reasons given by investigators. *PLoS One* 2014; **9**(10):e110418.

25. van Lent M, Overbeke J, Out HJ. Role of editorial and peer review processes in publication bias: analysis of drug trials submitted to eight medical journals. *PLoS One* 2014; **9**(8):e104846.

26. Doshi P. Neuraminidase inhibitors—the story behind the Cochrane review. *BMJ* 2009; 339:b5164.

27. Cowley AJ, Skene A, Stainer K, Hampton JR. The effect of lorcainide on arrhythmias and survival in patients with acute myocardial infarction: an example of publication bias. *Int J Cardiol* 1993; **40**(2):161–166.

28. Chalmers I. The true lorcainide story. *BMJ* 2015; 350:h287.

29. Psaty BM, Kronmal RA. Reporting mortality findings in trials of rofecoxib for Alzheimer disease or cognitive impairment: a case study based on documents from rofecoxib litigation. *JAMA* 2008; **299**(15):1813–1817.

30. Garner P, Taylor-Robinson D, Sachdev HS. DEVTA: results from the biggest clinical trial ever. *Lancet* 2013; **381**(9876):1439–1441.

31. Adams B. The pioneers of transparency. *BMJ* 2015; 350:g7717.

32. Montori VM, Wilczynski NL, Morgan D, Haynes RB. Optimal search strategies for retrieving systematic reviews from Medline: analytical survey. *BMJ* 2005; **330**(7482):68.

33. Haynes RB, McKibbon KA, Wilczynski NL, Walter SD, Werre SR. Optimal search strategies for retrieving scientifically strong studies of treatment from Medline: analytical survey. *BMJ* 2005; **330**(7501):1179.

34. Lindholm LH, Carlberg B, Samuelsson O. Should beta blockers remain first choice in the treatment of primary hypertension? A meta-analysis. *Lancet* 2005; **366**(9496):1545–1553.

35. Glass J, Lanctot KL, Herrmann N, Sproule BA, Busto UE. Sedative hypnotics in older people with insomnia: meta-analysis of risks and benefits. *BMJ* 2005; **331**(7526):1169.

36. Shang A, Huwiler-Muntener K, Nartey L, Juni P, Dorig S, Sterne JA, et al. Are the clinical effects of homoeopathy placebo effects? Comparative study of placebo-controlled trials of homoeopathy and allopathy. *Lancet* 2005; **366**(9487):726–732.

37. Lafranca JA, IJzermans JN, Betjes MG, Dor FJ. Body mass index and outcome in renal transplant recipients: a systematic review and meta-analysis. *BMC Med* 2015; **13**:111.

38. Fleiss JL, Gross AJ. Meta-analysis in epidemiology, with special reference to studies of the association between exposure to environmental tobacco smoke and lung cancer: a critique. *J Clin Epidemiol* 1991; **44**:127–139.

39. **Committee on Government Operations**. *Misused Science: The National Cancer Institute's Elimination of Mammography Guidelines for Women in their Forties*. Washington, DC: U.S. Government Printing Office; 1994.

40. Elwood JM. Breast cancer screening in younger women; the need for evidence based medicine. *N Z Med J* 1995; **108**(1002):239–241.

41. Zhou H, Chen G, Chen C, Yu Y, Xu Z. Association between extremely low-frequency electromagnetic fields occupations and amyotrophic lateral sclerosis: a meta-analysis. *PLoS ONE* 2012; **7**(11):e48354.

42. Sterne JA, Sutton AJ, Ioannidis JP, Terrin N, Jones DR, Lau J, et al. Recommendations for examining and interpreting funnel plot asymmetry in meta-analyses of randomised controlled trials. *BMJ* 2011; **343**:d4002.

43. Harbord RM, Egger M, Sterne JA. A modified test for small-study effects in meta-analyses of controlled trials with binary endpoints. *Stat Med* 2006; **25**(20):3443–3457.

44. Peters JL, Sutton AJ, Jones DR, Abrams KR, Rushton L. Comparison of two methods to detect publication bias in meta-analysis. *JAMA* 2006; **295**(6):676–680.

45. Egger M, Davey Smith G, Schneider M, Minder C. Bias in meta-analysis detected by a simple, graphical test. *BMJ* 1997; **315**(7109):629–634.

46. Juni P, Altman DG, Egger M. Assessing the quality of randomised controlled trials. In: Egger M, Davey Smith G, Altman DG (Eds). *Systematic Reviews in Health Care. Meta-Analysis in Context*, 2nd ed. London: BMJ Publishing Group; 2001:87–108.

47. Kaduszkiewicz H, Zimmermann T, Beck-Bornholdt HP, van den BH. Cholinesterase inhibitors for patients with Alzheimer's disease: systematic review of randomised clinical trials. *BMJ* 2005; **331**(7512):321–327.

48. Schulz KF, Chalmers I, Hayes RJ, Altman DG. Empirical evidence of bias. Dimensions of methodological quality associated with estimates of treatment effects in controlled trials. *JAMA* 1995; **273**(5):408–412.

49. Moher D, Pham B, Jones A, Cook DJ, Jadad AR, Moher M, et al. Does quality of reports of randomised trials affect estimates of intervention efficacy reported in meta-analyses? *Lancet* 1998; **352**:609–613.

50. Glasziou PP, Woodward AJ, Mahon CM. Mammographic screening trials for women aged under 50. A quality assessment and meta-analysis. *Med J Aust* 1995; **162**:625–629.

51. Hill D, White V, Jolley D, Mapperson K. Self examination of the breast: is it beneficial? Meta-analysis of studies investigating breast self-examination and extent of disease in patients with breast cancer. *BMJ* 1988; **297**:271–275.

52. **Grady D, Rubin S, Petitti DB, Fox C, Black D, Ettinger B, et al.** Hormone therapy to prevent disease and prolong life in postmenopausal women. *Ann Intern Med* 1992; **117**(12):1016–1037.

53. **Kerlikowske K, Grady D, Rubin SM, Sandrock C, Ernster VL.** Efficacy of screening mammography. A meta-analysis. *JAMA* 1995; **273**(2):149–154.

54. **Bown MJ, Sutton AJ, Bell PR, Sayers RD.** A meta-analysis of 50 years of ruptured abdominal aortic aneurysm repair. *Br J Surg* 2002; **89**(6):714–730.

55. **Law MR, Wald NJ, Thompson SG.** By how much and how quickly does reduction in serum cholesterol concentration lower risk of ischaemic heart disease? *BMJ* 1994; **308**(6925):367–372.

56. **Elwood JM.** Childhood leukemia and residential magnetic fields—are pooled analyses more valid than the original studies? *Bioelectromagnetics* 2006; **27**(2):112–118.

57. **INTERPHONE Study Group.** Brain tumour risk in relation to mobile telephone use: results of the INTERPHONE international case-control study. *Int J Epidemiol* 2010; **39**(3):675–694.

58. **Riboli E, Kaaks R.** The EPIC Project: rationale and study design. European Prospective Investigation into Cancer and Nutrition. *Int J Epidemiol* 1997; **26(Suppl 1)**:S6–14.

59. **Sheikh A, Hurwitz B, Cave J.** Antibiotics for acute bacterial conjunctivitis. *Cochrane Database Syst Rev* 2000; **2**:CD001211.

60. **Mantel N, Haenszel W.** Statistical aspects of the analysis of data from retrospective studies of disease. *J Natl Cancer Inst* 1959; **22**:719–748.

61. **Greenland S, Robins JM.** Estimation of a common effect parameter from sparse follow-up data. *Biometrics* 1985; **41**(1):55–68.

62. **Yusuf S, Peto R, Lewis J, Collins R, Sleight P.** Beta blockade during and after myocardial infarction: an overview of the randomized trials. *Prog Cardiovasc Dis* 1985; **27**:335–371.

63. **Greenland S, Salvan A.** Bias in the one-step method for pooling study results. *Stat Med* 1990; **9**:247–252.

64. **Early Breast Cancer Trialists' Collaborative Group.** Systemic treatment of early breast cancer by hormonal, cytotoxic, or immune therapy. Part 1. *Lancet* 1992; **339**(8784):1–15.

65. **Prentice RL, Thomas DB.** On the epidemiology of oral contraceptives and disease. *Adv Cancer Res* 1987; **49**:285–401.

66. **Greenland S.** Quantitative methods in the review of epidemiologic literature. *Epidemiol Rev* 1987; **9**:1–30.

67. **Elwood JM, Jopson J.** Melanoma and sun exposure: an overview of published studies. *Int J Cancer* 1997; **73**:198–203.

68. **Lewis S, Clarke M.** Forest plots: trying to see the wood and the trees. *BMJ* 2001; **322**(7300):1479–1480.

69. **Higgins JP, Thompson SG, Deeks JJ, Altman DG.** Measuring inconsistency in meta-analyses. *BMJ* 2003; **327**(7414):557–560.

70. **Deeks JJ, Higgins JPT, Altman DG, on behalf of the Cochrane Statistical Methods Group.** Analysing data and undertaking meta-analyses. In: Higgins JPT, Green S (Eds). *Cochrane Handbook for Systematic Reviews of Interventions version 5.1.0 [updated March 2011]*. Oxford: The Cochrane Collaboration; 2011.

71. **DerSimonian R, Laird N.** Meta-analysis in clinical trials. *Control Clin Trials* 1986; **7**:177–188.

72. **Sterne JAC, Egger M.** Funnel plots for detecting bias in meta-analysis: guidelines on choice of axis. *J Clin Epidemiol* 2001; **54**(10):1046–1055.

73. **ISIS-4 (Fourth International Study of Infarct Survival Collaborative Group).** ISIS-4: a randomised factorial trial assessing early oral captopril, oral mononitrate, and intravenous magnesium sulphate in 58 050 patients with suspected acute myocardial infarction. *Lancet* 1995; **345**(8951):669–685.

Chapter 10

The diagnosis of causation

What is more unwise than to mistake uncertainty for certainty, falsehood for truth?
—Cicero (106–43 BC): *De Senectute,* XIX

Introduction

We have now come to the point where we can assess whether a particular study or set of studies allows us to conclude that a relationship is causal. The question of absolute proof is irrelevant. No amount of data from past experience can ever allow us to predict with absolute certainty the outcome of situations in individuals we have not studied, such as future patients. In health care, there are few situations where there is not another factor that could be considered, another study that could be done, or a variation of the hypothesis which could be suggested. To balance this, we have to be able to make judgements in order to make decisions, whether these are decisions about the diagnosis and treatment of an individual patient, or whether they are policy decisions which may affect many people. These decisions must be made by a process of judgement, and that judgement must be based on an objective consideration of the evidence.

In this chapter we present a scheme for assessing causal relationships in human health. The approach is that the diagnosis of causation depends on the consideration of both causal and non-causal explanations for the association seen. A reasoned judgement must be reached as to whether the association is most likely produced by causality, rather than by any other mechanism. The conclusion as to whether a particular association reflects causation is not a simple yes or no, but requires reasoned and probabilistic judgements.

Part 1. The assessment of causation in one study or in a set of studies

An overall scheme to assess causality is shown in full in Box 10.1, and in a shorter form in Box 10.2. The questions shown will be dealt with in turn.

Box 10.1 Twenty questions relevant to the assessment of evidence relating to a causal relationship

A SCHEME FOR THE ASSESSMENT OF CAUSATION

A. *Description of the evidence*

    1. What was the exposure or intervention?

    2. What was the outcome?

    3. What was the study design?

    4. What was the study population?

    5. What was the main result?

B. *Internal validity: consideration of non-causal explanations*

    6. Are the results likely to be affected by observation bias?

    7. Are the results likely to be affected by confounding?

    8. Are the results likely to be affected by chance variation?

C. *Internal validity: consideration of positive features of causation*

    9. Is there a correct time relationship?

    10. Is the relationship strong?

    11. Is there a dose–response relationship?

    12. Are the results consistent within the study?

    13. Is there any specificity within the study?

D. *External validity: generalization of the results*

    14. Can the study results be applied to the eligible population?

    15. Can the study results be applied to the source population?

    16. Can the study results be applied to other relevant populations?

E. *Comparison of the results with other evidence*

    17. Are the results consistent with other evidence, particularly evidence from studies of a similar or more powerful study design?

    18. Does the total evidence suggest any specificity?

    19. Are the results plausible in terms of a biological mechanism?

    20. If a major effect is shown, is it coherent with the distribution of the exposure and the outcome?

Box 10.2 A scheme for the assessment of causation in note form

THE ASSESSMENT OF CAUSATION

A. *Description of the evidence*

   1. Exposure or intervention

   2. Outcome

   3. Study design

   4. Study population

   5. Main result

B. *Non-causal explanations*

   6. Observation bias

   7. Confounding

   8. Chance

C. *Positive features*

   9. Time relationship

  10. Strength

  11. Dose–response

  12. Consistency

  13. Specificity

D. *Generalizability*

  14. Eligible population

  15. Source population

  16. Other populations

E. *Comparison with other evidence*

  17. Consistency

  18. Specificity

  19. Plausibility

  20. Coherence

What evidence do we have?

Consider the practical situation with initially one set of evidence, such as a published study or raw data from our own or others' work. We must critically evaluate the methods used and the results given, and decide whether a causal relationship seems a likely explanation for the results. The questions to be asked are as follows.

Description of the study (Questions 1–5)

Question 1.   What was the exposure or intervention?

Question 2.   What was the outcome?

Question 3.   What was the study design?

Question 4.   What was the study population?

Question 5.   What was the main result?

The first and often overlooked step is to understand for the particular study exactly what relationship is being evaluated, or, to put it another way, what hypothesis is being tested. We can reduce (almost) every study to a consideration of a relationship between an *exposure* or intervention and an *outcome*. We should be clear about the *design* used; comparative studies of individuals will be intervention studies, randomized or non-randomized, or observational studies of the cohort, case–control, or survey designs. As was shown in Chapter 4, understanding the design shows what type of analysis is appropriate and which methodological issues will be most important. Then we need to consider the *subjects* studied, in terms of the source populations, the eligibility criteria, and the participation rates of the different groups compared, as was discussed in Chapter 5. More than occasionally, describing a published study in this way requires a careful assessment of the methods section rather than simply a glance at the title. The question which has actually been answered may be somewhat different from the one the investigators would like to have answered.

Two advantages arise from this systematic consideration. First, before getting caught up in the particular details of the study, which may be quite complex, reviewing these questions will give us a clear idea of the overall purpose and relevance of the study. Second, it will help us decide whether the study is sufficiently relevant and important for us to review it in more detail. Consideration of the study design and study population may show that this particular study is not relevant to the question we need to assess; for example, we may be interested in the primary treatment of a newly diagnosed cancer patient, but we may find that the study describes the use of a drug in palliation. Third, if there is a great deal of literature available on the topic, this may help us decide which studies are worthy of most attention. Later in this chapter, a system of classifying different types of study in order of their likely relevance will be given; for example, if the question has been addressed in several randomized trials, there is little value in reviewing an uncontrolled descriptive study in any detail.

Having defined the topic of the study, it is very useful to summarize the *main result*: what is the result in terms of the association between exposure and outcome? This step forces us to distinguish the main result from subsidiary issues, which should be considered only after the main result has been dealt with. It should be possible to express the main result in a simple table, and obtain from the paper or calculate ourselves the appropriate measure of association (usually relative risk, odds ratio, or a difference in proportions).

In much current literature, the main result will come from a complex analysis, such as a multivariate analysis. Even so, the raw data are usually available, from which a simple 2×2 table of the primary crude result can be generated. Although of course this crude result should not be used in preference to the published more complex analysis, assuming that the analysis is appropriate, it is often a great help in understanding the study and giving us some feeling for the essential content. Moreover, if the simply derived crude result differs dramatically from the published result based on a more complex analysis, it is useful to look at that more complex analysis very carefully.

Internal validity: consideration of non-causal explanations (Questions 6–8)

Having described the study, we assess its *internal validity*, that is, for the subjects who were studied, does the evidence support a causal relationship between the exposure and the outcome? This assessment is in two parts; first, we consider the three possible non-causal mechanisms which could produce the result seen. The questions are as follows:

Question 6.   Are the results likely to be affected by observation bias?

Question 7.   Are the results likely to be affected by confounding?

Question 8.   Are the results likely to be affected by chance variation?

These have been dealt with in detail in Chapters 6, 7, and 8. For each, we need to consider how the main result of the study may be influenced. It is useful to consider each separately, making our assessment of the likelihood of the study result being produced by that mechanism compared with a causal effect. Thus, for a study which shows an association between exposure and outcome, the questions can be summarized as follows:

- Could the results seen have arisen by observation bias, if there were no true difference between the groups being compared?

- Do the results show a true difference, but is it due to a confounding factor rather than to the putative causal factor?

- Do the results show a true difference, but one which has occurred through chance, there being no general association between exposure and outcome?

As mentioned previously, while our final assessment will take all these factors into account, and the problems in a particular study may involve all three, considering each in the extreme case of it alone explaining the results seen will often clarify our judgement. The order of these non-causal explanations is relevant. If there is severe observation bias, no manipulation of the data will overcome the problem. If there is confounding, an appropriate data analysis may be able to demonstrate it and control for it; we need to assess if such analysis has been done. The assessment of chance variation should be made on the main result of the study, after considerations of bias and confounding have been dealt with.

Internal validity: consideration of positive features of causation (Questions 9–13)

So far we have considered the recognition of a causal relationship only by the exclusion of non-causal explanations. The new material in this chapter is a consideration of features which when present can be regarded as positive indicators of causality. At this point we will discuss the assessment of these features within a particular study, and later we will discuss them with regard to all available information relevant to the hypothesis under assessment.

The relevant questions are as follows:

Question 9.   Is there a correct time relationship?

Question 10.   Is the relationship strong?

Question 11.   Is there a dose–response relationship?

Question 12.   Are the results consistent within the study?

Question 13.   Is there any specificity within the study?

Question 9. Time relationship

For a relationship to be causal, the putative exposure must act before the outcome occurs. In a prospective design comparing exposed and non-exposed subjects, this is established by ensuring that the subjects do not already have the outcome when the study is commenced. The ability to clarify time relationships is obviously weaker in retrospective studies, and care must be taken to avoid considering as possible causal factors events which took place after the outcome had developed. For this reason, in retrospective studies of disease it is best to enrol incident subjects (those who have just been found to have the outcome), to interview subjects fairly rapidly, and to record only information related to events preceding the outcome.

A difficulty in all study designs, but particularly in retrospective studies, is that the occurrence in biological terms of the outcome of interest may precede the recognition and documentation of that outcome by a long and variable time; often some arbitrary assumption about this time is used. For example, in the retrospective study described in Chapter 15, drug histories of case and control subjects were taken from medical records, but excluding the time period of 1 year prior to clinical diagnosis in the cases, and an equivalent time in the controls. In the cohort study described in Chapter 13, it is suggested that differences between studies may be due to the key association changing with the time since exposure.

A similar issue may arise in the definition of exposure. For example, in assessing an association between an occupational exposure and disease, it may be reasonable to define exposure as a minimum of, say, 5 years in a particular occupation. In that event, the follow-up period begins immediately the 5-year period is completed.

A study may show no association because the time scale is inadequate; a treatment comparison may give irrelevant results if based on a short follow-up, and long-term effects of an exposure factor such as radiation or oral contraceptive use will be missed by studies with a short time scale.

Question 10. Strength of the association

A stronger association, that is, a larger relative risk, is more likely to reflect a causal relationship. One reason is that as the measured factor approaches the biological event in the causal pathway more closely, the relative risks will become larger. The deterministic ideal is that the factor is the necessary and sufficient cause, which gives a risk of zero in the unexposed and 100 per cent in the exposed, and a relative risk of infinity. However, this is a very rare situation in health issues. Suppose that a rare disease is in fact caused totally by exposure to a specific chemical used in the manufacture of, for example, plastic pipes. In sequential studies, we might detect a weak association with employment in a plastics factory, a stronger one with working in the manufacture process for pipes, and a very strong association with heavy exposure to the particular chemical.

However, a true causal factor may be related to a small increase of risk, as the factor may be one of a number of such factors operating. Consider the role of air pollution in the causation of chronic bronchitis. Where there are few other factors operating to cause the disease, for example, in non-smoking subjects who are not exposed to occupational hazards, the role of air pollution may be major, producing a high relative risk which is relatively easy to demonstrate. However, in a heavy smoker, the smoking factor is of such overwhelming importance that the extra risk contributed by atmospheric air pollution will be relatively small; if the attributable risk of air pollution is similar to that in a non-smoker, the relative risk will be small because of the very high baseline risk produced by smoking. This does not alter the causal nature of the relationship, but it does make the strength of the relationship less and makes it more difficult to demonstrate.

The fact that a relationship is strong does not protect against certain non-causal relationships. Severe observational bias may produce very strong relationships (some examples are in Chapter 6). Suppose we identify mothers who have recently been delivered of babies with abnormalities, ask them about exposure to drugs in early pregnancy, and compare their responses with those of mothers of healthy babies. We should anticipate that bias in selective recall might be very considerable. If it operated at all, there is little reason to assume that the bias it could produce would be small; it could quite easily be very large. Similarly, strength does not protect against confounding caused by closely associated factors. An example of this is where a disease risk may be related to a previous drug exposure, or to the reason for that exposure. There may be a close relationship between the indication and the drug, and therefore if one of them is a true causal factor, the association of disease with the other factor will be strong despite the fact that it is due only to confounding.

However, if a strong relationship is due to bias, the bias must be large and so should be relatively easy to identify. If a strong relationship is due to confounding, either the association of the exposure with the confounder must be very close, or the association of the confounder with the outcome must be very strong. For example, the relative risk of lung cancer in heavy smokers compared with non-smokers is of the order of 30. It has been suggested that this relationship is due to confounding by a genetic predisposition to lung cancer, linked to a genetically determined personality trait leading to smoking. If so, that genetic predisposition factor must have a relative risk of about 30 for lung cancer. Even given the difficulties of assessing personality, it should be possible to demonstrate the existence of such a relationship.

Question 11. Dose–response relationship

The consideration of a dose–response relationship is similar to that of strength. The major issue which it does not protect against is the relationship being due to a confounding factor closely related to the exposure, such as in the drug versus indication for drug situation. In some circumstances, the demonstration of a smooth dose–response relationship may be a strong argument against the relationship being due to bias. For example, it could be argued that those who use a drug long term might be more likely to have symptoms recorded, simply because they visit their doctors more frequently than those not taking the drug. However, it is less likely that there would be a regular trend between the dose of the drug and the frequency of visits. Therefore, if the outcome under study shows a regular dose–response relationship with the dosage, this bias is less likely to be the explanation.

We usually expect unidirectional dose–effect relationships. Obviously other types of associations, such as a threshold or all-or-none effect, or a complex relationship, may occur. However, the general assumption that if a causal relationship holds, the frequency of the outcome should show a unidirectional increase with increasing exposure, even though the relationship may not be linear, is usually reasonable—so reasonable, that evidence that that is not the case should be considered carefully. For example, the age distribution of Hodgkin's disease does not show the common unidirectional increase of incidence with age as is seen in many other cancers, but instead shows a complex pattern with a peak at younger ages followed by a decrease followed by a further increase. On the general assumption that complex relationships are unlikely, this pattern suggested that there are two distinct diseases, of which one shows the steady increase of incidence with age characteristic of many other cancers, and the other shows a peak incidence at young ages. This suggestion, made in the 1950s simply from descriptive data [1], was later confirmed by the demonstration of differences in clinical and pathological features between the previously unseparated types of disease [2]. The demonstration of a dose–response relationship is an important component of the study presented in Chapter 15, and is one of the prime objectives of the study described in Chapter 16.

Question 12. Consistency of the association

A causal relationship will be expected to apply across a wide range of subjects. If a new pain killer is effective, it is likely to be effective in patients of both sexes and different ages, for a wide variety of causes of pain. In other circumstances, specificity (see Question 13) rather than consistency might be predicted; for example, a hormonal treatment for breast cancer might be expected to work best for cancers which are positive for hormone receptors. If an association within one study is seen to be consistent in different groups of subjects, that would generally support causality, particularly if the likely sources of bias and confounding are different in those subgroups. Similarly in reverse: when a new study showing a positive association between the consumption of artificial sweeteners (mainly saccharine) and bladder cancer was published, the association was seen only in males, and in the absence of a biological explanation for that lack of consistency, it weakened the case for causality [3]. The international trial described in Chapter 12 demonstrates consistency of the main effect with regard to different geographical areas and the main subtypes of the outcome.

The difficulty with consistency is that large data sets are required to compare the associations in different subgroups of subjects; the effective sample size is the number of observations in each subset. Even with adequate numbers, the subgroups to be compared need to be defined on a priori grounds, and not merely generated from the analysis. In a large analysis where many subgroups are defined, it is to be expected that some will show different results by chance alone, as discussed in Chapter 8. This has been a major problem in clinical trials; even where no overall benefit of a new treatment is shown, a benefit may be apparent in one subgroup of patients. Such post hoc analysis is misleading and best avoided; such findings should be regarded as new hypotheses which require testing.

Question 13. Specificity of association

It has been argued that a specific association between one causal factor and one outcome is good evidence for causality. This may be misleading; some took the view that the fact that smoking was shown to be associated with a number of cancers and other serious diseases, and so was not specific to one outcome, made the hypothesis of a causal link with lung cancer less likely. However, specificity is often contrived by definition. If we define tuberculosis as a clinical disease comprising various signs and symptoms which is produced by infection by the tubercle bacillus, we end up with a specific association between that disease so defined and the infectious agent. Without that definitional convenience, the associations between infection with tubercle bacillus and chronic meningitis, swollen joints, and lung disease do not appear to be specific.

However, in many situations demonstration of specificity may be valuable, as it may show that bias or confounding is unlikely to explain the results. For example, consider a retrospective study in which recently delivered mothers are interviewed, which shows that use of a certain drug is much more frequently reported by mothers of infants with cardiac malformations than by mothers of healthy babies. We would have to question whether recall bias is the explanation of that association. However, if mothers of babies with a range of other defects were also questioned, and their reported histories of drug use were similar to the mothers of the healthy babies, this would be a strong argument against recall bias being the explanation of the association seen with cardiac disease. In a study of birth defects in relation to vitamin A intake, an excess risk was found with high intakes only before pregnancy and in early pregnancy, but there was no association with high intake after 6 weeks of pregnancy; this specificity of exposure is consistent with causality and provides some protection against both confounding and observation bias [4]. The trial described in Chapter 12 was set up to distinguish the effects of two different exposures, and showed a result specific to one of the exposures. Previous observational studies could not separate the effects of these two related exposures. The study described in Chapter 16 also illustrates specificity, as an association between breast cancer and alcohol intake was found for only certain types of alcohol intake, but further work on this result has produced conflicting evidence.

A hospital-based study showed that women who had developed endometrial cancer had a higher frequency of past use of oestrogenic drugs than did patients who had cervical cancer [5]. Endometrial cancer is more common in high socioeconomic groups, while cervical cancer is less common. The use of this drug is likely to be greater in the higher socioeconomic groups, and so the association seen may be due to confounding. However, patients with ovarian cancer, which has a similar socioeconomic distribution to endometrial cancer, were also assessed, and their usage of oestrogen drugs was also much lower than that of the endometrial cancer patients. This makes confounding by socioeconomic status a less likely explanation for the association seen.

Therefore specificity may be useful if we do not make it an absolute criterion, as one causal agent may in truth produce various outcomes, and one outcome may result from various agents. The concept is often useful in study design; as a check on response bias we may deliberately collect information on factors which we expect to be the same in the groups compared, as similar results will indicate a lack of observation bias. We may choose control groups to capitalize on similar effects, as noted previously.

Summary of internal validity

By this point, we should be able to decide whether the internal validity of the study is adequate. A positive decision means that we accept the results to be a valid measure of the true association in the subjects studied, and if an association between exposure and outcome is present, we regard it as likely to be due to a causal relationship.

A negative decision means that we decide that one or more of the non-causal explanations is likely to hold; the association seen is due to observation bias, to confounding, or to chance, and we should be able to specify the likely biases or confounding factors. Often we will be able to eliminate some but not all of the options, and decide, for example, that the result is likely to be due to either causation or to confounding; such a conclusion is very valuable as it makes clear what further information is necessary.

Observation bias is discussed in all the studies presented in the later chapters, but is of particular interest in the studies described in Chapters 12, 13, and 15; all these studies demonstrate efforts to minimize observation bias. In the studies described in Chapters 13 and 15, the major question of interpretation is whether the association is causal or is due to confounding; for the studies discussed in Chapters 11 and 14, the main issue is whether the result is causal or due to chance variation.

External validity: generalization of the results (Questions 14–16)

If the internal validity of the study is very poor, there is no point in proceeding further, for if the study result is not valid even for the subjects studied, its application to other groups of subjects is irrelevant. However, if we conclude that it is a reasonably valid result and that a causal relationship is a reasonably likely explanation, we need to go on to consider the external validity of the result. The relevant questions are as follows:

Question 14. Can the study results be applied to the eligible population?

Question 15. Can the study results be applied to the source population?

Question 16. Can the study results be applied to other relevant populations?

The relationship between the study participants and the population of eligible subjects should be well documented. Losses due to non-participation have to be considered carefully as they are likely to be non-random, and the reasons for the losses may be related to the exposure or to the outcome. These issues were discussed in Chapter 5.

Beyond this, it is unlikely that the study participants will be a 'representative sample' of a definable source population, and even if they were, we would want to extrapolate the results further, for example, to our own community, future patients, and so on. The issue is not whether the subjects studied are 'typical' or 'representative', but whether the *association* between outcome and exposure given by the study participants is likely to apply to other groups. In assessing the applicability of results, we need to be specific about the factors which are likely to affect the association. Most clinical trials are done on patients in teaching hospitals. If a new therapy for breast cancer is shown to be effective in such a trial, we would readily apply the results to patients in a district hospital who had a similar stage and type of tumour and were of similar age, even though the trial patients cannot be said to be 'representative' of district hospital patients in a general or statistical sense. Similarly, women in the United States and Japan have very different incidence rates of breast cancer, and very different diets; but if a causal relationship exists between saturated fat intake and breast cancer incidence, we should expect to see it in both populations, even though its strength might be modified by the relative importance of other factors. However, other considerations may apply. If we read of a clinical trial of a new drug therapy used for severe depression in a well-known teaching centre, we should not apply the results to patients in general practice uncritically; the general practice patients, even with the same diagnosis, are likely to be different (e.g. in the severity and duration of disease) from those in the teaching centre, and the effects of the therapy may well differ between inpatients and community patients. In general, the difficulties of applying results from one group of subjects to another will be minimal for issues of basic physiology and genetics, and maximal for effects in which cultural and psychosocial aspects are dominant. The generalizability of the results is important for all the studies discussed in subsequent chapters, but is particularly interesting for the trial discussed in Chapter 12, where generalization from a high-risk population to a general population is a major issue. The applicability of the results of the trial described in Chapter 11, and of the cohort study described in Chapter 13, are important issues in the interpretation.

Comparison of the results with other evidence (Questions 17–20)

We have now made a critical assessment of the evidence presented by one study. We have assessed the internal validity, and come to a reasoned judgement as to whether the results of the study are consistent with a cause and effect relationship. We have explored the external validity of the study, and come to a decision concerning how far we can generalize the result beyond the subjects who participated in the study.

We can now move to the issue of comparing the result of this particular study with the evidence from other studies and other types of experience. As we did with the evidence from within the study, we shall make these comparisons with specific questions in mind. In comparing the results of a particular study with those of other studies, we will ask the following questions:

Question 17.　Are the results consistent with other evidence, particularly evidence from studies of a similar or more powerful study design?

Question 18.　Does the total evidence suggest any specificity?

Question 19.　Are the results plausible in terms of a biological mechanism?

Question 20.　If a major effect is shown, is it coherent with the distribution of the exposure and the outcome?

Question 17. Consistency with other studies

This is the most important characteristic used in the judgement that an association is causal. To say that the result is consistent requires that the association has been observed in a number of different studies, each of which individually can be interpreted as showing a causal explanation, and which have enough variation in their methodology and study populations to make it unlikely that the same biases or confounding factors apply in all the studies. For example, when a British case–control study demonstrated a new relationship between hormone replacement therapy and venous thromboembolism [6], the interpretation of this was aided by the simultaneous publication, because of cooperation between investigators, of a case–control study and a cohort-based study from the United States [7,8] with consistent results.

Consistency of results between studies, each of which is individually unsatisfactory, is of little value, as is consistency between studies which all suffer from the same design defect. For example, it is difficult to assess the effect of breast self-examination in producing early diagnosis of breast cancer from observational studies, because women who practise self-examination are likely to have many other characteristics which may lead them to an earlier diagnosis of a tumour. A meta-analysis of such studies has been performed [9], but it is still open to the alternative explanation of confounding due to other factors associated with earlier diagnosis. Lack of consistency argues against causality, but care must be taken in its assessment also. The failure to find an association in a study which is limited in its methodology and size so that it has very little power to detect an association, if one were present, is of no value. When a new and controversial result is published, weak, badly designed, and small studies which show no association are often presented to refute it; these studies have to be examined with the same critical approach as is applied to the original.

Consistency is assessed statistically within meta-analyses by the assessment of heterogeneity, testing by methods such as those described in Chapter 9 whether the results for each study are consistent with the overall pooled result. The difficulty arises when there is significant heterogeneity. Often, the studies with outlying results are simply noted and then removed from the overall analysis, and a summarized result based on the rest is published. It is more satisfactory if the reasons for these discrepancies can be explored, as was discussed in Chapter 9. Consideration of the quality of the studies and their specific characteristics, using meta-regression methods if appropriate, may be valuable.

Question 18. Specificity

Specificity relates closely to consistency. Whether a difference in results between two studies is interpreted as inconsistency or specificity depends on whether the difference is anticipated by a hypothesis set up before the comparison is made. If not, but a plausible mechanism can be found or if the difference is itself found consistently, then the hypothesis may be modified to take into account the specificity which has been shown. This creates a new hypothesis which should be assessed by a further independent study.

For example, the two congenital defects of spina bifida and anencephalus have similar embryological and epidemiological features, and both are prevented by folic acid, as discussed in Chapter 12. However the antiepileptic drug valproic acid shows a strong and apparently specific association with spina bifida, while no excess of anencephalus has been recorded. If this is not due to some observation bias, it suggests a specificity of effect, showing one substantial difference in the aetiology of the two conditions [10]. A highly specific association is easier to recognize; an example quoted by Bradford Hill in a celebrated paper [11] was that of nickel miners in South Wales, where there were 16 deaths from lung cancer and 11 from cancer of the nasal sinuses, compared with expected numbers of about 1 and much less than 1, respectively; deaths from all other causes numbered 67, similar to the expected number of 72, pointing to a risk specific to these two cancer types.

Question 19. Plausibility

Plausibility refers to the observed association being biologically understandable on the basis of current knowledge concerning its likely mechanisms. The consideration of plausibility is useful, particularly as it may indicate biases or confounding factors which should be considered. The interpretation of the positive association between ice-cream sales and drowning at summer holiday resorts is an example, as a consideration of its plausibility will suggest a confounding factor.

However, any dramatically new observation may be in advance of current biological thinking and its lack of plausibility may reflect deficiencies in biological knowledge rather than an error in the observation. John Snow effectively prevented cholera in a district of London 25 years before the isolation of the cholera bacillus and acceptance of the idea that the disease could be spread by water. Percival Pott demonstrated the causal relationship between exposure to soot and scrotal cancer some 150 years before the relevant carcinogen was isolated and the mechanism further understood. The greatest value of the concept of plausibility is to emphasize that where an association does not match a known biological mechanism, further studies are indicated to clarify this, but these need not necessarily delay appropriate action if the evidence for causality is strong enough.

There has been considerable debate on the possible relationship between exposure to electric and magnetic fields from electric power sources and the occurrence of childhood leukaemia. Meta-analyses of several epidemiological studies show an empirical association [12,13], but there is a lack of plausibility. Even after extensive research, there is little evidence from cellular or animal studies that indicates a mechanism for a carcinogenic effect. It is unclear whether these epidemiological findings are the first indication of an important effect, with the elucidation of a biological mechanism to follow, or whether these observations are explicable by non-causal relationships such as confounding and selection biases.

The dramatic reduction in the frequency of a major developmental defect by a relatively low dose of a common vitamin is described in the study in Chapter 12. Although plausible in general terms, this empirical demonstration of effect preceded specific knowledge of a mechanism, but has stimulated extensive work to identify the key biochemical process and its genetic aspects [14].

Lists of the expected features in causality often include the concept of *analogy*, meaning that a relationship is regarded as more acceptable if it is analogous to some other well-established relationship, but clearly this concept comes within the overall concept of plausibility.

Question 20. Coherence

An association is regarded as coherent if it fits the general features of the distribution of both the exposure and the outcome under assessment; thus if lung cancer is due to smoking, the frequency of lung cancer in different populations and in different time periods should relate to the frequency of smoking in those populations at relevant earlier time periods. The concept of coherence has several limitations: it will apply only if the exposure and the outcome are the same in different populations, if a high proportion of the outcome is caused by the exposure, and if the frequency of the outcome is fairly high in those exposed. If the factor causes only a small proportion of the total disease, the overwhelming influence of other factors may make the overall pattern inconsistent. A comparison of an exposure such as smoking in different countries, or a general category of disease such as lung cancer, may not take sufficient note of differences in types of smoking and in types of lung cancer.

As an example of an argument based on coherence, it was suggested some years ago that neural tube defects were caused by a teratogen in damaged potatoes. In support, the high frequency of the defects in Ireland and the strong association with low social class were quoted, on the argument that these populations had a high consumption of potatoes. However, it was also noted that the condition is fairly common in Taiwan, and is also more common in the poor, although potato consumption is probably higher in the upper social classes [15]. The case–control study described in Chapter 15 shows an association between a drug and a disease outcome, and in this instance the question of coherence is of great importance in separating a causal relationship from the alternative explanation of confounding. However, in the other studies described in subsequent chapters, coherence is not particularly helpful, either because the association suggested is not strong enough, or the information on the distribution of the relevant exposure and outcome is inadequate.

Assessing causal relationships and making decisions

A general method has now been set out which should assist the reader to assess written evidence, his or her own experience, and the experience of colleagues. The system is only a framework, and issues specific to each subject will influence the relative importance of different aspects of the process; a minor issue in one subject may be a major issue in others. The entire process is summed up in Figure 10.1. Presented with new results from a study of a putative causal relationship, the question we ask is: 'Does the evidence given in this study support a causal relationship?' This involves the assessment of the internal and external validity of the study, and its relationship to other evidence, as expressed in the scheme given in this chapter.

If our judgement is that the evidence does support a causal relationship, we should be able to reinforce this by answering the question: 'What is this relationship, in terms of the causal agent, the outcome, and the population to which it applies?'

If the answer to our question is in the negative, we need to be able to answer the question: 'What other explanation is there for the results observed?' The results we have been presented with do not go away; they are the facts from which we are arguing. If we reject a causal explanation, we must be able to propose an alternative hypothesis. The specification of the alternative hypothesis, or hypotheses, will help us to see the weaknesses in the evidence we have and guide us in how to search for better information.

THE DECISION PROCESS

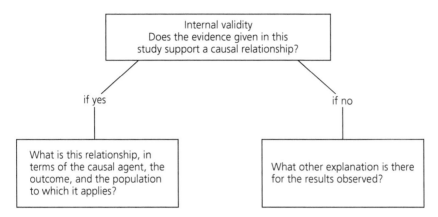

Figure 10.1 Assessment of causal relationships: the decision process.

Some further applications of the assessment of causality

In this book, we have concentrated on the assessment of cause and effect relationships, and almost exclusively on evidence provided by studies of groups of individuals. There are many important relationships which are not necessarily of a cause and effect type, and there are other types of data which can be considered. While there is no intention to go into these fully, a few comments on the relevance of the concepts expressed in this approach to these other questions may be helpful.

Associations can be useful even if not causal

If we can establish that an association exists, even if it is not causal, this information may be very valuable. For example, the diagnosis of a disease is based on the features associated with that condition; whether they are causal is irrelevant. Diagnostic symptoms, signs, and laboratory-measured abnormalities may be features produced by the disease process. Despite that, many of the principles outlined in this volume are applicable to the study of diagnostic concepts, particularly the issues of observation bias and external validity.

Similarly, many studies assess associations between factors, for example, whether attitudes to health care are different in different social groups, without considering cause and effect relationships. Often, however, assumptions and judgements about cause and effect relationships lie not far below the surface, and again the principles set forth in this volume should be of assistance in assessing such questions.

Application to studies of populations, and of physiological or biochemical parameters

This book is primarily about studies of individuals, where each contributes one exposure and one outcome event. Studies comparing different population groups also give comparisons between rates of exposure and rates of outcome. While such studies are inherently weaker than studies of individuals, they can be analysed in the same way.

Most can be considered as cross-sectional surveys or cohort studies. For example, it was shown that populations (Canadian provinces) with more intense programmes of cervical cytology (the exposure) showed a larger decrease in mortality from uterine cancer (the outcome) [16]. The comparisons of firearm-related outcomes in Seattle and Vancouver [17], noted in Chapter 4 in Table 4.10 is similar. The interpretation of these associations is conceptually the same as for a study of individuals: is the association likely to be due to bias, confounding, or chance? Does it show the positive features of causation? The same logical approach can be applied.

Similarly, many studies are based on series of physiological or biochemical measurements within an individual. Thus, to show the causal relationship between external temperature and peripheral blood flow, measurements could be made in different subjects at different temperatures, but it is much more efficient to compare the same individuals, making a series of measurements of peripheral blood flow while varying the external temperature. The logic of causal inference presented here is totally applicable: bias, confounding, and chance must be considered, and the positive indicators of causality sought. Such studies can be considered as matched cohort studies, with each group of subjects under one set of conditions being one study cohort.

Often the outcome, exposure factors, or both, will be continuous rather than discrete variables, such as temperature, peripheral blood flow, and morbidity rate. The statistical methods applicable are those for continuous variables, including Student's t-test, correlation and regression methods, analysis of variance, multiple linear regression, and non-parametric methods such as rank correlation techniques. Such methods are well described in most statistical textbooks.

Applications in designing a study

This scheme can also be used in the design of studies. A useful general approach to the design of a study is that the investigator should attempt a *forward projection* to the point where the study has been completed and the results have been compiled [18]. It is useful for the investigator to consider all possible results, that is, a positive association or one in the direction expected, no association or a negative one, or an association in the opposite direction from that expected. The investigator can then ask the question, given that those results arise, 'How will I assess this study in terms of its internal and external validity?' or in simpler terms, 'Will I believe the results that I have obtained?' A good test of a well-designed study is that the investigator will be willing to accept and act on the results, even if they are different from the anticipated result. This is also a useful question to ask colleagues who wish you to be involved in their research. By projecting yourself to the point of assessing the possible results of the study, you as investigator can consider the major issues of bias, confounding, and chance variation, and consider methods by which these issues can be recognized and dealt with. You can also consider the desirability of being able to demonstrate strong associations, dose–response effects, specific relationships, and so on. By doing this, you give yourself the opportunity to incorporate into the design of the study the potential for demonstrating such features. The discussion of the study design with colleagues who are prepared to adopt a similar critical approach and who bring to bear specialist knowledge of the issues involved will be a major safeguard against embarking on a study which is inadequately designed.

Part 2. The application of causal reasoning to questions of clinical care and of health policy

Hierarchies of evidence

In appraising the science relevant to an issue, each piece of evidence has three relevant dimensions: What type of study is it? Is it a high-quality study? Is it relevant to the question? So far in this text we have concentrated on assessing the quality of studies within the major study types, and in assessing their external validity, which will determine whether they are relevant to a particular question.

For most clinical and policy questions, a large amount of evidence from different types of study is available, and so it is useful to consider a hierarchy of evidence. Given that the studies are adequately performed within the limitations of the design used, the reliability of the information from them can be ranked in the manner shown in Table 10.1. Most generally accepted classifications follow this format.

At the top are randomized intervention trials, if properly performed on adequate numbers of subjects and, of course, in the human situation. Evidence from such studies should be given the greatest weight because of the unique advantages of these studies in overcoming the problems of bias and confounding.

Second come observational studies of appropriately selected groups of subjects, that is, the cohort and case–control designs. There is logic in placing cohort studies somewhat ahead of case–control studies because, if well performed, cohort studies should have less observation bias, give clearer evidence of the time relationships of the association, and have a comparison group whose results are more easily interpreted. However, both these observational designs can have severe problems, and a well-performed case–control study may be of more value than a poorly performed cohort study.

As we have seen in Chapter 9, the data from many randomized trials can be summarized in a meta-analysis, and meta-analyses can also be done for cohort and case–control studies, although they are generally more difficult as there are usually greater methodological differences between the studies. Thus, in categories 1 and 2 in Table 10.1, we can give higher ranking to an appropriately performed meta-analysis which combines the results of several relevant trials. The best possible evidence relating

Table 10.1 A simple hierarchy of types of evidence relevant to human health studies. As well as the level of evidence, the consistency or otherwise of the results, the quality and detail of the studies, and the relevance of the studies to the situation and question of interest have to be assessed.

Level 1:	Randomized trials	1m: Results from a meta-analysis of trials
		1s: One or more individual trials
Level 2:	Cohort and case–control studies	2m: Results from a meta-analysis of such studies
		2s: One or more individual studies
Level 3:	Other comparative studies	
Level 4:	Case series, descriptive studies, professional experience, etc.	

to an intervention would come from a clear result from a well-performed meta-analysis of all available randomized trials.

The third level of evidence comes from studies comparing groups of subjects not chosen specifically for the purpose of the study but representing different population or subject groups. This includes correlation studies of populations in which data on each individual are not assessed separately, and also informal comparisons between patients in different hospitals, patients treated at different time periods, and so on.

In the fourth category there is evidence which is largely anecdotal, based on the unsystematic recollection of personal or group experience (sometimes referred to as 'clinical judgement' or 'experience'), conclusions based on traditional practice, and information derived from other species, *in vitro* testing, physiological principles, and other indirect assessments. Meta-analyses may also be applied to evidence in the third and fourth categories.

It is sensible to concentrate on the best possible evidence. If there are randomized trials available on the question, they should be evaluated first, and if they provide strong evidence for or against causality, the results of the other types of study may add little. For many topics, randomized trial evidence will not be available, and therefore we must look particularly at the results of well-performed cohort and case–control studies.

This general hierarchy of evidence is followed in the now numerous specific versions of hierarchies, some of which are becoming quite complicated. Terms may be used such as 'level 1 evidence', meaning randomized trials, 'level 2 evidence', meaning comparative observational studies, but the use of such terms varies and can be confusing. For example, because the best source of evidence for studies of the effects of hazardous exposures comes from cohort and case–control studies, some refer to these studies as level 1 evidence in this context. Many systematic reviews, including many Cochrane clinical reviews, use an even simpler ranking system, concentrating solely on randomized trials and ignoring other evidence.

Examples of critical appraisal processes

We have considered how to appraise one study or a set of studies, concentrating on whether the evidence supports a causal relationship between defined cause, and the defined effect. This is the essential first step in any process using that information for many specific purposes; we will comment on three such applications.

Clinical and policy recommendations: the US Preventive Services Task Force

The US Preventive Services Task Force (USPSTF) is a government supported, but independent, group created in 1984 that is recognized internationally as providing high-quality evidence-based recommendations. It deals with services including screening, counselling, and preventive interventions, orientated its recommendations to primary care in the United States. It was set up by Congress and relates to the Agency for Healthcare Research and Quality (AHRQ). It sets itself key criteria to ensure integrity: transparency, accountability, consistency, and independence [19]. In reviewing a particular intervention, it conducts systematic reviews of relevant literature on both benefits and

Table 10.2 Assessment of 'level of certainty' from evidence reviews by the US Preventive Services Task Force. They define this as 'likelihood that the USPSTF assessment of the net benefit of a preventive service is correct.' The net benefit is defined as benefit minus harm of the preventive service as implemented in a general, primary care population

Level of certainty	Description
High	The available evidence usually includes consistent results from well-designed, well-conducted studies in representative primary care populations. These studies assess the effects of the preventive service on health outcomes. This conclusion is therefore unlikely to be strongly affected by the results of future studies
Moderate	The available evidence is sufficient to determine the effects of the preventive service on health outcomes, but confidence in the estimate is constrained by such factors as: • The number, size, or quality of individual studies • Inconsistency of findings across individual studies • Limited generalizability of findings to routine primary care practice • Lack of coherence in the chain of evidence As more information becomes available, the magnitude or direction of the observed effect could change, and this change may be large enough to alter the conclusion
Low	The available evidence is insufficient to assess effects on health outcomes. Evidence is insufficient because of: • The limited number or size of studies • Important flaws in study design or methods • Inconsistency of findings across individual studies • Gaps in the chain of evidence • Findings not generalizable to routine primary care practice • Lack of information on important health outcomes. More information may allow estimation of effects on health outcomes

Reproduced with permission from US Preventive Services Task Force (USPSTF), *Grade Definitions*, revised July 2012, available from http://www.uspreventiveservicestaskforce.org/Page/Name/grade-definitions [21].

harms, considering six key questions [20]. These are very similar to the scheme set item this book in Box 10.1, and are to consider study design, internal validity, and external validity applied to the US population; and to ask how many studies, their size, the consistency of the results, and other factors such the Bradford Hill guidelines.

From the evaluation and the consideration of the balance between benefits and harms, the 'level of certainty' of the evidence is classified into three groups (Table 10.2). Then based on the certainty and on the estimated size of the net benefit, recommendations are made in five 'grades' of the level of certainty (Figure 10.2): they define this as 'likelihood that the USPSTF assessment of the net benefit of a preventive service is correct' [21]. The net benefit is defined as benefit minus harm of the preventive service

Grade	Definition	Suggestions for Practice
A	The USPSTF recommends the service. There is high certainty that the net benefit is substantial.	Offer or provide this service.
B	The USPSTF recommends the service. There is high certainty that the net benefit is moderate or there is moderate certainty that the net benefit is moderate to substantial.	Offer or provide this service.
C	The USPSTF recommends selectively offering or providing this service to individual patients based on professional judgment and patient preferences. There is at least moderate certainty that the net benefit is small.	Offer or provide this service for selected patients depending on individual circumstances.
D	The USPSTF recommends against the service. There is moderate or high certainty that the service has no net benefit or that the harms outweigh the benefits.	Discourage the use of this service.
I Statement	The USPSTF concludes that the current evidence is insufficient to assess the balance of benefits and harms of the service. Evidence is lacking, of poor quality, or conflicting, and the balance of benefits and harms cannot be determined.	Read the clinical considerations section of USPSTF Recommendation Statement. If the service is offered, patients should understand the uncertainty about the balance of benefits and harms.

Figure 10.2 The US Preventive Services Task Force (USPSTF) grades of recommendations: based on the strength of evidence and magnitude of net benefit (benefits minus harms). Reproduced with permission from US Preventive Services Task Force (USPSTF), *Grade Definitions*, revised July 2012, available from http://www.uspreventiveservicestaskforce.org/Page/Name/grade-definitions [21].

as implemented in a general, primary care population. Thus, a simple and clear scheme for final recommendations and summaries of the evidence comes from the extensive background work. Many other groups make such recommendations, in different countries, relating to different topics and different levels of care, but the methods of the USPSTF are often regarded as a model of good practice.

Clinical guidelines: the GRADE process

Clinical guidelines in the past were often produced by small groups of experts, perhaps in one medical speciality in one country or one hospital, using very variable methods of little or no documentation of the assessments made. The GRADE system—Grading of Recommendations Assessment, Development and Evaluation—has arisen from the voluntary efforts of practitioners and academic groups in many countries, and has achieved a high reputation, for example, being recommended by the *BMJ* since 2006 [22]. They categorize the overall evidence in four categories of high, moderate, low, and very low quality, defining these by whether the evidence is likely to change: thus high-quality evidence is unlikely to be changed by further research, whereas low-quality evidence is very likely to be changed [22]. The process pays considerable attention to patient choice and shared decision-making, and they summarize the factors that affect strength of a recommendation (Table 10.3). These include 'values and preferences', meaning the attitude of the patient; as many therapeutic choices involve a balance between different harms of different benefits, for example, a small long-term benefit compared to an immediate risk of side effects, these guidelines accept that people will vary in their consideration of these choices. The factors also include some degree of economic consideration.

The GRADE system advises that recommendations be placed in four categories of continuum (Figure 10.3), with a further category for interventions that should only be used in research. They define a 'strong' recommendation as applying where 'they believe that all or almost all informed people would make the recommended choice for or against an intervention', and a weak recommendation 'when they believe that most informed people would choose the recommended course of action, but a substantial number may not' [23].

The GRADE system is designed to assist physicians and patients in the individual care situation. For wider policy decisions, involving costs to society and affecting the care of whole populations, more importance will be paid to factors including the

Table 10.3 Factors that affect the strength of a recommendation, on the GRADE system

Factor	Examples of strong recommendations	Examples of weak recommendations
Quality of evidence	Many high quality randomised trials have shown the benefit of inhaled steroids in asthma	Only case series have examined the utility of pleurodesis in pneumothorax
Uncertainty about the balance between desirable and undesirable effects	Aspirin in myocardial infarction reduces mortality with minimal toxicity, inconvenience, and cost	Warfarin in low risk patients with atrial fibrillation results in small stroke reduction but increased bleeding risk and substantial in convenience
Uncertainty or variability in values and preferences	Young patients with lymphoma will invariably place a higher value on the life prolonging effects of chemotherapy than on treatment toxicity	Older patients with lymphoma may not place a higher value on the life prolonging effects of chemotherapy than on treatment toxicity
Uncertainty about whether the intervention represents a wise use of resources	The low cost of aspirin as prophylaxis against stroke in patients with transient ischemic attacks	The high cost of clopidogrel and of combination dipyridamole and aspirin as prophylaxis against stroke in patients with transient ischaemic attacks

Strength of recommendation on a continuum: categorical terminology

Figure 10.3 Suggested format by GRADE group for recommendations, as a continuum divided into categories.
Reprinted from the *Journal of Clinical Epidemiology*, Volume 66, Issue 7, Andrews J et al., 'GRADE guidelines: 14. Going from evidence to recommendations: the significance and presentation of recommendations,' pp. 719–725, © 2013 Published by Elsevier Inc., with permission from Elsevier, http://www.sciencedirect.com/science/journal/08954356 [23].

prevalence of the health problem, equity considerations, total costs and feasibility of implementation and acceptance. Groups such as the National Institute for Health and Care Excellence (NICE) in the United Kingdom have this orientation [24]. Further, many countries have Health Technology Assessment (HTA) procedures, usually applied where the evidence of the benefits and hazards of an intervention have been assessed, so that cost and implementation are the key elements; so such processes often include formal economic assessments. There is an international network of HTA agencies (http://www.inahta.org/).

The assessment of environmental hazards: the International Agency for Research on Cancer (IARC)

The International Agency for Research on Cancer is an independent scientific group which is part of the World Health Organization, and supported by 24 member countries (http://www.iarc.fr/). The programme to assess carcinogenic hazards produced its first monograph in 1972; a recent paper describing and supporting the work was authored by 123 independent scientists from 16 countries [25]. The choice of which potentially hazardous exposures are chosen for review is an open system, and any person or organization can make proposals. For each group of exposures to be assessed, a Working Group is set up, composed of scientists with appropriate expertise who have to be free of conflicts of interest; their names and disclosures of conflicts of interest are posted publicly on a website. All the relevant literature has to be accessed the evidence review; IARC staff have expertise in identifying and retrieving the scientific papers, for each scientist to assess. This process can take a year or more. The final report is produced by consensus, usually after much debate, usually in the 1- or 2-week meeting at IARC in Lyon, France. Working Group members are not paid for their time.

The IARC uses only four categories for the final decisions by; again a very extensive evaluation of evidence results in a simple summary (Table 10.4). Details of the criteria are given in the preamble to each of the monographs and on their website (http://

Table 10.4 Classification scheme for exposures assessed by the International Agency for Research on Cancer. Table shows the numbers of exposures assessed up to April, 2015 (total 970)

Classification	Number of exposures (up to 2015)	Examples
Group 1: the agent is carcinogenic to humans	114	Asbestos, alcoholic drinks, ionizing radiation, tobacco smoke
Group 2A: the agent is probably carcinogenic to humans	69	Indoor emissions from wood burning; shiftwork with circadian rhythm disruption; work as a hairdresser
Group 2B: the agent is possibly carcinogenic to humans	283	Gasoline; welding fumes; low frequency magnetic fields; radiofrequency electromagnetic fields
Group 3: the agent is not classifiable as to its carcinogenicity to humans	504	Chlorinated drinking water; polystyrene; selenium
Group 4: the agent is probably not carcinogenic to humans	1	Caprolactam (an organic compound used in the manufacture of Nylon-6)

Source: data from International Agency for Research on Cancer (IARC), *IARC Monographs on the Evaluation of Carcinogenic Risks to Humans*, IARC, Lyon, France, © IARC 2006, available from http://monographs.iarc.fr/ENG/Preamble/index.php

monographs.iarc.fr/ENG/Preamble/index.php). These final ratings are based on a consideration of epidemiological evidence in humans, studies in experimental animals, and other studies including effects on reproduction and development and genetic-related effects, including laboratory tests for carcinogenic actions. These areas are evaluated separately, and for each the evidence is classified as being 'sufficient' if 'a causal relationship has been established' between exposure and cancer production in humans or animals, with weaker evidence classified as 'limited evidence', 'inadequate evidence', or 'evidence suggesting a lack of carcinogenicity'. In keeping with the terminology used in this book, for epidemiological studies, sufficient evidence is described as 'a positive relationship between the exposure of cancer in studies in which chance, bias and finding could be ruled out with reasonable confidence'. The equivalent for animals is that a causal relationship between the exposure and an increased incidence of malignant neoplasms has been shown in '(a) two or more species of animals or (b) two or more independent studies in one species carried out at different times or of different laboratories or hundred different protocols'. For the overall evaluation, both the human and animal evidence is used.

Up to 2015, the IARC had considered 970 different exposures [25]. Group 1, 114 classed as 'carcinogenic to humans', are established as carcinogenic, with both epidemiological and animal evidence to support that. Group 2A, 'probably carcinogenic' is a fairly small group including 69 exposures. Group 2B is a much larger group, 283 grouped 'possibly carcinogenic'. This means that there is some scientific evidence suggesting a carcinogenic effect, but other evidence against that, or there are major limitations in the quality or extent of information available. Group 3 is the largest group (504), defined as 'not classifiable', meaning that neither the epidemiological nor the experimental evidence is substantial enough, clear enough, or consistent enough, to come to any reasonable conclusion. Group 4 is exposures that have been considered by the process, but categorized as 'probably not carcinogenic'. There is only one substance in this category, because of course this IARC assessment procedure is resource-intensive and not used unless there is a substantial suspicion of a hazard.

The IARC does not make recommendations for how to deal with carcinogens, leaving that to the environmental and regulatory agencies in each country. For the substances reported on, the monographs are often the best single source of information on the exposure itself and studies relating to carcinogenicity. While concentrating on cancer, if an exposure has effects on other diseases, those also may be covered. The IARC process has been imitated by many other systems of evaluation of hazards, although these are often less thorough.

References

1. **MacMahon B**. Epidemiological evidence on the nature of Hodgkin's disease. *Cancer* 1957; **10**(5):1045–1054.
2. **Glaser SL, Jarrett RF**. The epidemiology of Hodgkin's disease. *Baillieres Clin Haematol* 1996; **9**(3):401–416.
3. **Howe GR, Burch JD, Miller AB, Morrison B, Gordon P, Weldon L, et al**. Artificial sweeteners and human bladder cancer. *Lancet* 1977; **2**:578–581.
4. **Rothman KJ, Moore LL, Singer MR, Nguyen US, Mannino S, Milunsky A**. Teratogenicity of high vitamin A intake. *N Engl J Med* 1995; **333**(21):1369–1373.
5. **Smith DC, Prentice R, Thompson DJ, Herrmann WL**. Association of exogenous estrogen and endometrial carcinoma. *N Engl J Med* 1975; **293**(23):1164–1167.
6. **Daly E, Vessey MP, Hawkins MM, Carson JL, Gough P, Marsh S**. Risk of venous thromboembolism in users of hormone replacement therapy. *Lancet* 1996; **348**:977–980.
7. **Jick H, Derby LE, Myers MW, Vasilakis C, Newton KM**. Risk of hospital admission for idiopathic venous thromboembolism among users of postmenopausal oestrogens. *Lancet* 1996; **348**:981–983.
8. **Grodstein F, Stampfer MJ, Goldhaber SZ, Manson JE, Colditz GA, Speizer FE, et al**. Prospective study of exogenous hormones and risk of pulmonary embolism in women. *Lancet* 1996; **348**:983–987.
9. **Hill D, White V, Jolley D, Mapperson K**. Self examination of the breast: is it beneficial? Meta-analysis of studies investigating breast self-examination and extent of disease in patients with breast cancer. *BMJ* 1988; **297**:271–275.
10. **Elwood JM, Little J, Elwood JH**. *Epidemiology and Control of Neural Tube Defects*. Oxford: Oxford University Press; 1992.
11. **Hill AB**. The environment and disease: association or causation? *Proc R Soc Med* 1965; **58**:295–300.

12. Greenland S, Sheppard AR, Kaune WT, Poole C, Kelsh MA. A pooled analysis of magnetic fields, wire codes, and childhood leukemia. *Epidemiology* 2000; **11**:624–634.

13. Zhao L, Liu X, Wang C, Yan K, Lin X, Li S, et al. Magnetic fields exposure and childhood leukemia risk: a meta-analysis based on 11,699 cases and 13,194 controls. *Leuk Res* 2014; **38**(3):269–274.

14. Mitchell LE, Adzick NS, Melchionne J, Pasquariello PS, Sutton LN, Whitehead AS. Spina bifida. *Lancet* 2004; **364**(9448):1885–1895.

15. Emanuel I, Sever LE. Questions concerning the possible association of potatoes and neural-tube defects, and an alternative hypothesis relating to maternal growth and development. *Teratology* 1973; **8**:325–332.

16. Miller AB, Lindsay J, Hill GB. Mortality from cancer of the uterus in Canada and its relationship to screening for cancer of the cervix. *Int J Cancer* 1976; **17**(5):602–612.

17. Sloan JH, Kellermann AL, Reay DT, Ferris JA, Koepsell T, Rivara FP, et al. Handgun regulations, crime, assaults, and homocide. *N Engl J Med* 1988; **319**(19):1256–1262.

18. Elwood M. Forward projection—using critical appraisal in the design of studies. *Int J Epidemiol* 2002; **31**:1071–1073.

19. Guirguis-Blake J, Calonge N, Miller T, Siu A, Teutsch S, Whitlock E. Current processes of the U.S. Preventive Services Task Force: refining evidence-based recommendation development. *Ann Intern Med* 2007; **147**(2):117–122.

20. Sawaya GF, Guirguis-Blake J, Lefevre M, Harris R, Petitti D. Update on the methods of the U.S. Preventive Services Task Force: estimating certainty and magnitude of net benefit. *Ann Intern Med* 2007; **147**(12):871–875.

21. U.S. Preventive Services Task Force. *Grade Definitions*. 2014. Available from: http://www.uspreventiveservicestaskforce.org/Page/Name/grade-definitions

22. Guyatt GH, Oxman AD, Vist GE, Kunz R, Falck-Ytter Y, onso-Coello P, et al. GRADE: an emerging consensus on rating quality of evidence and strength of recommendations. *BMJ* 2008; **336**(7650):924–926.

23. Andrews J, Guyatt G, Oxman AD, Alderson P, Dahm P, Falck-Ytter Y, et al. GRADE guidelines: 14. Going from evidence to recommendations: the significance and presentation of recommendations. *J Clin Epidemiol* 2013; **66**(7):719–725.

24. National Institute for Health and Care Excellence (NICE). *Developing NICE Guidelines: The Manual.* 2015. Available from: http://www.nice.org.uk/article/pmg20/resources/non-guidance-developing-nice-guidelines-the-manual-pdf

25. Pearce NE, Blair A, Vineis P, Ahrens W, Andersen A, Anto JM, et al. IARC monographs: 40 years of evaluating carcinogenic hazards to humans. *Environ Health Perspect* 2015; **123**(6):507–514.

Chapter 11

Critical appraisal in action

Introduction to Chapters 12–17

The following six chapters present examples of the application of the scheme for critical appraisal to six studies of different types: randomized trials of interventions, observational cohort studies, and case–control studies.

These studies have been chosen because they were published in prominent medical journals (*The Lancet, The New England Journal of Medicine*, and the *Journal of the National Cancer Institute*), and the summaries and usually the full text can be obtained through the Internet. An extract from each study has been reproduced, with the permission of the journal and the first author. The main elements of the study and the key results are described in these appraisals, and so it is possible to follow the study from the material presented here.

However, to gain most value from these appraisals, you are urged to find the original paper and work through it, applying the scheme for critical appraisal presented in this book, and summarized in Chapter 10 in Box 10.1. You should prepare a summary of your own appraisal, with brief answers to each of the questions in Box 10.1. This includes summarizing the key result of the study in as simple a table as possible. You are encouraged to calculate for yourself the key measure of effect and an appropriate statistical test, even if a more sophisticated analysis is given in the original paper. You should be able to summarize the main conclusions in terms of the internal and external validity of the study: What does it show? Is it true? Is it relevant? You can then compare your appraisal with the one given here; you will likely note several points that may not be covered here.

The assessment of any study involves specific subject matter knowledge as well as a methodological framework. The subject matter issues of these various studies are not dealt with here in any detail, although some comments on their substantive importance are made. At the end of each of these chapters there is a brief summary of the situation since the study was published up to the time of writing (2015). The general system of critical appraisal is a framework which helps to identify the major strengths and weaknesses of any study, so that you can then concentrate on the particular issues of critical importance.

These studies have been chosen for their accessibility, because they address important issues, and because they are good examples of the research methods. All represent important research contributions. In some of these chapters, the end conclusion will be that the association seen is due to either causation or confounding; for others, observation bias or chance variation are the main alternative explanations. All have questions of generalizability.

In each of the following six chapters, we will go through the 20 questions set out in Box 10.1 in sufficient detail to illustrate the key points. The approach is not exhaustive; the reader may be able to add more to each particular issue.

Chapter 12

Critical appraisal of a randomized clinical trial

Introduction

This randomized clinical trial was published in *The Lancet*, 2 July 2005, 366, 37–43 [1]. The summary is reproduced here, and the full paper can be accessed at http://www.thelancet.com or at http://www.sciencedirect.com/science/article/pii/ S0140673605667098.

Chloramphenicol treatment for acute infective conjunctivitis in children in primary care: a randomised double-blind placebo-controlled trial

Peter W Rose, Anthony Harnden, Angela B Brueggemann, Rafael Perera, Aziz Sheikh, Derrick Crook, David Mant

Summary

Background. One in eight schoolchildren have an episode of acute infective conjunctivitis every year. Standard clinical practice is to prescribe a topical antibiotic, although the evidence to support this practice is scarce. We undertook a randomised double-blind trial to compare the effectiveness of chloramphenicol eye drops with placebo in children with infective conjunctivitis in primary care.

Methods. Our study included 326 children aged 6 months to 12 years with a clinical diagnosis of conjunctivitis who were recruited from 12 general medical practices in the United Kingdom. We assigned 163 children to receive chloramphenicol eye drops and 163 to receive placebo eye drops. Eye swabs were taken for bacterial and viral analysis. The primary outcome was clinical cure at day 7, which was assessed from diaries completed by parents. All children were followed up for 6 weeks to identify relapse. Survival statistics were used for comparison, and analysis was by intention to treat.

Findings. Nine children were lost to follow-up (one in chloramphenicol group; eight in placebo group). Clinical cure by day 7 occurred in 128 (83 per cent) of 155 children with placebo compared with 140 (86 per cent) of 162 with chloramphenicol (risk difference 3.8 per cent, 95 per cent CI −4.1 per cent to 11.8 per cent). Seven (4 per cent) children with chloramphenicol and five (3 per cent) with placebo had further conjunctivitis episodes within 6 weeks (1.2 per cent, −2.9 per cent to 5.3 per cent). Adverse events were rare and evenly distributed between each group.

Interpretation. Most children presenting with acute infective conjunctivitis in primary care will get better by themselves and do not need treatment with an antibiotic.

Reprinted with permission from *The Lancet*, Volume 366, Number 9479, Peter W Rose et al., 'Chloramphenicol treatment for acute infective conjunctivitis in children in primary care: a randomised double-blind placebo-controlled trial', pp. 37–43, © 2005 Elsevier Ltd, with permission from Elsevier, http://www.sciencedirect.com/science/journal/01406736.

A. Description of the evidence

1. What was the exposure or intervention?
2. What was the outcome?
3. What was the study design?
4. What was the study population?
5. What was the main result?

As stated in the summary, this trial was undertaken to assess whether using antibiotic eye drops (chloramphenicol) in children with conjunctivitis is any more effective than a placebo. The background explained in the paper is that conjunctivitis in children is a common complaint presenting to general practitioners, and it is usually treated with antibiotic eye drops although there is no strong evidence that such treatment is beneficial. This results in extensive prescribing of antibiotics at considerable costs, and some schools require children to be treated before they return to school. It is noted that there has been a Cochrane systematic review of the treatment of conjunctivitis in adults and children, which showed superiority of antibiotic treatment to placebo, but it is noted that all the trials included in that review were based on hospital populations, with patients who are likely to have more severe infections. It is not stated if the review was of all ages, and if results specific to children are available.

The intervention tested was regular use of 0.5 per cent chloramphenicol eye drops, compared with placebo eye drops containing water, boric acid, and borax, which could have a soothing effect.

The definition of the outcome is important. The primary outcome measure, decided in advance, was the clinical cure rate at 7 days, as stated by the parents who were asked to keep a diary. The time of cure was defined as the first recorded time in the diary after which none of the three symptoms of pain, redness, or discharge was recorded. There was also an assessment by a research nurse at study entry and at 7 days, and the nurse took two conjunctival swabs from the more affected eye at these times; microbiological cure or improvement was defined on these results. So, clinical cure was the primary end point.

The study design was a randomized controlled trial, comparing the active agent with a placebo, and the study was double-blind, with neither the treating doctors nor the children or their parents being aware of whether the active drug or placebo was used. Although the family doctors identified the eligible patients, they were then seen by a research nurse either at the doctor's premises or at home. The study was explained to parents and children old enough to understand, with standard information sheets designed for children being used, and written consent was obtained. The full paper has quite a long section describing the procedures. A research nurse assessed the clinical severity of the conjunctivitis, assessing the degree of redness by comparison with validated photographs, and then the active drug or placebo was provided. These had been prepared to be in identical bottles, labelled A or B, with the persons knowing the code not participating in the trial. Parents were given instructions for administration of the drugs, and also given a symptom sheet to fill in every time drops were given. The research nurse saw the children again at 7-day follow-up, and further swabs were taken for laboratory examination. Finally, parents were telephoned 6 weeks after the trial had started to identify any further problems or recurrences. Further details of the laboratory techniques are given, which need not concern us here.

The study population, as is usual in clinical trials, is specified in detail and has some restrictions. The target population comprises children in the United Kingdom or a similar country presenting to a primary care practitioner with conjunctivitis. The source population was 12 general practices in Oxfordshire, UK. Eligible subjects were children aged between 6 months and 12 years, who presented during office hours and had a diagnosis of acute infective conjunctivitis. There were some exclusions for clinical reasons—children allergic to chloramphenicol, those with evidence of severe infection that would necessitate active treatment, those who were immunocompromised, and those who were taking an antibiotic currently or within the previous 48 hours—to avoid modification of the intervention. The restriction to children who presented during office hours was for logistical reasons. The study was done over the winter period of October to April in three consecutive years from 2001 to 2004. Participants are those eligible children who were identified, and whose parents gave written consent to their participation.

The main result of the study is the proportion of children clinically cured, that is, symptom free, at 7 days, as assessed by the parents' diaries. Nine children had an unknown outcome, and were excluded from the results shown in the summary: this will be discussed later. The key results are shown in Box 12.1. This shows that 140 of the 162 children randomized to treatment with chloramphenicol were clinically cured (86.4 per cent) compared with 128 out of the 155 children randomized to placebo (82.6 per cent). Thus there is a slightly higher cure rate in the actively treated group, but this is not statistically significant. The result shown in the paper (summary, and in Table 3) is the risk difference, 3.8 per cent, and its 95 per cent confidence limits, which were –4.1 per cent and 11.8 per cent. The number needed to treat, which is the inverse of the risk difference of 3.8 per cent, is 26: thus from these results, 26 children would need treated for one extra child being clinically cured at 7 days. Also shown in Box 12.1 are the full calculations for this 2 × 2 table, using the methods described in Chapters 4 and 8.

Box 12.1 Main outcome of trial comparing antibiotic treatment with placebo for conjunctivitis in children

RESULTS OF A RANDOMIZED TRIAL

Result shown in summary, for primary outcome of clinical cure at day 7

(Nine participants lost to follow-up and excluded)

	Clinical cure	Not cured	Total assessed	Proportion cured	Percentage cured
Chloramphenicol	**140**	22	**162**	0.864	86.4
Placebo	**128**	27	**155**	0.826	82.6
Total	268	49	317	0.845	84.5

Risk calculations

Relative risk	= 0.864/0.826	1.05
Odds ratio	= (140 × 27)/ (128 × 22)	1.34
Risk difference	= (0.864 – 0.826) × 100	3.84 per cent
Number needed to treat = 1/(risk difference)		26.0

Statistical test (Mantel–Haenszel)

$a = 140$	$E = 136.9589905$	$V = 10.38417$
$\chi^2 = 0.89$	$\chi = 0.94$	$P = 0.345$

Confidence limits are calculated based on the standard deviation of ln RR, ln OR, or RD, following Table A2.2

	Value	ln	Std dev	95% confidence limits	
Relative risk	1.05	0.0454	0.0483	0.95	1.15
Odds ratio	1.34	0.2944	0.3122	0.73	2.48
Risk difference (%)	3.839		4.065	–4.1	11.8%
Number needed to treat = 1/(risk difference)				8.5	infinity

Source: data from Peter W Rose et al., 'Chloramphenicol treatment for acute infective conjunctivitis in children in primary care: a randomised double-blind placebo-controlled trial', *The Lancet*, Volume 366, Number 9479, pp. 37–43, © 2005 Elsevier Ltd [1].

The relative risk is 1.05, and the odds ratio is 1.34; these differ because the frequency of the outcome is high; relative risk is easier to interpret here.

This outcome examines only if children had a clinical cure or not at one point in time, that is, 7 days. The first time at which the children were symptom free could be assessed from the parents' diaries, and Figure 3 of the paper shows the cumulative proportion of children with clinical cure at each day after recruitment. This is presented as a cumulative incidence curve for clinical cure, using the Kaplan–Meier calculation shown in Chapter 8. This shows that the time to cure, that is, the duration of the conjunctivitis, tended to be shorter in the group receiving chloramphenicol; for example, the median time, at which 50 per cent of the children were cured, was around 3.5 days for the chloramphenicol group and around 4 days for the placebo group.

Further outcome data are given for the subgroup of children with confirmed bacterial pathogens and full follow-up, in whom the risk difference was in fact smaller than in the intention-to-treat analysis (Table 12.1). This shows that there was no larger effect in confirmed bacterial cases. Results for 'microbiological cure', that is, the eye swabs at day 7 being free from pathogens, are also shown. These give a higher cure rate in the chloramphenicol group; the risk difference is 16.8 per cent, which is statistically significant. Further results are given in the original paper.

B. Internal validity: consideration of non-causal explanations

6. Are the results likely to be affected by observation bias?

Observation bias is a critical issue, as the primary outcome is defined as 'cure', based on observations by each child's parents, and is open to observer variation. Clinical cure was defined in advance as the absence of the key symptoms of pain, redness, or discharge, as recorded in the parents' diaries. The parents were asked to keep a regular record of symptoms, recording them each time the drops were given, rather than being asked to state when symptoms resolved. It might be thought that a more 'scientific' outcome would be, for example, the rate of bacteriological or viral clearance as detected by the eye swabs at day 7, or the clinical observations by the nurse at day 7, and these outcomes were also assessed, but there is wisdom in the definition of clinical cure used in the study. It allows constant observation; the parents are acting as unpaid researchers in recording the study end point. More importantly, this definition of clinical cure is what is used in normal practice in primary care, and is what affects activities such as return to school. In the paper there is discussion of this, and it is pointed out that the relationship between clinical state and bacteriological findings is mixed, as bacteria and viruses can be isolated from normal eyes, and are isolated from only a proportion of eyes with clinical conjunctivitis. Thus clinical cure can occur without microbiological clearance. Therefore the outcome chosen is clinically relevant, and can be observed continuously in time. However, it is still weak methodologically; the outcome is assessed by laypersons, and a different person makes the observations of outcome for each child in the study. There will be considerable observer variation, which may be random but could vary with the characteristics of the parents or the child (e.g. some parents will be health professionals, and the observations may be more difficult in younger children).

The chief defence against this is the fact that the study is randomized, a placebo is used, and the essential element is that the trial is double-blind. Some of the parents may have suspected or assumed that the treatment their child was receiving was either active or placebo, but as long as the blindness is preserved, it protects against any

Table 12.1 Several outcomes assessed in the randomized trial.

Outcome	Basis of comparison	Chloramphenicol			No. events	Placebo		Risk difference%	95% confidence limits	
		No. events	No. children assessed	Rate%		No. children assessed	Rate%			
Clinical cure at day 7	Intention to treat	140	163	85.9	128	163	78.5	7.4	−0.9	15.6
	Excluding lost to follow-up	140	162	86.4	128	155	82.6	3.8	−4.1	11.8
	Children with bacteria isolated, and full information	101	119	84.9	94	117	80.3	4.5	−5.1	14.2
Microbiological cure at day 7	Only subjects with information	50	125	40.0	29	125	23.2	16.8	5.5	28.1
Adverse clinical events, day 1 to 7	Excluding lost to follow-up	3	162	1.9	3	155	1.9	−0.1	−2.9	2.9
Further episodes of conjunctivitis within 6 weeks	Only subjects with information on 6 weeks' follow-up	7	157	4.5	5	150	3.3	1.1	−2.9	5.3

Source: data from Peter W Rose et al., 'Chloramphenicol treatment for acute infective conjunctivitis in children in primary care: a randomised double-blind placebo-controlled trial', *The Lancet*, Volume 366, Number 9479, pp. 37–43, © 2005 Elsevier Ltd [1].

systematic observation bias between the two groups. This method of recording the clinical outcome would be very inadvisable in a study which was not double-blind and placebo-controlled.

Results are also presented for microbiological cure, which interestingly enough show a statistically significant difference in favour of chloramphenicol, and the results for microbiological improvement, or for the combination of cure or improvement, while not statistically significant, show larger effects than the results based on the clinical cure. This could be because the drug is more effective at producing a biological cure than a clinical cure, or because of a larger degree of random observation error with respect to the clinical data. The children were also assessed clinically by the research nurse at the beginning of the study and to day 7, and those results would be interesting in this respect, but are not given. In later correspondence, the authors state that the clinical cure rate assessed by the nurses was 79 per cent in the chloramphenicol group and 78 per cent in the placebo group [2]. In summary, we must accept that there will be some random error in the clinical cure information, which might impact to reduce the observed difference, but bias in the clinical observations is unlikely to be important.

7. Are the results likely to be affected by confounding?

The prime protection against confounding is the randomized design, applied to a reasonably large number of study entrants, and the correct intention-to-treat analysis. Of course, randomization does not guarantee that the two groups are comparable on all relevant factors, and information is presented on demographic factors, clinical features, and results of microbiological assessment at baseline, in Tables 1 and 2 of the paper. These show very similar distributions, showing the value of the randomization. The group receiving chloramphenicol includes slightly more children with unilateral disease and a slightly higher social class distribution, but the distributions for other factors and bacterial and viral results are very similar. The relevant factors are those related to the outcome of acute conjunctivitis in children, and a literature review or specialist knowledge is needed to assess if there are other important relevant factors. If there had been substantial differences in recorded potential confounding factors despite the randomization, stratification or multivariate analysis could be used, as described in Chapters 7 and 8.

The randomization process is described. Family doctors identified eligible children and parents, and gave them an information sheet. Then a research nurse explained the study, and received consent from those who chose to participate. Identical numbered bottles of the active and the placebo agent had been prepared; the nurse contacted the randomization centre and gave a bottle to the family, chosen according to the assigned number. The randomization was in blocks of 10; so for each 10 children, five received active drug and five received placebo. The main analysis of the study was done before the randomization code was broken, so the study could be described as being triple-blind.

The protection against confounding requires an intention-to-treat analysis, that is, the group randomized to active treatment (not just the children who received the treatment) was compared with the group randomized to placebo, as discussed in Chapter 7. There is likely to be considerable variation in the actual regimen of treatment; some parents may be very rigorous, others less so. Again, this mirrors normal practice, and the double-blind trial design should ensure that such variations are similar in the two groups. Some children may have had very little treatment; others may have had other treatment in addition to the study treatment. One child was found not to fulfil the eligibility criteria (by being too old) after randomization, and was withdrawn from the study. This is acceptable, but if a large number of children were found to be ineligible after randomization, that would raise questions about the quality of the study process.

As would be expected in any trial, some participants entered the study but did not complete it, being 'lost to follow-up'. These children may be substantially different in factors which could be related to outcome. An intention-to-treat analysis can include these children, but assumptions must be made about their outcome. In this study only nine of the 326 children had missing outcome data; this small number testifies to the care taken in the practical aspects of this study. However, presumably simply by chance, one child was randomized to the active treatment group and eight to the placebo group. In the results shown in the summary and in Box 12.1, these nine children were excluded. The predetermined protocol was to that assume children lost to follow-up were failures of treatment; so, on an intention-to-treat analysis, the proportion in the placebo group with clinical cure falls to 128/163, 78.5 per cent, and is little changed in the treatment group, 140/163, 85.9 per cent. So the difference between the groups is larger, although still non-significant: the risk difference is 7.4 per cent, with 95 per cent limits of −0.90 to 15.6 per cent. If we make the opposite assumption, that all children lost to follow-up were cured, the cure rates would be 83.4 per cent in the placebo group and 86.5 per cent in the treatment group, with a smaller risk difference of 3.1 per cent, again non-significant. Given that the overall cure rate was high, at 83 per cent, an assumption that those lost to follow-up were cured would probably be more accurate than the assumption that they were treatment failures. Therefore although the numbers of children lost to follow-up are very small, because the numbers are unevenly distributed this does influence the results, and larger numbers lost to follow-up could make the results very difficult to interpret. Indeed, this type of analysis—considering the results based on different assumptions—is helpful; in all these analyses, the difference in outcome between the groups compared is not significant.

The fact that more children were lost to follow-up in the placebo group also raises a question about whether the blinding could have been compromised. Could families who received the placebo have guessed that, and therefore have lost interest in the study more readily than families with active treatment? We have the authors' assurance that the drops and bottles were identical and the same numbers were prescribed extra antibiotics (see next paragraph), and the overall results of the trial would suggest that the clinical course of the disease was similar, so the inequity of distribution of loss to follow-up is probably just chance variation.

Some children were prescribed antibiotic eye drops during the trial; presumably their parents or practitioners were concerned or impatient. These children were correctly included in the main analysis, as excluding them would compromise the randomization. This extra treatment could be associated with the outcome, and if unevenly distributed between the two groups, would be a confounding factor. However, this only applied to 12 children, 6 in each group. If a large number had received extra treatment outside the protocol, and if the numbers had been unequal in each group, this would raise questions of interpretation. The effect of an equal distribution of such extra treatment would tend to decrease any real difference in effectiveness between the chloramphenicol and placebo groups in the trial, but only if the extra treatment were effective; otherwise it would have no effect on the study.

Thus because the study was reasonably large, the groups compared were obtained by randomization, and losses to follow-up were few, confounding is unlikely to have any substantial influence on the results.

8. Are the results likely to be affected by chance variation?

These results show the problems of concentrating on a conventional significance level of 5 per cent. The results shown in Box 12.1 are not statistically significant. The analysis taking the time to cure into consideration gives a log-rank statistic (see Chapter 8) with a P-value of 0.025, which is statistically significant. Overall, the probability that the difference seen is due only to chance, and the real situation is that the clinical cure rate is the same with either active or placebo treatment, is reasonably substantial. However, the results do show an increased cure rate with chloramphenicol, and this may be the true situation.

The graph in Figure 3 of the paper also raises the question of whether the small difference in cure rate at 7 days persists. The telephone follow-up with the parents at 6 weeks showed that further episodes of conjunctivitis were experienced by 4 per cent of children with active treatment and 3 per cent of those on placebo. It is not clear whether the conjunctivitis resolved in all other children, or when it did.

In assessing chance variation we need to assess both whether appropriate tests have been used, and whether they have been done at the appropriate time. In clinical trials the issues of multiple testing, and perhaps publication of results or termination of studies on the basis of one of a series of tests, are relevant. With regard to this study, there is a clearly stated protocol setting the follow-up at 7 days, and there is no issue with interim or frequent analyses.

Thus we cannot exclude chance variation in this study, nor can we be sure that chance variation explains the results. The difference in outcome at 7 days and the more sensitive analysis of time to cure give results close to the conventional 0.05 significance level.

This raises a question of whether the trial had sufficient statistical power. The statistical design is well described. An earlier study had shown a 19 per cent improvement in outcome with antibiotics, regarded as clinically important. So, the study was designed to have 500 participants, based on 80 per cent power to detect a 19 per cent difference, a cure rate in the placebo arm of 72 per cent, using a two-sided test at the 5 per cent significance level; and it was further assumed that 60 per cent of children would have a bacterial aetiology, and only in these would a difference be seen. The method by which the sample size was calculated is not given. The relatively simple method described in Chapter 8 using the given figures gives a sample size of 124 in each group; increasing this by 100/60 gives 207 in each group, 414 in total. It is best to increase this to account for losses to follow-up and other issues, so the sample size of 500 seems reasonable. When the trial was started, there was bacterial infection in almost 80 per cent and an overall cure rate of more than 80 per cent. The higher bacterial component increases the power of the study; a recalculation showed that randomization of 326 children gave 80 per cent power to detect a 12–14 per cent difference, and therefore recruitment to the trial was stopped early. This trial took 3 years to complete recruitment, and was obviously difficult logistically, so this may be reasonable, but in fact the results are somewhat borderline in statistical terms and a larger sample size would have been advantageous.

C. Internal validity: consideration of positive features of causation

9. Is there a correct time relationship?

This is not a problem in an intervention study; the outcomes follow the randomization. An intention-to-treat analysis must include events from the time of randomization, even if they occur prior to the intervention. In this trial, the whole process was rapid. The children were identified by the family doctors, and seen by a research nurse usually within 4 hours. After informed consent, the treatment was allocated and started. There was active follow-up over 7 days and a 6-week telephone follow-up, completed for an impressive 307 children, 94 per cent of study entrants. All trials have time limitations; obviously, no statements can be made about events later than 6 weeks.

10. Is the relationship strong?

The value of a strong relationship in an observational study is largely because bias and confounding are usually more readily detected for a strong association. In a randomized double-blind trial, such issues can be dealt with firmly, and so the strength of the relationship is less crucial to internal validity, although still helpful. The relationship observed here is weak, with a small difference in clinical cure rate and somewhat larger differences in the time to cure and the microbiological cure rate. All these differences show better outcomes in the active treatment group, but the small size of the difference means that the differences could simply be due to chance. The weak association also means that small differences in confounding factors could be influential, despite the randomization. Observation bias can be excluded from the double-blind design, but a substantial amount of non-differential misclassification in the clinical outcome assessment may have occurred, which would diminish the observed difference if there were true difference in outcome between the two groups. The fact that the difference in microbiological cure rate was greater might be because of less non-differential error. The more important aspect in this study is the clinical implications of the size of the difference, as will be discussed.

11. Is there a dose–response relationship?

Only one fixed dose of the chloramphenicol eye drops was used. In other trials, more than one dose or time course of treatment may be used, and consideration of dose–response may be relevant. We could ask whether the children who received the drops according to the protocol, rather than in smaller amounts or perhaps not at all, had better outcomes, and if the drug is active it is logical that they should. However, children who accepted full doses of treatment are likely to be very different to those who did not (see Chapter 7). No information on compliance in the trial is presented in this paper, although the design allows assessment of compliance. The implication is that compliance was good, and perhaps the requirement of the parents both to give the treatment and to record symptoms in the diary every time treatment was given has ensured that.

12. Are the results consistent within the study?
And 13. Is there any specificity within the study?

As consistency and specificity are often related, they can be discussed together. Consistency is often a relevant issue in clinical trials, as we wish to know whether the intervention has different effects in some groups of patients. However, this requires the trial to be specifically designed to answer questions about subgroups of patients. The use of post hoc analysis looking at subgroups of patients defined after the trial has been done is open both to the problems of multiple comparisons and comparisons between non-randomized groups. Such analyses are appropriately avoided in this paper.

The one pre-planned subgroup analysis was in terms of microbiological cause, although this is limited because few children did not have a bacterial pathogen. The results for those who did (Table 12.1) are similar to the overall result; this excludes children lost to follow-up as they did not have the further swab taken. If the results for those without bacteria isolated are calculated by subtraction, the result is similar, with wider confidence limits as the numbers are small. This is consistent with no overall effect. It might be expected that if chloramphenicol were effective, this effect would be restricted to, or increased in, children in whom bacterial pathogens were isolated. The demonstration of such specificity would strengthen the evidence for a real effect. It would also depend on the validity of the isolation of pathogens as showing the aetiology of the child's condition; it cannot be assumed that children from whom bacteria were not isolated were in fact free from bacteria. The results compared are consistent within the trial in that there is reasonable consistency between microbiological and clinical cure, although the effect on microbiological cure is larger, and the pattern of time to cure shows a smooth trend.

Other relevant assessments of consistency could be by the age, sex, and social group of the children, or by different bacterial or viral results or different clinical features. However, such assessments have the major problem of being subgroup analyses in a relatively small study, and if any differences were seen they could well be due to chance.

Conclusions with regard to internal validity

This is a well-designed and carefully performed randomized trial, and so we can be reasonably confident about its internal validity. We can dismiss with considerable certainty observation bias and confounding as explanations of the differences seen. As is often the case with randomized trials, statistical variation is an issue, and we cannot firmly conclude whether the small differences in outcome between the active treatment and placebo groups are simply due to chance variation or are reflecting real differences.

D. External validity: generalization of the results

The next few questions relate to the generalizability of the results from the study participants to the populations from which they are derived, following the approach set out in Chapter 5. A profile of the trial, following the CONSORT principles [3], was given in the paper and is shown as Figure 12.1.

In the first question, we must first assess if there are any differences between the study participants—those who complete the study and provide data for the analysis—and the study entrants. Then we assess issues comparing the study entrants with the eligible population.

14. Can the study results be applied to the eligible population?

Almost all children entering the study completed it. There were 327 study entrants, that is, children who were randomized, and of these one was found after randomization to be too old to be eligible. Finding subjects to be ineligible after they have been randomized is not uncommon. In principle, any exclusions after randomization compromise the validity of the randomization, but keeping an ineligible subject in the trial analysis also breaches the protocol. With only one subject affected, the choice to withdraw that subject is reasonable. The remaining 326 children were divided equally by the randomization process, and all appear in the main analyses. However, nine were lost to follow-up and so the outcomes for these children were unknown. The remaining 317 completed the main trial, with outcomes assessed at 7 days. There was a telephone follow-up 6 weeks later, completed for 307 children, with 10 not assessed. The fact that very few study entrants did not complete this study is a major strength. If the study losses are similar equal in each group, that is also helpful. Here, there were five children in each group for whom the 6-week follow-up information was not available. However, of the nine children lost to follow-up earlier, one had been allocated to chloramphenicol and eight to placebo, and so the handling of these can affect the results.

A strong aspect of this study is that the generalizability is explicitly addressed in the study design. During 1 week of each month during active recruitment for the trial, the records of the practitioners involved in the study were audited to find all children in the eligible age group who presented with acute infective conjunctivitis, including those presenting out of working hours. Thus it was established that during the recruitment period, 29 per cent of all eligible children entered the study. It would also be helpful to know the reasons for non-participation: how many were out of hours? How

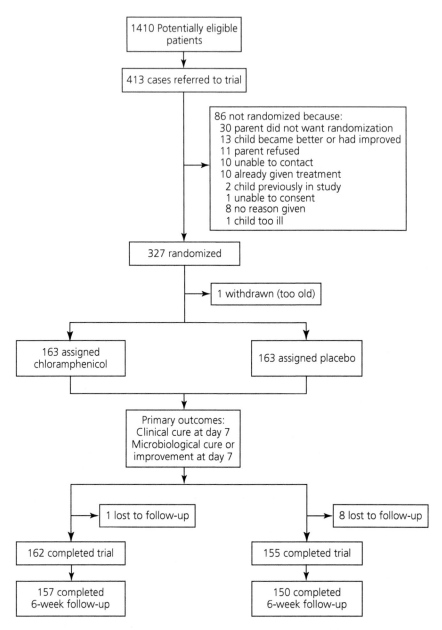

Figure 12.1 Flowchart of trial comparing antibiotic treatment with placebo for conjunctivitis in children.

Reprinted with permission from *The Lancet*, Volume 366, Number 9479, Peter W Rose et al., 'Chloramphenicol treatment for acute infective conjunctivitis in children in primary care: a randomised double-blind placebo-controlled trial', pp. 37–43, © 2005 Elsevier Ltd, with permission from Elsevier, http://www.sciencedirect.com/science/journal/01406736 [1].

many of the rest were not approached? How many were invited to participate but declined? The authors point out that children presenting out of working hours may have had more severe symptoms, and also that family doctors may have tended to exclude children with more severe symptoms, feeling that they required antibiotics; therefore the participants may have had less severe conjunctivitis than a representative sample. However, the fact that for 78 per cent of the children recruited, bacteria were cultured from the eye swabs shows that the participants had significant pathology. It is reasonable to assume that the results can be applied to the eligible population.

15. Can the study results be applied to the source population?

The source population is children coming to these 12 general practices in Oxfordshire, with a quite limited list of contraindications which are clinically justified. It is stated in the methods that the study was done in the winter months because conjunctivitis is more likely to be infectious than allergic in origin in the winter; so the results could be different at other times. However, with this proviso, the study results should be applicable to the source population.

16. Can the study results be applied to other relevant populations?

The diagnostic criteria used in this study are consistent with those used in normal clinical practice. The results are similar for the children with positive bacterial cultures, and so this study also applies to clinical practice where topical chloramphenicol is used only after laboratory tests. If the results of this study reflect a causal relationship with the intervention, it seems likely that such a relationship will hold in similar patients seen in other areas of the United Kingdom, and even in similar patients elsewhere in the world, at the current time and into the future. The authors point out that the study area had a more privileged social class distribution than the United Kingdom in general, but state that this is more likely to affect the transmission of the disease than change its causation or prognosis. Whether the ethnic background of the patient would influence the result is not mentioned. They conclude that the results are probably generalizable to most primary care settings in developed countries.

We should be cautious in applying the results to any groups in which the aetiology and natural history of conjunctivitis might be substantially different, such as older patients, patients with concomitant clinical conditions, and patients in different environments. The bacterial or viral agent present is important; Table 2 of the paper gives details of bacteria and viruses cultured, with a comparison to two other studies, presented as the prevalence ratio for the presence of specific bacteria in swabs from children with conjunctivitis compared with asymptomatic controls in the same population. This shows some consistency (e.g. for *Haemophilus influenza*) but also some substantial differences (e.g. in the frequency of different types of *Staphylococcus*); the authors suggest that the isolation rates of particular species will vary in different laboratories. To apply the results to a quite different population, for example, children in Africa, an assessment of the bacteriological and viral characteristics of acute conjunctivitis in that country would be useful.

The trial was restricted to one agent and one dose, 0.5 per cent chloramphenicol eye drops. This agent has broad-spectrum activity against several bacterial pathogens. The authors note that the other agent commonly used in the United Kingdom is fusidic acid, and clinical trials show similar effectiveness for this drug as for chloramphenicol. The results clearly may not apply to substantially different or new agents with different effectiveness.

E. Comparison of these results with other evidence

17. Are the results consistent with other evidence, particularly evidence from studies of similar or more powerful study design?

The consistency of information with other studies is not discussed in the paper, implying that there are no other relevant clinical trials. A Cochrane systematic review of antibiotic treatment of conjunctivitis is noted, dated 1999, but it is not stated if that incorporated many studies of children. If there are other relevant randomized trials, it would be useful to compare these results, with a meta-analysis if possible. Given that this is a well-designed randomized trial, non-randomized comparisons or case reports on similar topics are much less reliable.

18. Does the total evidence suggest any specificity?

No conclusions can be reached on this point. Meta-analysis of several studies could provide the large numbers of observations needed to assess specificity.

19. Are the results plausible in terms of the biological mechanism?

In clinical trials, the issue of a biological mechanism has usually been answered before the trial is initiated, and that certainly applies to this trial. The results are plausible in terms of biological mechanism, in that the main result is that most of these infections are self-limiting, with clinical cure of around 80 per cent within 7 days without active antibiotic intervention. The results show a small increase in this cure rate with an active antibiotic, which is a plausible result. There is still debate about the key pathogens in conjunctivitis.

20. If a major effect is shown, is it coherent with the distribution of exposure and the outcome?

In the context of a randomized trial, this is better applied as the question of whether the results will influence the outcome in a substantial way. If the results show a true effect, is the effect substantial enough to be clinically important?

The key issue in this study is whether the small difference in cure rate observed is a real difference or a chance finding, and, if real, whether this is clinically important and justifies the intervention. The difference in cure rates at 7 days was 3.8 per cent, giving a number needed to treat of 26. This means that for a patient being treated the probability that their cure is related to the treatment is small, and on a population basis it means that considerable numbers of children need to be treated for an extra cure by day 7. Whether this is valuable or not depends on the importance of an extra cure by day 7.

This is where the further information beyond day 7 would be very valuable. For example, the graph shown in Figure 3 of the paper suggests that the curves are parallel beyond day 7, meaning that children not cured by day 7 may have a long continuation of conjunctivitis; if so, an extra individual cured at day 7 may be quite important. On the other hand, those not cured at day 7 may well be cured at day 8 or 9, and therefore the extra advantage of a cure at day 7 would be small. The finding on the 6-week follow-up that the proportion of children with further episodes of conjunctivitis within the 6 weeks was small and similar in the two groups is reassuring in this regard. In terms of microbiological cure, the difference seen in the study is larger (16.8 per cent), and the number needed to treat is correspondingly smaller at around 6.

The result stressed by the authors is that most children presenting with acute infective conjunctivitis in primary care will recover by themselves and do not need treatment with an antibiotic. The authors' interpretation is that treatment should not be used routinely. Whether parents, or the older children, presented with the same data would come to that conclusion is uncertain. The coherence issue can be envisaged as stating that if, as the authors propose, routine treatment with antibiotics were greatly reduced, would that occur without any substantial increase in the complications of conjunctivitis in children, and perhaps in the incidence of conjunctivitis (which might represent cross-infection). The last point may be the more difficult issue, as a major effect of giving antibiotics may be to decrease parental or the child's own concern about the disease, and reassure them that cure will come quickly. In practice, this may be a major barrier to reducing antibiotic prescribing. In contrast, some parents may be aware of the dangers of using unnecessary antibiotics (e.g. the development of resistance) and may be pleased not to use them.

Summary of external validity

This study was carried out in a primary care setting in England, and the results should be applicable to children presenting to primary care facilities in that country. The results are likely to be applicable much more widely, the main issue being whether the causal agents and clinical progression of acute conjunctivitis in children differs substantially in different places and at different times. While children with severe infection such as periorbital cellulitis were excluded in the protocol, as noted, the more severe eligible cases may be under-represented.

Conclusions

In summary, this study illustrates both the strengths and weaknesses of randomized trials. A summary of the appraisal is shown in Table 12.2. The strengths are that, with reasonable confidence, we can exclude confounding and observation bias as explanations for the results seen. The eligibility criteria were clearly set out and relevant to clinical practice, and the trial results should be generalizable to children of this age seen in primary care in at least the UK. The main weakness is that, despite the enormous effort

Table 12.2 Assessment of causality in a randomized trial: trial of chloramphenicol eye drops, compared with placebo, in the treatment of acute infectious conjunctivitis in children, by Rose et al. [1].

Chloramphenicol eye drops for conjunctivitis in children: Rose et al. [1]

A. Description of evidence

1. Intervention	Chloramphenicol 0.5 per cent eye drops, compared with placebo drops
2. Outcome	Clinical cure at 7 days
3. Design	Double-blind randomized trial
4. Study population	Children aged 6 months to 12 years attending 12 general practices in England, with diagnosis of acute infective conjunctivitis
5. Main result	Clinical cure in 86 per cent of those randomized to antibiotic and 79 per cent of placebo group; relative risk 1.09, 95 per cent confidence limits 0.99 to 1.21

B. Non-causal explanations

6. Observation bias	Outcome based on parents' diaries—relevant outcome, probably some error, but double-blind design protects against bias; error would make the results conservative. Differences based on microbiological clearance greater; less error potential, but less relevant outcome
7. Confounding	Randomized design protects against confounding
8. Chance	Main result close to the 0.05 probability level; could be due to chance

C. Positive features of causation

9. Time relationship	The small difference in outcome is seen by day 2 and persists with little change. Further follow-up to 6 weeks shows no differences
10. Strength	Main result weak; not large enough to be clinically important, even if not due to chance
11. Dose–response	Not assessed as only one dose was used
12. Consistency	One subgroup defined in protocol, those with a bacterial pathogen isolated; showed similar result to whole group
13. Specificity	Not assessed as only one intervention-outcome combination is assessed

Summary of internal validity: high, result shows a small effect, which may be due to chance or causation. Effect may be weakened by error in observations of outcome. No likely confounders

D. External validity

14. To the eligible population	Very high completion rate by randomized subjects. Some 29 per cent of eligible subjects entered study; more severe cases possibly excluded, but main result should apply to eligible population
15. To the source population	Few contraindications to eligibility; result should apply to source population

(Continued)

Table 12.2 (Continued)

Chloramphenicol eye drops for conjunctivitis in children: Rose et al. [1]	
16. To other populations	Source population is children presenting in primary care in winter months. Likely to be applicable to similar contexts in other places. Extension of results to other age groups unknown
E. Other evidence	
17. Consistency	Few other studies; but result is consistent with most other less rigorous evidence
18. Specificity	Result may be generalizable to other antibiotic treatments, or may be specific to the treatment assessed—little evidence that other antibiotics would give different result
19. Plausibility	Shows that antibiotic clearance of bacteria is not necessary for clinical cure; plausible and suggests role of bacterial agents is minor
20. Coherence	Little information on coherence; size of effect suggests that clinical cure will vary with level of antibiotic treatment
Summary of external validity: study has been done in a relevant setting (primary care and home treatment), and result is widely generalizable; it suggests topical antibiotic treatment has only a small, or no, effect, and is unnecessary for cases similar to those included in this trial	

Source: data from Peter W Rose et al., 'Chloramphenicol treatment for acute infective conjunctivitis in children in primary care: a randomised double-blind placebo-controlled trial', *The Lancet*, Volume 366, Number 9479, pp. 37–43, © 2005 Elsevier Ltd [1].

involved, the study is still limited in terms of size, and the main results are close to the conventional 5 per cent cut-off for statistical significance.

The interpretation of this study is, however, not straightforward. For the primary outcome, clinical cure at 7 days, the intervention gave a small and non-significant benefit. This is probably best expressed by the results in absolute terms: the clinical cure rate was 83 per cent with the placebo, and 86 per cent with active treatment, an increase of 3.8 per cent, with 95 per cent limits of −4.1 to 11.8 per cent. The increase in cure rate was slightly larger, and statistically significant, for microbiological remission and for clinical cure assessed by cumulative analysis. So the cure rate with placebo is high and the additional cure rate with antibiotic treatment relatively small. The question therefore is whether this additional cure rate justifies the costs and potential complications of prescribing antibiotics; and this has to be considered from both a community policy and a clinical single-patient perspective. Thus, the paper challenged widely held normative practice at that time.

An interpretative exercise

Any study can be interpreted in different ways, some of which are more reasonable than others. Consider these different statements: are they accurate, and (more important) are they a fair and balanced interpretation?

- In children with acute conjunctivitis, treatment with antibiotic resulted in a 74 per cent increase in cure rates within 7 days, confirmed by laboratory testing (from Table 12.1, microbiological cure).

- If your child has a painful red eye, treatment with simple and safe antibiotic eye drops may decrease the risk of treatment failure by a third (including all subjects, comparing 14 to 21 per cent non-cure—Table 3 of paper).

- In children with conjunctivitis, treatment with antibiotic eye drops may increase the cure rate by 12 per cent (summary, using upper confidence limit).

- The use of antibiotic eye drops increases the clinical cure at day 7 from 83 per cent to 86 per cent (summary).

- In children with conjunctivitis, treatment with antibiotic eye drops has no effect on the cure rate (summary, using 'non-significance').

- Most children presenting with an acute infective conjunctivitis in primary care will get better by themselves and do not need treatment with an antibiotic (summary).

All these statements are factually accurate. The last statement is the authors' conclusion expressed in the summary of the paper, and approved by the peer review process. A paper published in a clinical journal needs to report both the factual results and the implications in practical terms. Not all the statements listed here are reasonable summaries of the study. You may wish to reflect on the different impacts of these statements, and how they could be used to support different points of view.

Influence of this paper

This paper was published in July 2005. In June 2005, chloramphenicol eye drops were approved for over-the-counter sales, being the first antibiotic available without a doctor's prescription in the UK. The regulatory authority knew about the results of this trial before they made this decision (P. Rose, personal communication). This implies that policy had been influenced by general practitioners' workloads and costs, but not by the danger of emerging antibiotic resistance; both these issues were noted in the paper. There followed an aggressive television marketing campaign from pharmaceutical companies promoting the use of chloramphenicol eye drops for conjunctivitis [4].

In correspondence in *The Lancet* following publication of this paper, several of the points discussed in this chapter were raised, and some more information was given, such as the data on the nurses' evaluation given under question 6. This paper and other relevant studies have given rise to a meta-analysis, a Cochrane collaboration review, and a GRADE review, illustrating various methods described in Chapters 9 and 10.

In 2011, an individual patient data meta-analysis (as described in Chapter 9) included randomized studies comparing antibiotics with placebo or no treatment, in primary care, for adults or children [5]: there were only three such studies, this paper and two others [6,7]. It was noted that since 2005, general practitioners' prescribing rates for acute conjunctivitis had reduced, but there had been a 48 per cent increase in the use of topical chloramphenicol. The meta-analysis had sufficient power to assess subgroups, and the conclusions were that acute conjunctivitis seen in primary care usually required no antibiotics, although a small benefit of antibiotics was seen, mainly in subgroups with purulent discharge or mild severity of red eye. A Cochrane review of antibiotics versus placebo for acute bacterial conjunctivitis identified 11 studies, most done in hospitals, with similar conclusions: that the condition is frequently self-limiting, but antibiotic eye drops give modestly improved rates of clinical and microbiological remission [8]. Interestingly, this Cochrane review documents the 'risk of bias' in each study, a measure of quality, and this study and one other primary care study [6] were assessed as the best studies. The GRADE review [9] for treatment of suspected bacterial conjunctivitis included more studies, as several comparing different antibiotics were included. The inclusion of studies in a variety of settings resulted in the conclusion that topical antibiotics may be more effective than placebo or no treatment, but the overall evidence was assessed as low quality; the overall recommendation was that topical antibiotics were 'likely to be beneficial', but the benefit was 'marginal'.

References

1. **Rose PW, Harnden A, Brueggemann AB, Perera R, Sheikh A, Crook D, et al**. Chloramphenicol treatment for acute infective conjunctivitis in children in primary care: a randomised double-blind placebo-controlled trial. *Lancet* 2005; **366**:37–43.
2. **Rose PW, Harnden A, Brueggemann AB, Perea R, Mant D**. Antibiotics for acute infective conjunctivitis in children. *Lancet* 2005; **366**:1431.
3. **Moher D, Hopewell S, Schulz KF, Montori V, Gotzsche PC, Devereaux PJ, et al**. CONSORT 2010 explanation and elaboration: updated guidelines for reporting parallel group randomised trials. *BMJ*. 2010; **340**:c869.
4. **Saha N**. Antibiotics for acute infective conjunctivitis in children. *Lancet* 2005; **366**:1432.
5. **Jefferis J, Perera R, Everitt H, van WH, Rietveld R, Glasziou P, et al**. Acute infective conjunctivitis in primary care: who needs antibiotics? An individual patient data meta-analysis. *Br J Gen Pract* 2011; **61**:e542–e548.
6. **Rietveld RP, ter Riet G, Bindels PJ, Bink D, Sloos JH, van Weert HC**. The treatment of acute infectious conjunctivitis with fusidic acid: a randomised controlled trial. *Br J Gen Pract* 2005; **55**:924–930.
7. **Everitt HA, Little PS, Smith PW**. A randomised controlled trial of management strategies for acute infective conjunctivitis in general practice. *BMJ* 2006; **333**:321.
8. **Sheikh A, Hurwitz B, van Schayck CP, McLean S, Nurmatov U**. Antibiotics versus placebo for acute bacterial conjunctivitis. *Cochrane Database Syst Rev* 2012; **9**:CD001211.
9. **Epling J**. Bacterial conjunctivitis. *BMJ Clin Evid* 2012; **2012**:0704.

Chapter 13

Critical appraisal of a randomized trial of a preventive agent

Introduction

In this chapter we will review an important randomized trial, published in *The Lancet*, 20 July 1991, 338, 131–137 [1]. In contrast with the trial reviewed in Chapter 12, this concerned a preventive strategy. The summary is reproduced and the full paper can be accessed at http://www.thelancet.com or at http://dx.doi.org/10.1016/0140-6736(91)90133-A.

Prevention of neural tube defects: results of the Medical Research Council Vitamin Study

MRC Vitamin Study Research Group

Summary

A randomized double-blind prevention trial with a factorial design was conducted at 33 centres in seven countries to determine whether supplementation with folic acid (one of the vitamins in the B group) or a mixture of seven other vitamins (A, D, B_1, B_2, B_6, C, and nicotinamide) around the time of conception can prevent neural tube defects (anencephaly, spina bifida, encephalocoele). A total of 1817 women at high risk of having a pregnancy with a neural tube defect, because of a previous affected pregnancy, were allocated at random to one of four groups—namely, folic acid, other vitamins, both, or neither. 1195 had a completed pregnancy in which the fetus or infant was known to have or not have a neural tube defect; 27 of these had a known neural tube defect, 6 in the folic acid groups and 21 in the two other groups, a 72 per cent protective effect (relative risk 0.28, 95 per cent confidence interval 0.12–0.71). The other vitamins showed no significant protective effect (relative risk 0.80, 95 per cent CI 0.32–1.72). There was no demonstrable harm from the folic acid supplementation, though the ability of the study to detect rare or slight adverse effects was limited. Folic acid supplementation starting before pregnancy can now be firmly recommended for all women who have had an affected pregnancy, and public health measures should be taken to ensure that the diet of all women who may bear children contains an adequate amount of folic acid.

A. Description of the evidence

1. What was the exposure or intervention?
2. What was the outcome?
3. What was the study design?
4. What was the study population?
5. What was the main result?

The *objective* of this study was to test whether dietary supplementation with different types of vitamins could reduce the recurrence risk of neural tube defects in pregnancies in women who had already had at least one affected birth. The background, described in the introduction, notes that two intervention studies for such high-risk women had been done, with inconclusive results. One of the studies [2] was large, and showed a large and statistically significant decrease in recurrence risk in women taking a combination of folic acid with seven other vitamins, but as the study was not randomized, the difference might have been due to selection factors or other confounding factors. The second study was randomized and used only folic acid [3], but was too small and showed a non-significant benefit when analysed in an intention-to-treat manner, although the published results, analysed by compliance with treatment, showed a significant effect. Thus, from these trials, it was uncertain whether there was a true preventive action of dietary supplementation, and it was not clear if folic acid as a single agent or in combination with other vitamins was the more effective agent. As a result, a large randomized trial of high-risk women was designed.

The *intervention* was a dietary supplementation. Two types of supplement were tested: folic acid alone, 4 mg per day, and several vitamins other than folic acid. An efficient design to test two different interventions, a 2 × 2 *factorial design,* was used, where the women were randomized into four groups, and then received folic acid, other vitamins, both folic acid and other vitamins, or neither. Four identical sets of capsules were prepared; three sets contained the three combinations of supplementation, and the capsules for the fourth group contained only ferrous sulphate and calcium phosphate, which were also included in all the other groups and are regarded as a placebo.

The *outcome* was the occurrence of a further neural tube defect. There are a set of these congenital defects of the nervous system, which can usually be recognized easily in live births and still births, and in induced and spontaneous abortuses if appropriate examination is done. The expected frequency of such outcomes in pregnancies to women who have already had an affected baby is around 2–5 per cent.

The *study design* was a prospective, double-blind, randomized trial. A study size calculation showed that approximately 2000 pregnancies would be needed, and therefore the study was international, involving 33 centres in seven countries. The *eligible population* comprised women with a previous pregnancy with an 'isolated' neural tube defect, that is, excluding defects associated with Meckel's syndrome. This syndrome includes neural tube defects, but because it has an autosomal recessive inheritance pattern, it has a substantially higher recurrence risk than the more common situation of an isolated neural tube defect. Because folic acid interacts with drugs used to control epilepsy, women with epilepsy were excluded from this study.

The main result (Table 13.1) consists of two comparisons: between all women randomized to take folic acid and all women randomized not to take folic acid, and between all women randomized to take other vitamins and all those randomized not to take other vitamins. The outcome variable is prevalence at birth of any neural tube defect, that is, the number of affected babies divided by the total number of births. The results are shown in 2 × 2 tables, and the relative risk calculated as the ratio of the prevalence rates. A Mantel–Haenszel analysis is appropriate.

The main result is that six of the 593 births to mothers allocated folic acid were affected (1.0 per cent) compared with 21 of 602 births in those not receiving folic acid (3.5 per cent), giving a relative risk of 0.29 with 95 per cent confidence limits of 0.12–0.71 (see Table A2.2 for the calculations). The prevalence in births to women receiving other vitamins was 2.0 per cent compared with 2.5 per cent in those not receiving other vitamins, giving a relative risk of 0.80; this modest reduction in risk is not statistically significant, with 95 per cent confidence limits of 0.37–1.72.

Table 13.1 Results of Medical Research Council trial: main treatment comparisons.

	Neural tube defects	Total pregnancies	Rate (%)	Relative risk	95% CI
Results in the four groups by supplement assigned in factorial design					
Folic acid and multivitamins	4	295	1.36		
Folic acid, no multivitamins	2	298	0.67		
No folic acid, multivitamins	8	302	2.65		
No folic acid, no multivitamins	13	300	4.33		
Comparisons for each treatment contrast					
Allocated folic acid	6	593	1.01	0.29	0.12–0.71
No folic acid	21	602	3.49		
Relative risk for folic acid adjusted for stopping rule					
Allocated other vitamins	12	597	2.01	0.33	0.06–0.80
No other vitamins	15	598	2.51	0.80	0.37–1.72

Source: data from MRC Vitamin Study Research Group, 'Prevention of neural tube defects: Results of the Medical Research Council Vitamin Study', *The Lancet*, Volume 338, Number 876, pp. 131–137, © 1991 Published by Elsevier Ltd [1].

B. Internal validity: consideration of non-causal explanations

6. Are the results likely to be affected by observation bias?

We must first assess if the recorded results in terms of pregnancy outcome are likely to be accurate, or whether they could be influenced by observation bias. There are two main issues. First, is the outcome of the pregnancy observable? A major problem with any study of birth defects is that what is observed is the net result of two processes: the occurrence of the birth defect, very early in pregnancy, and the survival of the affected fetus *in utero*. If affected fetuses do not survive, but are expelled as spontaneous abortuses early in the pregnancy, then the outcomes of pregnancy will not be measurable in a routine study. If they survive to present as later spontaneous abortions, as stillbirths, or as live births, then they can be observed. For these reasons, the information on all pregnancies occurring, and whether these were 'informative', that is, they could be examined to ascertain if a neural tube defect was present, is important and is shown in Table 3 of the paper. Overall, 75 per cent of the women randomized had a pregnancy known to the study, and 88 per cent of these pregnancies were informative; most non-informative pregnancies were miscarriages (11 per cent). The important issue is that the mothers allocated folic acid and those not allocated folic acid were extremely similar. There was a considerably higher number of terminations of informative pregnancies in mothers not receiving folic acid. This will include pregnancies terminated after recognition of a neural tube defect following antenatal diagnosis, as this service was available to all women in this study. There is also a somewhat higher number (three compared with none) of non-informative terminations, that is, a termination of pregnancy for which information was not available to the study authors; these may include some neural tube defects.

Overall, it seems unlikely that any differences in the ascertainment of pregnancy outcomes would influence the result.

The second issue is the completeness and accuracy of ascertainment of neural tube defects in informative pregnancies. In general, neural tube defects are severe abnormalities that can be accurately recognized and classified if careful examination is performed, although this is more difficult for a termination than it is for a live birth. There are also minor and even subclinical forms of the condition, so that some biological occurrences of defects may not be recognized. The trial protocol called for independent corroboration of a report of the neural tube defect. The necropsy report or a description of the lesion was sent to the trial centre for independent review, and this was done without knowledge of the allocated group. A total of 27 neural tube defects were reported, and in the discussion the authors comment that in 23 cases the women had a termination of pregnancy after antenatal diagnosis, and in four there was a live birth, two of which survived. For 18 of the 25 dead cases there was a necropsy report, and there were confirmatory descriptions in the remaining seven. The authors state that they are confident about the reliability of the diagnoses. The reports of neural tube defects are likely to be valid. The main limitation is that it is difficult to be certain that all neural tube defects were counted; some may have occurred in non-informative pregnancies, some may not have been recognized at all, and some could have been missed in informative pregnancies, although that seems unlikely.

The main potential problem is less complete ascertainment in mothers allocated folic acid, as that direction of bias would contribute to the observed result. If the reported frequency of other abnormalities were also lower in pregnancies to women allocated folic acid, it would suggest general under-ascertainment or that folic acid prevents other abnormalities. In fact, the number of other abnormalities was slightly higher in the group allocated folic acid, suggesting that under-ascertainment did not occur.

7. Are the results likely to be affected by confounding?

The primary strength of the randomized trial design is in protection against confounding. The previous large non-randomized trial of vitamin supplementation showed a statistically significant benefit [2], but because the women allocated the supplement were self-selected by their attendance at a specialized unit, that group may have had other features which put them at a lower risk of recurrence of neural tube defects. From the general epidemiology of these defects, factors such as higher social class, residence in low-risk geographical areas, lower parity, or younger age could reduce risk. In this study, randomization was used on a substantial number of mothers. In Table II of the paper the four groups resulting from the randomization are compared in terms of age, previous pregnancy history, and the number of previous pregnancies affected by neural tube defect, and information is also given on social class for the women within the UK; all of these show almost identical distributions between the four groups. The randomization was done within each centre, so that the distribution of mothers receiving or not receiving folic acid is similar over the different centres. This design provides good reassurance that the baseline characteristics of the different groups of mothers were the same.

Another major problem with the previous non-randomized study was that the women allocated the supplement were aware of it, and had probably received more information about the disease and their pregnancy than had the comparison women. Therefore the women receiving the supplement may have actively made other changes, such as improving their own diet in other ways, which may have confounded the effect of the supplement. The randomized trial used a double-blind design, so that all women involved were given the same information, and were given identical capsules. They were not given any special advice about diet. Many of the women involved in the trial may have taken other actions, such as modifying their diet, changing their consumption of substances such as alcohol, or changing their lifestyle in terms of exercise and occupation, and so on. The strength of the double-blind design is that all women received the same information, and therefore the extent to which they made other modifications should have been the same irrespective of the supplementation they received. The one danger that still remains, even with the double-blind design, is the possibility that all the women in the trial would make dramatic differences to other aspects of their diet, so that their total vitamin intake would increase to the point where the marginal effect of the supplementation would be irrelevant. Partially as a protection against this, and more directly to assess whether women actually took the allocated tablets, serum folic acid levels were assessed from blood samples at various times. These results (Table VII of the paper), show substantially higher serum folic acid levels in those allocated folic acid than in others, which both indicates compliance and shows that the folic acid levels were not increased in the whole group to the extent of removing the effect of the supplement.

8. Are the results likely to be affected by chance variation?

As noted earlier, the simple analysis of the results shows that the reduction in risk associated with folic acid supplementation is very unlikely to have recurred by chance, whereas the small reduction in risk associated with other vitamins is well within the likely range of chance variation. The results of this study were monitored by an independent review group, using a sequential method of analysis which is described in the paper. The trial was terminated when the cumulative difference between the number of neural tube defects in the folic-acid group compared with the non-folic-acid group reached a preset boundary (Figure 13.1). Because the trial was stopped at a point that depended on the results at that time, the relative risk estimate produced by standard

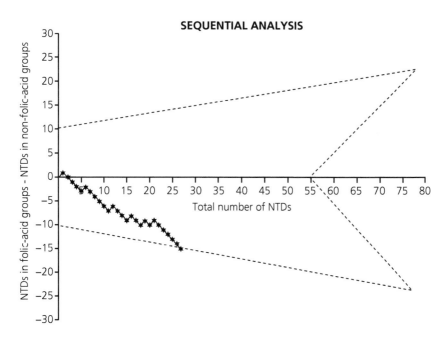

Figure 13.1 Sequential analysis, showing cumulative difference between number of neural tube defects (NTDs) in the folic acid and non-folic acid groups plotted against total number of NTDs occurring in the trial. The boundaries of the diagram define the stopping points of the study. The methods used to determine the boundaries are described in the paper.

Source: data from MRC Vitamin Study Research Group, 'Prevention of neural tube defects: Results of the Medical Research Council Vitamin Study', The Lancet, Volume 338, Number 876, pp. 131–137, © 1991 Published by Elsevier Ltd [1].

methods is somewhat exaggerated. The relative risk needs to be calculated by a different method which allows for this early stopping; this gives a result of 0.33, with 95 per cent confidence limits of 0.06–0.80. This is not quite as extreme as the more simply calculated relative risk of 0.29. As the simpler estimate is very similar, it can be used to explore the results of this study further.

The relative risks and confidence limits shown in Table 13.1 can be reproduced by applying the formulae in Table A2.2, using the variance formulae in section 4A.

C. Internal validity: consideration of positive features of causation

9. Is there a correct time relationship?

The time relationship is clear in this prospective intervention trial. It is stated that 7 per cent of women with informative pregnancies had stopped taking their capsules before they became pregnant, usually because they lost interest in participation. Specific results are not reported for these women; if the number were larger, the results specifically in these women would be of interest.

10. Is the relationship strong?

The overall relationship here is strong, with a 67 per cent reduction in risk. The result of the previous non-randomized trial was similar, but that did not adequately deal with the possibility of uncontrolled confounding. Indeed, an even larger variation in risk was seen in an observational study comparing the recurrence risks in women grouped by the hospital which they had previously attended, and these large differences in risk remained unexplained by any known differences in supplementation, diet, or other factors [4]. Therefore, while the strength of the relationship is of critical importance in terms of the implementation and impact of these results, in terms of the interpretation of causality, it assists, but the main strength comes from the double-blind randomized design in reducing the possibility of confounding or observation bias.

11. Is there a dose–response relationship?

There is no opportunity here to assess any dose–response relationship, as only a single dose was used. The questions of whether a lower dose would be equally effective, or a higher dose would be more effective, are not resolved.

12. Are the results consistent within the study?

Consistency within the study can be looked at in a number of ways (Table 13.2). The geographical distribution breaks down primarily into centres within and outside the United Kingdom, and the results are virtually identical for each of these groups. There are two major types of neural tube defect, anencephalus and spina bifida. The results show a protective effect for each defect, and although the relative risk is lower for spina bifida than it is for anencephalus, the confidence limits overlap. A major difference between the results for the two defects would raise a question of differences in ascertainment, or indicate a true biological difference. It would be possible to analyse the results

Table 13.2 Results of Medical Research Council trial: main treatment comparison within subgroups.

	Neural tube defects	Total pregnancies	Rate(%)	Relative risk	95% CI
Comparison specific to anencephalus					
Allocated folic acid	3	593	0.51	0.44	0.11–1.67
No folic acid	7	602	1.16		
Comparison specific to spina bifida and encephalocoele					
Allocated folic acid	3	593	0.51	0.22	0.06–0.75
No folic acid	14	602	2.33		
Comparison specific to centres within the UK					
Allocated folic acid	3	261	1.15	0.38	0.11–1.40
No folic acid	8	262	3.05		
Comparison specific to centres outside the UK					
Allocated folic acid	3	332	0.90	0.24	0.07–0.82
No folic acid	13	340	3.82		

Source: data from MRC Vitamin Study Research Group, 'Prevention of neural tube defects: Results of the Medical Research Council Vitamin Study', *The Lancet*, Volume 338, Number 876, pp. 131–137, © 1991 Published by Elsevier Ltd [1].

by other characteristics such as maternal age or previous pregnancy history, but this is not done in this paper.

13. Is there any specificity within the study?

The most important specificity is that the protective effect was shown for folic acid, but not for multivitamins. This specificity in results is based on a specific hypothesis set up in advance, and therefore can be accepted as valid. The authors conclude that the result is specific to folic acid supplementation, a conclusion of considerable practical importance. However, the results did show some reduction in risk with the other vitamins, although it was not statistically significant, and so some benefit of the other vitamins cannot be ruled out. Although the numbers are insufficient for confident results, there is no evidence that the risk was lower in those who received both folic acid and other vitamins than in those who received folic acid alone (Table 13.1). There is no evidence of specificity in terms of the particular defect, as discussed previously.

Conclusions with regard to internal validity

The internal validity of this study is extremely high. It is difficult to make a good argument for any explanation of the main result other than that of causality. Because of the randomization, the groups of women being compared are very similar in several documented factors related to their risk. The occurrence of informative pregnancies and the documentation of defects have been assessed consistently and in identical fashion for all women in this study. The main result is consistent with the pre-defined hypothesis and is strong, and the possibility of it occurring by chance variation is extremely remote. The results are consistent within different subgroups.

D. External validity: generalization of the results

14. Can the study results be applied to the eligible population?

The eligible population consists of the next occurring pregnancy in each woman identified as eligible in the participating centres. The fact that a high proportion of pregnancies were informative is an important strength of the study. The study was designed to ensure that each woman contributed no more than one informative event, so that each informative pregnancy is an independent observation. Each woman remained in the trial until she had an informative pregnancy, or until the end of the trial; women who had an uninformative pregnancy remained in the study in the same randomization group until an informative pregnancy resulted or the trial ended.

The relationship between the participants and the total eligible population is not clear. Women invited to join the trial were given a week to decide if they wished to take part. There is no information given on how eligible women were identified, what proportion of them were invited to participate, or what proportion of those invited to participate did so. Therefore the participants were a selected subgroup of all eligible women. This is relevant only if the effect of the supplementation could be different in eligible women who did not participate; it is difficult to see how this would occur. We might expect that the participants would be more interested and more knowledgeable about the pregnancy and their risk state than non-participants, and so might be more active in making other changes such as other dietary alterations. Such an effect would apply to all the randomized groups, and its effect, if any, would be to reduce the effect of supplementation. Therefore the results should apply to the eligible population.

15. Can the study results be applied to the source population?

The source population consists of all women who had a previous affected pregnancy who were seen in any of the participating centres. The eligibility criteria were to be planning another pregnancy, not be already taking vitamin supplements, and not to have epilepsy. The first two criteria may exclude women who are both least and most prepared for a further pregnancy. As with the previous issue, the relevant question concerns the generalizability of the result of the study, and these exclusion criteria do not seem likely to limit that.

16. Can the study results be applied to other relevant populations?

The generalization of the result to appropriate target populations is a very important issue. The underlying biological hypothesis being tested was that folate or vitamin supplementation reduces the *recurrence* risk of these defects in the reproductive population in general, that is, on a worldwide basis. We have to ask to what extent are the women who had the opportunity to take part in the trial likely to be representative of all at-risk women, that is, those who have had a previous affected child. Neural tube defects have a complex epidemiological pattern, and are much more common in some countries than others. Their aetiology may differ in different societies. They are less common in Oriental, Asian, and African populations, and much more common in European populations, particularly those of British origin [5]. The centres participating were in Britain, Australia, and Canada, which have substantial British populations, and in Hungary and Israel, which have lower population risks of neural tube defects. It seems unlikely that there were many mothers of Asian or African origin in this study, and there could be differences in the aetiology of these defects in such women.

Therefore the results are likely to apply, on a worldwide basis, to mothers of European origin who have had a previous affected pregnancy. Direct information for non-European ethnic groups would be useful, but in its absence it is reasonable to generalize the results to such groups in addition. This is particularly so as the application of these results may have a high benefit-to-cost ratio. The results suggest that a dietary supplement, which does not appear to have any major toxic consequences and is readily available and cheap, can produce a substantial reduction in risk for high-risk mothers, but antenatal diagnosis where culturally and legally acceptable would still be offered as a further protection. It seems very reasonable to apply these results to high-risk mothers, on a worldwide basis.

The more challenging question is whether these results show that supplementation with folic acid will reduce the frequency of neural tube defects occurring *for the first time* in births to mothers without any previous history. A reasonable case is made in this paper that the results would apply. It is generally thought that neural tube defects have an environmental and a genetic component in their causation. We can consider these two factors as joint causes, under the simple models described in Chapter 4. If their joint effect is multiplicative, the relative risk for the environmental cause will be the same in recurrences as in first affected births, and the absolute effect (risk difference) will be greater. If the joint effect is additive, the absolute effect will be the same, and the relative risk for the environmental cause will be less in recurrences than in first affected births. Therefore on these models, the result from this study is either a valid estimate or an underestimate of the relative risk from folate supplementation for general population low-risk pregnancies. The situation in which it could be an overestimate is that of synergy, where the benefit of folate supplementation is particularly great, or even confined to, mothers with a genetic factor which also increases their overall risk. That would apply, for example, if high-risk mothers had a genetic defect hampering their folate metabolism, such that the supplement is beneficial even with normal dietary intakes.

However, the application of the result to the prevention of first occurrences of neural tube defects involves more than accepting the argument of causality. Even if the causal relationship applies, with the same relative risk, the balance of potential benefit to potential harm is dramatically different. These defects occur very early in embryological development, before the pregnancy is recognized, and so folic acid supplementation would have to be offered on a population basis to all women who could become pregnant, raising a unique public health challenge. While the risk without supplementation for women who have had a previous abnormal baby is around 2–5 per 100, the corresponding risk in mothers without such a history is around 1–2 per 1000. Therefore the number of women who would need supplementation to prevent one defect (the number needed to treat (NNT)) would rise from around 50 to 5000. Issues of cost, any possibility of side effects, and the social and ethical issues related to mass medication all become relevant.

E. Comparison of these results with other evidence

17. Are the results consistent with other evidence, particularly evidence from studies of similar or more powerful study design?

This is the most powerful study design applied to this problem. The results are generally consistent with earlier studies using weaker designs. In the discussion the authors review the previous small randomized trial and the large non-randomized intervention study, which both showed a benefit, and also mention unpublished interim results of a further trial which will be discussed later. They also note six observational studies using cohort or case–control designs, of which all but one showed an association consistent with protection from increased folic acid consumption. However, the consistency question is not particularly relevant, as this study has the strongest design and is much more rigorous than any of the previous work. Therefore if the results of this trial had shown no benefit, the previous results from non-randomized trials or observation studies would not have offset that null result.

18. Does the total evidence suggest any specificity?

The specificity of the result with regard to folic acid alone is important. In the previous work, the large non-randomized study used several vitamins including folic acid. The observational studies are understandably very weak in separating the effects of different vitamins. Some are concerned with total dietary intakes, and women who consume high folate levels also tend to have high intakes of a wide range of other vitamins; others assess supplementation, which is rarely specific to particular preparations, or used and recalled consistently enough to assist. The previous randomized study used folic acid alone and suggested a benefit, but was too small to be conclusive. Therefore the factorial design of the trial, designed to evaluate this specificity, is very important.

19. Are the results plausible in terms of the biological mechanism?

There is no discussion of biological plausibility or the mechanisms of the effect in this paper. These defects had been produced in experimental animals by folic acid deficiency and by folate antagonists, but as they could also be produced by a wide range of other dietary changes or external agents, these results did not appear particularly striking or important. When this trial was published in 1991 there was no accepted mechanism by which folic acid would protect against these defects. It seemed surprising to many that supplementation with a relatively low dose of a common vitamin could produce a dramatic reduction in the frequency of a common and severe congenital defect, whose occurrence had been studied intensively for several decades. However, this trial is a good example of an empirical advance preceding knowledge of mechanisms. These results stimulated research to discover a mechanism by which the protective effect is produced.

20. If a major effect is shown, is it coherent with the distribution of exposure and the outcome?

The results show a major effect, and so coherence can be anticipated. However, there is little information available on recurrence rates in different populations. Nevertheless, if the results also apply to the primary prevention of defects, then the descriptive epidemiology of neural tube defects should fit with this new result. The frequency (prevalence at birth) of these defects varies greatly by geography, time, season, maternal social circumstances, and so on. However, there was little information at this time on how folic acid consumption or tissue levels in pregnant women vary by place, time, or personal or social factors. The demonstration that women in the lower social classes in Britain had low folate intakes was one of the factors leading to the hypothesis, but this association was very non-specific, as such women have lower intakes of many nutrients. The authors note two issues of coherence. The United Kingdom has one of the highest rates of neural tube defects in the world, and yet is not known to be particularly deficient in folic acid; the authors suggest that the UK population may indeed have low folic acid intakes, or that the types of folic acids in foods eaten there may be relatively poorly absorbed. They also suggest there could be an interaction with a genetically controlled disturbance of folic acid metabolism, a hypothesis which could of course explain much of the other variability of neural tube defect occurrence. They also note that studies of serum or red cell folate levels in women with affected and unaffected pregnancies have not in general shown substantial differences, and suggest that this may be because the range of values within a population is too narrow to demonstrate such differences easily.

Since the study was done and folate supplementation became routine in many countries, coherence can be shown as rates of neural tube defects have reduced; this is discussed later under 'Influence of this study'.

Summary of external validity

In summary, the primary result that folic acid reduces the recurrence rates of these defects can be applied on a worldwide basis. The size of the effect may vary, as the contribution of folic acid deficiency to aetiology may vary in different communities, because of differences in both the defect and the background level of folic intake.

The main issue in generalizability is whether these results on recurrences can be applied to first occurrences of these defects. A reasonable case on both biological and epidemiological grounds is made by the authors, but more direct evidence would be useful. The results are consistent with most observational studies of first occurrences of the defect. At the time of publication, the mechanism for the effect was basically unknown.

Conclusions

This large individually randomized trial has produced a result with extremely high internal validity, with observation bias and confounding being ruled out as alternative explanations (Table 13.3). The result for folic acid is very unlikely to be due to chance, although the precision of the result is still modest, as shown by the fairly wide confidence limits. The association has an appropriate time relationship, is strong, and is consistent by the type of defect and geographical area, and the benefit appears to be specific to folic acid rather than to other multivitamins. Generalization of the result to other high-risk women for the prevention of recurrence is reasonable. Generalization of the result to the situation of the first occurrence of these defects raises further questions, but is certainly strongly suggested by this study.

Table 13.3 Summary of assessment of the randomized trial of prevention of recurrence of neural tube defects.

A. Description of the evidence	
1. Exposure	Folic acid 4 mg, or multivitamins, daily
2. Outcome	Recurrence of neural tube defects
3. Design	Individually randomized prospective double blind trial; 2 × 2 factorial design
4. Study population	Mothers with a previous neural tube defect; international, 33 centres
5. Main result	Reduction in recurrences after folic acid, relative risk 0.33; small reduction after multivitamins, *RR* 0.8
B. Non-causal explanations	
6. Observation bias	Double-blind design, independent review of records on outcome, high proportion of informative pregnancies virtually rule out observation bias
7. Confounding	Randomized design on large numbers protects against confounding; data show comparability on several factors
8. Chance	Result for folic acid significant, 95% limits 0.12–0.71; result for multivitamins non-significant, limits 0.32–1.72
C. Features consistent with causation	
9. Time relationship	Appropriate; controlled by prospective design
10. Strength	Folic acid result strong
11. Dose–response	Not assessed; fixed dose
12. Consistency	Consistent by type of defect, geographical area
13. Specificity	Benefit specific to folic acid

D. External validity

14.	Eligible population	Participants represent eligible women
15.	Source population	Selection factors for study entry undefined, but no reason not to generalize the result
16.	Target populations	Application to high-risk mothers and recurrence clear, except perhaps non-European subjects. Extension to first occurrences likely but additional direct evidence would be desirable

E. Comparison with other evidence

17.	Consistency	Consistent with earlier intervention studies and with most observational studies
18.	Specificity	No other studies can assess specificity to folic acid
19.	Plausibility	Supported by animal evidence, but mechanism unknown
20.	Coherence	Limited data on distribution of dietary folate; social class gradient coherent, but not specific to folic acid

Source: data from MRC Vitamin Study Research Group, 'Prevention of neural tube defects: Results of the Medical Research Council Vitamin Study', *The Lancet*, Volume 338, Number 876, pp. 131–137, © 1991 Published by Elsevier Ltd [1].

Influence of this study

This is the strongest study of the six discussed in this section of the book. The study answered an important question and gave a definite result, which was accepted worldwide as relevant and important. This acceptance comes from the strengths of the study: a large, international, randomized, double-blind trial of a feasible intervention. The publication of this study in July 1991 led to rapid changes in clinical and public health practice. The primary result, that supplementation with 4 mg of folic acid per day would reduce the recurrence rate of these defects, was accepted quickly by health care authorities and professional associations worldwide as accepted clinical practice for high-risk women; for example, within a month, recommendations for high-risk women were issued by the US Centers for Disease Control (CDC) and by the Chief Medical Officer in England. This contrasts with the reception of the non-randomized trial by Smithells and colleagues in 1981 [2], although that study showed an even stronger protective effect with a relative risk of 0.15. Although it may have given some clinical adoption of supplementation for high-risk women, most health authorities and professional associations did not advocate a clear policy because of the limitations of the non-randomized study, as discussed in this chapter.

The greater issue was the prevention of first occurrences of these defects. Could the results of this randomized trial on recurrences be applied to first occurrences? If not, another, even larger, trial would be needed to answer that question. This was resolved by the publication in 1992 of a randomized trial of primary prevention in Hungary, showing no neural tube defects in births to 2104 women randomized to receive a multivitamin supplement including 0.8 mg folic acid daily, compared to 6 in 2052 comparison women (P = 0.03) [6]. So, before the end of 1992 both the CDC and the Chief Medical Officer in England issued recommendations that all women capable of becoming pregnant should take a supplement of 0.4 mg folic acid per day, in addition to ensuring a good diet. This dose was based on the three trials mentioned, but is still somewhat arbitrary. Similar recommendations were made in many other countries. In 2000, the Kennedy Foundation International award for scientific achievement was awarded jointly to Professors Smithells, Wald, and Czeizel.

Thus, it was quickly accepted that folate supplementation reduces the risk of these defects [7,8]. Discussion then concentrated on how best to apply this new knowledge, with the main challenge being that advice given once a woman knows she is pregnant is too late. The main approaches have been health education messages to encourage women in the reproductive age groups to take folic acid in anticipation of a possible pregnancy, and increasing the folic acid content of food stuffs such as flour and cereals ('fortification'), by permissive or compulsory legislative moves, to increase the total folic acid consumption on a community basis [9]. Canada and the United States introduced requirements to fortify flour and grain products in 1998, followed by many other countries. Guidelines for optimal folate levels for reproductive age women were produced by the World Health Organization in 2015 [10]. Some potential hazards of an increased folate intake have been identified, including possible increases in some cancers, but these need more assessment [11]. 'Coherence' now becomes a relevant test—has the prevalence at birth of neural tube defects reduced following preventive programmes? Indeed it has; this has been shown in several countries [12], although of course other factors are also relevant. The reduction has explained some of the previously noted features: for example, the strong east-to-west decline in prevalence at birth in Canada shown in the older studies has almost disappeared in recent years [13].

This trial also raises several general issues about the conduct of research. As pointed out in an editorial accompanying the trial result [14], Smithells and his colleagues wished to carry out a randomized trial in the 1970s, but permission was refused by an ethics committee which insisted that all women at increased risk should be offered the supplement. This led to the non-randomized trial, giving results which, while strong and statistically significant, were not regarded as definitive by most authorities. Therefore this ethical committee decision delayed the development of a fully randomized trial by some 10 years, and the considerable debate about it delayed recruitment into the MRC trial, so that it took 8 years to accumulate enough participating women to produce the results discussed in this chapter. This highlights the need for ethical committees to assess the scientific and ethical consequences of their decisions. On the other hand, the results of the non-randomized trial were correct; they demonstrated a large benefit for vitamin supplementation. Should this evidence from the non-randomized trial, in addition to the considerable number of observational studies, have been accepted as showing the preventive action of vitamin supplementation? By delaying public health policy until the results of the randomized trial came in 10 years later, many preventable defects must have occurred. This situation can be contrasted with the situations where randomized trials have produced results contradicting the conclusions from earlier studies, such as with beta-carotene, discussed in Chapter 7.

This trial also stimulated much more work on the biochemistry of folic acid and the mechanisms of this preventive action, relating to metabolic processes relating to folic acid, vitamin B_{12}, and DNA production, and many genetic factors and interactions [15]. Other issues include whether folic acid supplementation can prevent other congenital abnormalities, such as congenital heart disease or cleft lip and palate, or have benefits for chronic diseases such as heart disease and colon cancers. The evidence for the routine use of folic acid or multivitamin supplementation for such prevention is still unclear [16–18].

References

1. **MRC (Medical Research Council) Vitamin Study Group**. Prevention of neural tube defects: results of the Medical Research Council Vitamin Study. *Lancet* 1991; **338**:131–137.

2. **Smithells RW, Sheppard S, Schorah CJ, Seller MJ, Nevin NC, Harris R, et al**. Apparent prevention of neural tube defects by periconceptional vitamin supplementation. *Arch Dis Child* 1981; **56**:911–918.

3. **Laurence KM, James N, Miller MH, Tennant GB, Campbell H**. Double-blind randomised controlled trial of folate treatment before conception to prevent recurrence of neural-tube defects. *BMJ* 1981; **282**:1509–1511.

4. **MacCarthy PA, Dalrymple IJ, Duignan NM, Elwood JH, Guiney EJ, Hanratty TD, et al**. Recurrence rates of neural tube defects in Dublin maternity hospitals. *Ir Med J* 1983; **76**:78–79.

5. **Elwood JM, Little J, Elwood JH**. *Epidemiology and Control of Neural Tube Defects*. Oxford: Oxford University Press; 1992.

6. **Czeizel AE, Dudas I**. Prevention of the first occurrence of neural tube defects by periconceptional vitamin supplementation. *N Engl J Med* 1992; **327**:1832–1835.

7. **Toriello HV**. Policy statement on folic acid and neural tube defects. *Genet Med* 2011; **13**:593–596.

8. **Figo Working Group On Best Practice In Maternal-Fetal Medicine**. Best practice in maternal-fetal medicine. *Int J Gynaecol Obstet* 2015; **128**:80–82.

9. **Crider KS, Bailey LB, Berry RJ**. Folic acid food fortification-its history, effect, concerns, and future directions. *Nutrients* 2011; **3**:370–384.

10. **Cordero AM, Crider KS, Rogers LM, Cannon MJ, Berry RJ**. Optimal serum and red blood cell folate concentrations in women of reproductive age for prevention of neural tube defects: World Health Organization guidelines. *MMWR Morb Mortal Wkly Rep.* 2015; **64**:421–423.

11. **Choi JH, Yates Z, Veysey M, Heo YR, Lucock M**. Contemporary issues surrounding folic acid fortification initiatives. *Prev Nutr Food Sci* 2014; **19**:247–260.

12. **Blencowe H, Cousens S, Modell B, Lawn J**. Folic acid to reduce neonatal mortality from neural tube disorders. *Int J Epidemiol.* 2010; **39**(Suppl 1):i110–121.

13. **De Wals P.**, Tairou F, Van Allen MI, Uh SH, Lowry RB, Sibbald B, et al. Reduction in neural-tube defects after folic acid fortification in Canada. *N Engl J Med* 2007; **357**:135–142.

14. **Anonymous**. Folic acid and neural tube defects. *Lancet* 1991; **338**:153–154.

15. **Greene ND, Copp AJ**. Neural tube defects. *Annu Rev Neurosci* 2014; **37**:221–242.

16. **De-Regil LM, Fernandez-Gaxiola AC, Dowswell T, Pena-Rosas JP.** Effects and safety of periconceptional folate supplementation for preventing birth defects. *Cochrane Database Syst Rev* 2010; **10**:CD007950.

17. **Moyer VA.** Vitamin, mineral, and multivitamin supplements for the primary prevention of cardiovascular disease and cancer: U.S. Preventive services Task Force recommendation statement. *Ann Intern Med* 2014; **160**:558–564.

18. **Qin X, Cui Y, Shen L, Sun N, Zhang Y, Li J, et al.** Folic acid supplementation and cancer risk: a meta-analysis of randomized controlled trials. *Int J Cancer* 2013; **133**:1033–1041.

Chapter 14

Critical appraisal of a prospective cohort study

This chapter deals with the assessment of an interesting prospective cohort study, published in *The Lancet*, 21 September 2002, 360, 901–907, and available at http://www.thelancet.com or http://www.sciencedirect.com/science/article/pii/S0140673602110257 [1].

Long-term relation between breastfeeding and development of atopy and asthma in children and young adults: a longitudinal study

Malcolm R Sears, Justina M Greene, Andrew R Willan, D Robin Taylor, Erin M Flannery, Jan O Cowan, G Peter Herbison, Richie Poulton

Summary

Background. Breastfeeding is widely advocated to reduce risk of atopy and asthma, but the evidence for such an effect is conflicting. We aimed to assess long-term outcomes of asthma and atopy related to breastfeeding in a New Zealand birth cohort.

Methods. Our cohort consisted of 1037 of 1139 children born in Dunedin, New Zealand, between April 1972 and March 1973, and residing in Otago province at age 3 years. Children were assessed every 2–5 years from ages 9 to 26 years with respiratory questionnaires, pulmonary function, bronchial challenge, and allergy skin tests. History of breastfeeding had been independently recorded in early childhood.

Findings. Five hundred and four (49 per cent) of 1037 eligible children were breastfed (4 weeks or longer) and 533 (51 per cent) were not. More children who were breastfed were atopic at all ages from 13 to 21 years to cats ($p = 0.0001$), house dust mites ($p = 0.0010$), and grass pollen ($p < 0.0001$) than those who were not. More children who were breastfed reported current asthma at each assessment between age 9 ($p = 0.0008$) and 26 years ($p = 0.0008$) than those who were not.

Breastfeeding effects were not affected by parental history of hayfever or asthma. Multifactor analysis controlling for socioeconomic status, parental smoking, birth order, and use of sheepskin bedding in infancy, showed odds ratios of 1.94 (95 per cent CI 1.42–2.65, $p < 0.0001$) for any allergen positive at age 13 years, 2.40 (1.36–4.26, $p = 0.0003$) for current asthma at 9 years, and 1.83 (1.35–2.47, $p < 0.0001$) for current asthma at 9–26 years by repeated-measures analysis.

Interpretation. Breastfeeding does not protect children against atopy and asthma and may even increase the risk.

Reprinted from *The Lancet*, Volume 360, Number 9337, Malcolm R Sears et al., 'Long-term relation between breastfeeding and development of atopy and asthma in children and young adults: a longitudinal study,' p. 901–907, © 2002 Elsevier Ltd, with permission from Elsevier, http://www.sciencedirect.com/science/journal/01406736 [1].

A. Description of the evidence

1. What was the exposure or intervention?

2. What was the outcome?

3. What was the study design?

4. What was the study population?

5. What was the main result?

The exposed group comprised 504 children who had been breastfed for 4 weeks or longer and entered this prospective cohort study at age 3 years. The comparison group comprised 533 children who were not breastfed for as long as 4 weeks and entered the study at the same time.

This paper is one of many resulting from this prospective study, which incorporated detailed assessments of physical, psychological, and social factors for a cohort of children. An assessment of the results of skin prick tests to several allergens (with positive tests referred to as atopy) at age 13 years and at age 21, and to asthma ascertained at various examinations from the age of 9 years up to the age of 26 is presented. For the purpose of this chapter we will concentrate on the outcome of *current asthma at the age of 9*. This was the first age at which a comprehensive questionnaire on asthma was used.

This is a prospective cohort study with active and intensive follow-up [2, 3], and has produced over 1000 scientific papers. It started as a study of all 1661 children born at the main maternity hospital in the small university city of Dunedin, New Zealand, between April 1972 and March 1973. All these children were included in a neonatal study. Later, a prospective cohort study was developed, and children eligible for this study were the members of that birth cohort who were still resident in the province of Otago, which includes Dunedin, at age 3 years; there were 1139 eligible children. These families were invited to participate and 91 per cent (1037 children) joined the study and so formed the study cohort. The study used very active assessment, with the subjects being asked to visit the study centre for a series of questionnaires and clinical and psychosocial assessments within a month of their birthday at ages 3, 5, 7, 9, 11, 13, 15, 18, 21, and 26 years. The study is still continuing, now with extension to the children of members of the original cohort. Out of the 1037 study entrants at age 3 years, 815 (78.6 per cent) participated in the assessment at age 9. The numbers participating then decreased gradually to 735 participating at age 13. Then an increase in funding allowed larger numbers to participate in further assessments, with 980 (94.5 per cent) of the original cohort participating at age 26. This involved considerable effort, including providing airfares for subjects outside Dunedin and even outside New Zealand to participate, and carrying out some assessments in other centres. This prospective study, carried out in a community with a population of about 120 000, has become an interesting social phenomenon, with members of the group being actively involved and kept informed of the results of the study by newsletters and other means; information on the study can be found on the website at http://dunedinstudy.otago.ac.nz.

The assessment of asthma at age 9 years used a standardized questionnaire and respiratory tests, giving the prevalence of asthma at this age. As shown in Box 14.1, of those children who were breastfed, 43 (10.8 per cent) of the 398 assessed at age 9 had asthma, compared with 19 (4.6 per cent) of the 417 who were not breastfed. Therefore breastfeeding is associated with an increase in asthma, with an odds ratio of 2.54, 95 per cent confidence limits of 1.45–4.44, and a P-value of 0.0008.

A relative risk (the ratio of the prevalence rates) also can be calculated, which is 2.37, similar to the odds ratio as the frequency of the outcome is reasonably low. The risk difference is 6.2 per cent, and if we assume causality, the attributable proportion in the exposed is 58 per cent, that is, the proportion of cases of asthma in breastfed children that are associated with breastfeeding. The attributable fraction in the population is 40 per cent; this is given as 'population attributable risk' in the paper. If this were an intervention study we would also calculate the number needed to treat, as the inverse of the risk difference. In an aetiological study, this calculation is better described as the number exposed for each additional case of asthma, which is 16. Box 14.1 also shows the derivation of a Mantel–Haenszel statistical test following the methods described in Chapter 8, and the confidence limits for the results; these are identical to those published in this paper.

Errors can occur even in high-profile journals like *The Lancet*, and in this publication the summary and the text state that 504 eligible children were breastfed and 533 were not breastfed, whereas in the headings in 1 and 2 of the paper these numbers are reversed. The numbers in the headings of the published tables are wrong, but the detailed results in these tables, including the numbers of children at later examinations, are correct.

B. Internal validity: consideration of non-causal explanations

6. Are the results likely to be affected by observation bias?

The study shows a higher recorded prevalence of asthma in children who were breastfed than in those who were not. As in any study, there are questions of non-differential error and of bias. Neither the classification of children as breastfed or not, nor the classification of children as having asthma at age 9, will be totally accurate. Some degree of error is likely with both these assessments. If this error is substantial, but non-differential, it will act to reduce the association towards the null value. One simple issue to be checked is: is there any possibility of miscoding of data? The general care and quality control of this study would seem to make such an explanation untenable, and the authors did check this thoroughly (M. Sears, personal communication).

Box 14.1 Main outcome of cohort study comparing asthma at age 9 years in breastfed and non-breastfed children

RESULTS OF A COHORT STUDY

Result for primary outcome of asthma current at age 9 years

	Asthma	No asthma	Total assessed	Proportion affected	Percentage affected
Breastfed	43	355	398	0.108	10.8
Not breastfed	19	398	417	0.046	4.6
Total	62	753	815	0.076	7.6

Prevalence of breastfed 0.49

Risk calculations

Relative risk	$= 0.108/0.046$	2.37
Odds ratio	$= 43 \times 398/(19 \times 355)$	2.54
Risk difference	$= (0.108 - 0.046) \times 100$	6.25 per cent
Number exposed per additional case $= 1/($risk difference$)$		16.0
Assuming causality, attributable proportion in exposed group $= 6.25/10.8$		57.8 per cent
Also $= (2.37 - 1)/2.37$ and attributable proportion in population $= (7.6 - 4.6)/7.6$		
Also $= 0.49 \times (2.37 - 1)/[0.49 \times (2.37 - 1) + 1]$		40.1 per cent

Statistical test (Mantel–Haenszel)

$a = 43$	$E = 30.27730061$	$V = 14.33066$
$\chi^2 = 11.30$	$\chi = 3.36$	$P = 0.001$

Confidence limits are calculated based on the standard deviation of RR, ln OR, or RD, following Table A2.2

	Value	ln	Std dev	95% confidence	limits
Relative risk	2.37	0.8634	0.2664	1.41	4.00
Odds ratio	2.54	0 9311	0.2850	1.45	4.44
Risk difference (%)	6.248		1.861	2.6	9.9%
Number exposed per additional case $= 1/($risk difference$)$			infinity	10.1

Source: data from Malcolm R Sears et al., 'Long-term relation between breastfeeding and development of atopy and asthma in children and young adults: a longitudinal study,' *The Lancet*, Volume 360, Number 9337, p. 901–907, © 2002 Elsevier Ltd [1].

Is there observation bias? The extreme case would be that the excess prevalence observed is not a true excess, but an artefact. Such bias could only occur if the validity of the assessment of asthma at age 9 is different in children who were breastfed and in those who were not, or if the validity of the assessment of breastfeeding was different in those children who later developed asthma compared with those who did not.

The protection is that the two assessments, of breastfeeding and of asthma, were made independently, and were both made in standardized ways. The history of breast-feeding was documented by interviews with the parents when the children were aged 3 years, and this information was validated by comparison with the records maintained by child health nurses. Some children who later had asthma may have had related con-ditions earlier in life, but these would only influence the history taken on breastfeeding if they were generally accepted as being related to breastfeeding at the time of the as-sessment at age 3.

In the assessment at age 9, a trained interviewer used a comprehensive standardized questionnaire and respiratory function tests were performed, including spirometry and a methacholine challenge test, which assesses airway hyper-responsiveness. The definition of current asthma used in the study was 'a positive response to the question "Do you (does your child) have asthma?" together with symptoms reported within the previous 12 months'. This is somewhat unclear, as it is not stated what symptoms or how many symptoms were required. It is stated that the definition was not dependent on whether treatment was prescribed or used. As we will see later, the association between breastfeeding and asthma is very controversial, and studies vary in their definitions of both breastfeeding and asthma, so that variations in definitions are important in interpretation.

Because the assessment of the exposure was made several years before the assess-ment of the outcome, and both were made by standardized methods, observation bias can be reasonably dismissed as contributing to these results. Non-differential error in the assessment of both outcome and exposure will be present. The details of the defini-tions of outcome and exposure may affect the generalizability of the study and com-parisons with other studies.

7. Are the results likely to be affected by confounding?

Do breastfed and non-breastfed children differ in factors that could affect the preva-lence of asthma? In the results section of the paper, it is noted that the children who were breastfed were more likely to be first born, have parents of higher socioeconomic status, have non-smoking mothers, and have had a sheepskin on their bed in infancy. Whether these factors are confounding will depend on whether they are independently associated with asthma. Girls and boys had similar proportions of being breastfed, and a history of hayfever or asthma in either mother or father was not related to breast-feeding, so these factors will not be confounding. For parental history, Box 14.2 shows that compared with the crude odds ratio of 2.54 relating asthma to breastfeeding, the Mantel–Haenszel odds ratio corrected for parental history is very similar at 2.43, and its confidence limits are also similar, confirming the absence of confounding. There is also no effect modification; the odds ratio is 2.26 where the family history is positive and 2.66 where the family history is negative, and this variation is well within the range of the confidence limits. A statistical test of heterogeneity shows a chi-square statistic of only 0.02.

Confounding is addressed in this paper by a multivariate analysis. The precise mul-tivariate model is not described, but is likely to be similar to the logistic regression model described in Chapter 8. From Table 4 of the paper, for breastfeeding, compared to the crude odds ratio of 2.54, the odds ratio controlled for family history, father's smoking, and cat ownership is similar, 2.40. The other associations were also little changed by the multivariate analysis, showing that these factors, while associated with asthma, were not strongly associated with breastfeeding and therefore were not confounding.

Should 'cat ownership' have been included in the multivariate model? This is 'cat ownership to 9 years', which presumably means the family ownership of a cat at any time before the child's ninth birthday, and it shows a strong negative association, with an odds ratio for asthma of 0.56 after control for other factors. If this is causal, it means that cat ownership prevents asthma, and this could be a useful and practical method of prevention! However, given the lack of information on the time relationships, it is likely that some families with a child with asthma would avoid owning a cat because of the generally held belief that contact with cats can produce allergies and respiratory effects. Therefore this association may be due to reverse causation: the child's asthma may prevent cat ownership. If that is true, it is not an independent risk factor for asthma, and should not be included in the multivariate model. However, it was probably anticipated that cat ownership could be an independent risk factor, associated with an expected *increase* in risk, in which case its inclusion in the model would be important. As its inclusion does not affect the association between breastfeeding and asthma, this is an intriguing issue but one that does not affect the interpretation of this study.

The relationship between asthma and breastfeeding has an odds ratio of 2.54. This association is stronger than the other associations seen in the study, with odds ratios of 1.6 for family history in relationship to asthma and also for father's smoking in relationship to asthma, and weaker relationships for the other variables assessed. This makes it unlikely that more careful control for any of the factors already included in the study would change the results.

Thus the key association is unlikely to be affected by confounding by any of the factors considered in this study. The main limitation is that there could be other factors associated with both asthma and breastfeeding that have not been assessed in this study.

8. Are the results likely to be affected by chance variation?

The association shown here is moderately strong, with odds ratio 2.54, with 95 per cent confidence limits of 1.45–4.44. These change very little after multivariate analysis, and observation bias is unlikely. The statistical methods used are appropriate, and we can conclude that chance variation is a very unlikely explanation for the results seen.

In summary, the study is acceptable in terms of observation bias and chance variation being unlikely explanations of the results, and we proceed with the knowledge that both a causal association, or an association due to confounding by factors not addressed in the study, are viable hypotheses to explain the results seen.

Box 14.2 Analysis of association between asthma and breastfeeding, stratified for family history of asthma or atopy

ASSOCIATION OF ASTHMA WITH BREASTFEEDING, STRATIFIED BY FAMILY HISTORY OF ASTHMA OR ATOPY

Overall association

	Asthma at 9 years	Not affected	Total cohort	Prevalence rate	Prevalence per cent	% by exposure	Odds ratio
Breastfed > 4 weeks	43	355	**398**	0.108	10.8	48.8	2.54
Not breastfed	19	398	**417**	0.046	4.6	51.2	
Total 62	62	753	815	0.076	7.6	100.0	

Stratum 1: family history positive

	Asthma at 9 years	Not affected	Total cohort	Prevalence rate	Prevalence per cent	% by exposure	Odds ratio
Breastfed >·4 weeks	23	151	**174**	0.132	13.2	50.0	2.26
Not breastfed	11	163	**174**	0.063	6.3	50.0	
Total	34	314	348	0.098	9.8	100.0	

Stratum 2: family history negative

	Asthma at 9 years	Not affected	Total cohort	Prevalence rate	Prevalence per cent	% by exposure	Odds ratio
Breastfed > 4 weeks	19	197	**216**	0.088	8.8	48.5	2.66
Not breastfed	8	221	**229**	0.035	3.5	51.5	
Total	27	418	445	0.061	6.1	100.0	

Crude and stratified analyses

	95% confidence limits			ln *OR*	dev *OR*
Overall crude odds ratio	2.54	1.45	4.44	0.9311	0.2850
Mantel–Haenszel odds ratio	2.43	1.39	4.26	0.8881	0.2869
Heterogeneity χ^2	0.0217	d.f. = 1	$P = 0.9$		

Missing data

	Asthma at 9 years	Not affected	Total cohort
Breastfed > 4 weeks	1	7	8
Not breastfed	0	14	14
Total	1	21	22

Source: data from Malcolm R Sears et al., 'Long-term relation between breastfeeding and development of atopy and asthma in children and young adults: a longitudinal study,' *The Lancet*, Volume 360, Number 9337, p. 901–907, © 2002 Elsevier Ltd [1].

C. Internal validity: consideration of positive features of causation

9. Is there a correct time relationship?

The exposure, breastfeeding, is time limited and occurs substantially before the assessment of outcome at 9 years old. However, we have no information on the age at first occurrence of asthma, as earlier assessments did not include it. As the outcome assessed is prevalence, influences on the incidence, progression, and regression of the disease are all relevant. Information on current asthma in subsequent years from 11 through to 26 is given in the paper, and shows a slowly increasing prevalence in both breastfed and non-breastfed individuals (Box 14.1); the association strengthens until age 13 when the odds ratio is 2.93, and then diminishes somewhat, but remains increased and statistically significant at all ages. In this study with repeated time-dependent measurements on individuals, more specialized statistical methods were also used to take this regular testing into account, and these gave consistent results.

Could children who develop asthma have earlier related conditions? If children later diagnosed with asthma had allergic conditions in very early life which led to the avoidance or early discontinuation of breastfeeding, this would be a protopathic bias, where an earlier related condition could influence the exposure (see Chapter 7). However, no evidence is given to suggest this.

10. Is the relationship strong?

The relationship is reasonably strong with an odds ratio of 2.54. As noted, this association is stronger than the other associations seen in the study, with odds ratios of 1.6 for both family history and father's smoking in relationship to asthma, and weaker relationships for the other variables assessed. Whether there is another unmeasured factor which could produce confounding is still an open question, but such a factor would have to have at least as strong an association with asthma to explain the association seen. As the exposure—being breastfed—was very common, the attributable risk in the population is high.

11. Is there a dose–response relationship?

If breastfeeding increases asthma, a dose–response relationship might be expected with the duration of breastfeeding representing the dose. Data are given on the numbers of children with durations of breastfeeding from 1 to 3 weeks up to over 26 weeks. In Figure 14.1 confidence limits are shown, which were not shown in the paper. There is no dose–response seen above 4 weeks. The lower prevalence with 1 to 3 weeks' breastfeeding could suggest a minimum duration of breastfeeding necessary to produce the increase in asthma, that is, a threshold effect, but this is based on very small numbers and is insecure. Aspects of dose–response can also apply to the severity of outcome. There are some further details given on the asthma, whether it was accompanied by airway hyper-responsiveness, and whether there was current significant wheeze. These results were consistent with the main association shown between breastfeeding and asthma.

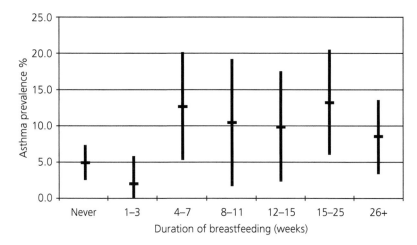

Figure 14.1 Prevalence of asthma at age 9 years, by duration of breastfeeding (weeks): data show the point estimate and 95 per cent confidence limits.

Source: data from Malcolm R Sears et al., 'Long-term relation between breastfeeding and development of atopy and asthma in children and young adults: a longitudinal study,' *The Lancet*, Volume 360, Number 9337, p. 901–907, © 2002 Elsevier Ltd [1].

12. Are the results consistent within the study?
And 13. Is there any specificity within the study?

The key result, the relationship of breastfeeding to asthma at age 9 years, is consistent with similar increased risks being observed subsequently in the study from the ages of 11 to 26, and is consistent with increased risks of atopy assessed at age 13 and age 21 by allergen testing to five different exposures. The elevated odds ratios for current asthma are consistent with increased risks of current wheeze with airways hyperresponsiveness. The association with asthma was similar in children with a parental history of hayfever or asthma and those without such a history, and no variation with duration of breastfeeding was seen.

The factors included as confounders in the multivariate analysis are listed. Results to assess if the main association varied with any of these factors (effect modification rather than confounding) are not given. Given the relatively small number of cases of asthma, subdividing the data into numerous subgroups is not a reliable form of analysis, as has been discussed in Chapter 8.

Conclusions with regard to internal validity

The prospective study design used here has great strength. The information on the exposure was collected independently from the assessment of outcome. The results at this assessment, at age 9 years, were consistent with outcomes assessed later up to age 26, and the internal consistency of the findings adds to the strength of these results.

There are two reasonable explanations for the results seen: (i) they reflect a causal relationship between being breastfed and asthma, and (ii) they are due to confounding by some unidentified factor or factors. A general problem with observational studies is whether further confounding factors can be excluded with confidence. Breastfeeding is a complex social behaviour, so other factors could be related to breastfeeding. Is there any evidence that any such factors would also be related to asthma? To contribute to these results, the direction of this association would need to be positive, that is, a factor would need to be more common in breastfed children and also more common in asthmatic children, or less common in breastfed children and less common in asthmatic children. We now proceed, with that conclusion in mind, to consider the external validity of the study.

D. External validity: generalization of the results

14. Can the study results be applied to the eligible population?

These results apply to the 815 children assessed for asthma at the age of 9 years, who comprised 79 per cent of the 1037 children who joined the cohort at age 3 years. The proportions participating were 398/504 (79 per cent) in breastfed and 417/533 (78 per cent) in non-breastfed children, so there is no variation in follow-up by exposure. These 1037 cohort entrants were 91 per cent of the eligible population of 1139 children at that age, and it is stated in the results that the childhood characteristics of the participants (based presumably on medical records) did not differ significantly from the 102 children who did not participate. The children in the eligible population who were available for assessment at age 9 might differ from the rest in ways which could influence the prevalence of asthma, and so the overall prevalence of asthma in those assessed could be different than in the entire eligible group. However, the fact that this selection effect was similar in breastfed and non-breastfed children makes it unlikely that it would influence the association between breastfeeding and asthma. Therefore the result can be applied to the eligible population.

15. Can the study results be applied to the source population?

The difference between the eligible population and the source population relates to the cohort study being based on 3-year-old children, the 1139 eligible, that is, those who were resident in the region at age 3 years, who comprised 69 per cent of the originally identified birth cohort of 1661 newborns. This is a reasonable criterion, although inclusion from birth would be better and is used in some other studies. Selection factors would have to be related to both breastfeeding and asthma to alter the associations seen. Therefore, although the participants in the asthma assessment represent only 815/1661 (i.e. 49 per cent of the original neonatal source population), it is reasonable to apply the results to the source population.

16. Can the study results be applied to other relevant populations?

This is much more difficult. The factors related to breastfeeding may well differ in different communities and at different time periods. Asthma is a multifactorial disease, which shows considerable variations between different populations, and can be associated with a multitude of environmental, including climatically related, factors. It is a complex disease with a number of subtypes that may have differing aetiological components. Whether the results of this study are likely to apply to other centres in New Zealand, to children in other countries, or to different time periods (these children were born in the early 1970s) are all issues open to discussion. It is pointed out in the paper that the families represented the full range of socioeconomic status in New Zealand, but they were predominately of European ancestry. The application of these results to the Maori population of New Zealand would be questionable without further evidence. The test of generalizability will be whether consistent associations are seen in studies in different communities.

Summary of external validity

Our conclusions on external validity must be cautious. Within the study, generalization of the key result to the eligible population and to the entire source population is appropriate. The source population is essentially a whole community, and there seems no reason why the results would not be applicable to other generally similar communities. However, the results are different from those of a number of other studies based in other countries and other time periods, and so the wider applicability of these results is unclear. The essential issue is whether these differences in results of different studies are due to true differences in the association, or differences in what has been assessed, or other differences in the methods used in the studies.

E. Comparison of the results with other evidence

We have gone about as far as we can in assessing this particular paper. Further discussion will take into account other relevant information, and will require an up-to-date review of the literature. It is not appropriate to consider such issues in detail here. We will consider the other evidence available at the time of publication of this paper. We can also use our assessment of the paper to identify the particular questions that need to be answered by other work.

As noted earlier, this prospective cohort study has high internal validity for an observational study, but we have identified confounding by other unidentified factors as the main issue in interpretation. The fact that the study results may not be generalizable to other populations has been noted. Both the discussion in this paper, and an assessment of subsequent studies, shows that this is indeed a controversial topic. There are many other studies, including other prospective cohort studies and meta-analyses.

17. Are the results consistent with other evidence, particularly evidence from studies of similar or more powerful study design?

The only more powerful study design would be an intervention trial. Clearly, an intervention trial of breastfeeding on a large representative general population of newborns would be difficult to perform and would be unethical, as there are many other reasons to support breastfeeding as superior. There have been intervention trials in high-risk groups, such as children born to parents with strong histories of allergic conditions, but based understandably on shorter-term end points. For example, the first such trial compared low-birthweight infants randomized to human breast milk or cows' milk, and showed no difference in the prevalence of allergic reactions at 18 months overall, although in the subgroup of infants with a positive family history of allergy, those given cows' milk had a higher frequency of allergies, mainly eczema [4].

The other relevant method of investigation is a case–control study comparing children with asthma with unaffected controls, gathering information on breastfeeding and other factors retrospectively. This is a weaker design as there is potential recall bias, although this might be alleviated if previous records were available to document breastfeeding. The advantage of such a case–control study is that further consideration could be given to a wider range of potential confounders, and to other clinical and laboratory aspects. Several case–control studies have been done, with inconsistent results.

Thus the major issue is consistency between this and other prospective cohort studies. In the discussion in the paper, the authors state that when the study was done, breastfeeding was widely advocated to reduce the risk of asthma, and they note that these results surprised them, as their working hypothesis was that breastfeeding would protect against asthma in childhood. The authors suggest that inconsistent results from different studies may arise if breastfeeding protects against asthma and similar conditions in early childhood, but increases the risks in later childhood. Few of the cohort studies went beyond 6 years. Developments after this study are noted at the end of this chapter.

18. Does the total evidence suggest any specificity?

As mentioned, the authors propose that the association between breastfeeding and asthma may be different at different ages. Other suggestions are that the association may depend on the duration of the breastfeeding, whether breastfeeding is exclusive with no exposure to cows' milk products, or on the family history of atopy or the personal history of atopy in the child. This study did assess length of time of breastfeeding and family history, without showing variations, but the breastfeeding used cannot be assumed to be exclusive.

19. Are the results plausible in terms of a biological mechanism?

This study shows the weakness of plausibility as a criterion in the assessment of the likely validity of findings. The authors point out that the most accepted belief before their study was that breastfeeding reduced asthma. A great deal has been written on the biological mechanisms behind this, related to protection against the development of inappropriate immune reactions. Indeed there is the impression that belief in this underlying mechanism is very strong amongst certain authorities, and this belief might be very little influenced by the results of this or other studies. However, the possible mechanisms are complex, so it is not difficult to come up with plausible biological mechanisms that would explain either an increase or a decrease in asthma related to breastfeeding. The authors consider several such mechanisms in their discussion.

20. If a major effect is shown, is it coherent with the distribution of the exposure and the outcome?

This study does show a major effect. If causal, and if the risk estimate is correct, in this population 40 per cent of all cases of asthma at the age of 9 years are caused by breastfeeding for more than 4 weeks. This is based on the attributable proportion in the population, as shown in Box 14.1. The authors state that in the early 1970s, when these children were born, the rate of breastfeeding, at around 50 per cent, was relatively low; by 1980 it had increased to over 80 per cent. We can calculate approximately what effect this would have on asthma prevalence. With an odds ratio of 2.5 and prevalence of exposure of 0.5, the frequency of asthma in the whole population, compared with the frequency in the low risk group, is $(0.5 \times 2.5) + (0.5 \times 1) = 1.75$. If the prevalence of exposure rises to 0.8, this becomes $(0.8 \times 2.5) + (0.2 \times 1) = 2.2$. Since $2.2/1.75 = 1.25$, the frequency of asthma at age 9 would be increased by 25 per cent, which should be measurable. This result is only approximate, and assumes both causality for this association and that all other aetiological factors and diagnostic criteria stay constant. Also, if the result from this study does apply to different populations, there should be a positive association, comparing populations, between the prevalence of breastfeeding and the prevalence of asthma 9 years later. In more general terms, there seems no doubt that the frequency of breastfeeding, at least for a few weeks, has increased in most developed countries from the 1970s, but the incidence of asthma in childhood has also greatly increased, at least to the 1990s [5]. This is consistent with the current study, but inconsistent with the general opinion that breastfeeding reduces asthma, so either this study is correct, or other factors are dominant, or the trends reflect changes in classification or recording.

Conclusions

Working through this critical appraisal shows that this is a substantial and carefully performed prospective cohort study, in which the information on outcome, asthma at the age of 9 years, is very clear, and the information on breastfeeding is almost equally clear. The results show a substantial association, which is statistically significant. Observation bias and chance variation are unlikely explanations for the results seen. Although several major factors were adequately controlled, the possibility of uncontrolled confounding remains, as there are many factors which could be confounding in this situation.

The external validity in terms of the application of the results to the source population is also high. The major question is: if these results are valid, why are they not consistently seen in other studies from different places in the world? Could the difference be in relationship to the age at onset of asthma, as these authors have suggested, or to some specificity in the type of asthma, or to some confounding factor or cofactor which is involved in the causal process and which varies in different places?

So we are left with two reasonable hypotheses to explain the observations seen (Table 14.1). One is that they do show a causal relationship. This may be specific to asthma at age 9 years (or close to it), and may not apply to asthma assessed at younger ages. The other is that the association is due to confounding, most likely by factors not measured in this study.

Subsequent development

This study generated considerable controversy, because the results were in the opposite direction to those expected. Among the criticisms of this study [6] were that in this cohort exclusive breastfeeding was unusual, and so the breastfed children could have had some exposure to cows' milk. However, that should only produce a bias towards a null result by misclassification of the exposure (unless mixed feeding is the key factor). The absence of dose–response was also noted as a weakness, as was the lack of interaction with a family history of atopy, but these are not essential elements of causation. A more serious criticism was that the information on feeding patterns in infancy could be biased because the information was collected only at age 3 years. However, the authors showed that the maternal recall at that age was supported in more than 98 per cent of instances by the records of infant care nurses, which were completed concurrently with early childhood [7]. The fact that only 69 per cent of the original cohort of neonates were included in this cohort has also been given as a criticism, and while it is a limitation in comparison with other cohorts starting from birth, it would only affect the results if the selection into the prospective cohort was related to both breastfeeding and the prevalence of asthma much later at age 9, which seems unlikely. The study's authors responded in detail to these criticisms [7].

The main difficulty in accepting the results of this study is that few other studies have shown an increased risk. For example, in another prospective study in a birth cohort in two other cities in New Zealand, asthma was assessed at several intervals up to the age of 6 years, and a protective effect of breastfeeding was seen, with a dose–response showing that more months of breastfeeding and exclusive breastfeeding gave greater protection [8]. Several other studies show protective effects at similar ages, leaving open the question of whether asthma at older ages has a different relationship with breastfeeding.

The relationship between breastfeeding and asthma is still uncertain in 2015. An authoritative review of the prevention of asthma states that the association is unclear, and randomized trials of the delayed introduction of solid food in infancy, and of the promotion of long-term and exclusive breastfeeding, have not shown benefits; but despite that, 'encouraging breastfeeding' is still one of the potential preventive strategies supported [9].

Table 14.1 Assessment of causality in a prospective cohort study. Study of breastfeeding and asthma and atopy in later childhood, by Sears et al. [1].

Breastfeeding and asthma: Sears et al. [1]	
A. Description of evidence	
1. Exposure	Breastfeeding for at least 4 weeks; controls less than 4 weeks' breastfeeding or none
2. Outcome	Asthma, from history and clinical assessment at age 9 years
3. Design	Cohort study, prospective from age 3 years
4. Study population	Children born in one hospital in Dunedin, New Zealand, from April 1972 to March 1973 and resident in the area at age 3 years
5. Main result	Current prevalence of asthma 10.8% if breastfed; 4.6% controls. Odds ratio 2.54, 95% confidence limits 1.45–4.44
B. Non-causal explanations	
6. Observation bias	Outcome assessment based on combination of clinical histories and respiratory tests. Breastfeeding data recorded at age 3 years, consistent with nurses' records made throughout infancy. Observation bias unlikely
7. Confounding	Several factors, including sex, birth order, socioeconomic status, parental smoking, cat ownership, family history of atopy, have been controlled, but other confounders are possible
8. Chance	Unlikely to be due to chance: main result has P-value less than 0.001
C. Positive features of causation	
9. Time relationship	Compatible with causation; no data on time of onset of asthma prior to age 9 years; data at later ages consistent
10. Strength	Main result strong; large enough to be clinically important
11. Dose–response	Data insufficient to assess a relationship with number of months of breastfeeding; no clear variation with severity of asthma
12. Consistency	Association with asthma consistent with later assessments at ages 11–26, and with associations with atopy
13. Specificity	No variation seen with family history or duration of breastfeeding
Summary of internal validity: result shows substantial effect, unlikely to be due to chance; observation bias unlikely; but there may be effects of unknown confounders.	
D. External validity	
14. To the eligible population	Participants represent 79% of cohort participants at age 3, and 72% of eligible population. Loss to follow-up is independent of exposure. Main result applies to eligible population
15. To the source population	Eligible population was 62% of the original birth cohort, but eligibility depends on place of residence only. Result should apply to source population
16. To other populations	Source population is births in one community in southern New Zealand in 1972–73. Applicability of results to other communities and time periods unknown. Extension of results to other age groups unknown

(Continued)

Table 14.1 (Continued)

E. Other evidence	
17. Consistency	Several other large prospective cohort studies, and meta-analyses. Several studies support opposite association, with lower asthma risk if breastfed. Effect may vary with age at assessment of asthma; some support from other studies of an increased risk in later childhood
18. Specificity	Association for asthma may be shared with other atopy outcomes. Variation in length of breastfeeding, whether breastfeeding is exclusive, and with family history of asthma or atopy may be relevant. Association may change with age
19. Plausibility	Despite general view that breastfeeding may protect against atopy, mechanisms are complex and any effect can be supported
20. Coherence	Population attributable risk is high because prevalence of breastfeeding is high, so if causal and generalizable should show coherence in time and place. Asthma and breastfeeding both increasing in time. Geographical coherence not assessed

Summary of external validity: study is done in one community, and other data from different places often seem conflicting, so external validity is limited and depends on the emergence of supporting data from other studies. Age at assessment may be critical.

Source: data from Malcolm R Sears et al., 'Long-term relation between breastfeeding and development of atopy and asthma in children and young adults: a longitudinal study,' *The Lancet*, Volume 360, Number 9337, p. 901–907, © 2002 Elsevier Ltd [1].

A 2015 review using GRADE principles is restricted to asthma at ages above 5 years, the authors stating that at younger ages it is easily misclassified with transient wheeze [10]. They found that more versus less breastfeeding was associated with a reduced risk of asthma at ages from 5 to 18, greater in medium- and low-income than in high-income countries, although this estimate had high heterogeneity and low quality. A meta-analysis including 13 cohort studies, two case–control studies, and 14 cross-sectional studies give an odds ratio of 0.90, with 95 per cent limits of 0.84–0.97. The study discussed in this chapter had the highest increased risk of all the studies, although two other cohort studies showed statistically significant increased risks. A large international study of asthma symptoms at ages 6–7 years in over 200 000 children in 31 countries reported no association between breastfeeding and symptoms of severe asthma [11]; the odds ratio was 0.95, with 95 per cent confidence limits of 0.87–1.05, so in fact a small and non-significant protective effect was seen, which is not inconsistent with the meta-analysis just mentioned. Most other reviews conclude that a small protective effect of breastfeeding applies, at least for young children [12, 13].

Of course, the use of breastfeeding goes much beyond this topic, and even the present authors do not use their data to suggest that the current approach of encouraging breastfeeding should be changed. A major Cochrane systematic review of the optimal duration of exclusive breastfeeding, with an emphasis on developing countries, led to a World Health Assembly resolution to recommend exclusive breastfeeding for 6 months, based mainly on a reduction in gastrointestinal tract infections, although noting that no reduction in atopic outcomes or asthma had been demonstrated in studies from Finland, Australia, and Belarus [14].

References

1. **Sears MR, Greene JM, Willan AR, Taylor DR, Flannery EM, Cowan JO, et al**. Long-term relation between breastfeeding and development of atopy and asthma in children and young adults: a longitudinal study. *Lancet* 2002; **360**:901–907.

2. **Poulton R, Moffitt TE, Silva PA**. The Dunedin Multidisciplinary Health and Development Study: overview of the first 40 years, with an eye to the future. *Soc Psychiatry Psychiatr Epidemiol* 2015; **50**:679–693.

3. **Silva PA, Stanton W**. *From Child to Adult: The Dunedin Multidisciplinary Health and Development Study*. New York: Oxford University Press; 1996.

4. **Lucas A, Brooke OG, Morley R, Cole TJ, Bamford MF**. Early diet of preterm infants and development of allergic or atopic disease: randomised prospective study. *BMJ* 1990; **300**:837–840.

5. **Pearce N, Douwes J**. The global epidemiology of asthma in children. *Int J Tuberc Lung Dis* 2006; **10**:125–132.

6. **Peat JK, Allen J, Oddy W, Webb K**. Breastfeeding and asthma: appraising the controversy. *Pediatr Pulmonol* 2003; **35**:331–334.

7. **Sears MR, Taylor DR, Poulton R**. Breastfeeding and asthma: appraising the controversy—a rebuttal. *Pediatr Pulmonol* 2003; **36**:366–368.

8. **Silvers KM, Frampton CM, Wickens K, Pattemore PK, Ingham T, Fishwick D, et al**. Breastfeeding protects against current asthma up to 6 years of age. *J Pediatr* 2012; **160**:991–996.

9. **Beasley R, Semprini A, Mitchell EA**. Risk factors for asthma: is prevention possible? *Lancet* 2015; **386**:1075–1085.

10. **Lodge CJ, Tan DJ, Lau M, Dai X, Tham R, Lowe AJ, et al**. Breastfeeding and asthma and allergies: a systematic review and meta-analysis. *Acta Paediatr* 2015; **104**:38–53.

11. **Bjorksten B, Ait-Khaled N, Innes AM, Clayton TO, Robertson C**. Global analysis of breast feeding and risk of symptoms of asthma, rhinoconjunctivitis and eczema in 6–7 year old children: ISAAC Phase Three. *Allergol Immunopathol (Madr)* 2011; **39**:318–325.

12. **Yong SB, Wu CC, Wang L, Yang KD**. Influence and mechanisms of maternal and infant diets on the development of childhood asthma. *Pediatr Neonatol* 2013; **54**:5–11.

13. **Ip S, Chung M, Raman G, Trikalinos TA, Lau J**. A summary of the Agency for Healthcare Research and Quality's evidence report on breastfeeding in developed countries. *Breastfeed Med* 2009; **4**(Suppl 1):S17–30.

14. **Kramer MS, Kakuma R**. Optimal duration of exclusive breastfeeding. *Cochrane Database Syst Rev* 2012; **8**:CD003517.

Chapter 15

Critical appraisal of a retrospective cohort study

Introduction

This study was published in *The Lancet*, 26 October 1991, 338, 1027–1032 [1], and is available at http://www.thelancet.com or at http://www.sciencedirect.com/science/journal/01406736/338/8774.

Cancer mortality in workers exposed to chlorophenoxy herbicides and chlorophenols

Rodolfo Saracci, Manolis Kogevinas, Pier-Alberto Bertazzi, Bas H. Bueno de Mesquita, David Coggon, Lois M Green, Timo Kauppinen, Kristan A. L'Abbé, Margareta Littorin, Elsebeth Lynge, John D Mathews, Manfred Neuberger, John Osman, Neil Pearce, Regina Winkelman

Abstract

Epidemiological studies have revealed an increased risk of cancer, notably soft-tissue sarcomas and non-Hodgkin's lymphomas, in people occupationally exposed to chlorophenoxy herbicides, including those contaminated by 2,3,7,8-tetrachlorodibenz o-*p*-dioxin (TCDD). We report here a historical cohort study of mortality in an international register of 18 910 production workers or sprayers from ten countries.

Exposure was reconstructed through questionnaires, factory or spraying records, and job histories. Cause-specific national death rates were used as reference. No excess was observed in all-cause mortality, for all neoplasms, for the most common epithelial cancers, or for lymphomas. A statistically nonsignificant two-fold excess risk, based on 4 observed deaths, was noted for soft-tissue sarcoma with a standardised mortality ratio (SMR) of 196 and 95 per cent confidence interval (CI) 53–502; this was concentrated as a six-fold statistically significant excess, occurring 10–19 years from first exposure in the cohort as a whole (SMR = 606 [165–1552]) and, for the same time period, as a nine-fold excess among sprayers (SMR = 882 [182–2579]). Risks appeared to be increased for cancers of the testicle, thyroid, other endocrine glands, and nose and nasal cavity, based on small numbers of deaths.

The excess of soft-tissue sarcomas among sprayers is compatible with a causal role of chlorophenoxy herbicides but the excess does not seem to be specifically associated with those herbicides probably contaminated by TCDD.

Reprinted from *The Lancet*, Volume 338, Issue 8774, Rodolfo Saracci et al., 'Cancer mortality in workers exposed to chlorophenoxy herbicides and chlorophenols', p. 1027–32, © 1991 Published by Elsevier Ltd, with permission from Elsevier, http://www.sciencedirect.com/science/journal/01406736 [1].

A. Description of the evidence

1. What was the exposure or intervention?
2. What was the outcome?
3. What was the study design?
4. What was the study population?
5. What was the main result?

The objective was to assess various possible effects of a specific exposure: *chlorophenoxy herbicides*. As described in the introduction, these chemicals have been widely used since the 1950s for controlling unwanted plant growth, and formed a component of the notorious 'agent orange' used in the Vietnam War for defoliation. The closely related *chlorinated phenol* compounds are intermediates in the production of these herbicides, and are also used themselves for wood preservation. Both sets of compounds may be contaminated during production by a range of other compounds, including tetrachlorodibenzo-dioxin (TCDD). This study is based on exposure to these compounds, defined through holding an occupation likely to involve such exposure.

The outcome was mortality, from all causes, with particular attention given to mortality from specified types of cancer.

Being exposure based, this is a cohort study, and is a retrospective (historical) cohort study. The study population was identified through current and past employment records, which were linked to mortality records to give outcome information.

The study population were workers identified through the 'International Register of Workers Exposed to Phenoxy Herbicides and their Contaminants', which was set up by an international and a US group. This consisted of 20 separate cohorts representing different employers, workplaces, and countries, involving in total 18 390 workers (16 863 male, 1527 female) from 10 countries. The derivation of the study participants is shown in Box 15.1.

Information on where each employee in the register worked and when, and a more detailed job history for most workers, was available. Job histories were categorized by levels of exposure, using the experience of industrial hygienists and workers. The employees were grouped into '*exposed*' workers, who had jobs regarded as very likely to involve exposure to chlorophenoxy herbicides or chlorinated phenols, '*probably exposed*' workers, which included all workers in two cohorts where no detailed job information was available, a group of workers with '*unknown exposure*', where there was no information, and a group of '*non-exposed*' workers. The last group comprised workers who had been employed in workplaces within the registry, but who had never been

Box 15.1 Derivation of the cohort of workers contributing to the analysis of Saracci et al. [1]

DESIGN OF A RETROSPECTIVE COHORT STUDY

	Total group	
	In study	**Excluded**
Source population, from Register (SP)	18 972	% of source
Found ineligible		62	0.3
Died or lost to follow up before 1955		220	1.2
Total excluded		282	1.5
Eligible population (EP)	18 690	% of eligible
Unknown year of birth		131	0.7
Unknown year of first exposure		105	0.6
Unknown sex		1	0.0
Other missing information		63	0.3
Total not approached		300	1.6
Included in study cohort	18 390	
Participants in study	18 390	
Loss to follow-up*		Unknown '<5%'
Participants in analysis (PA)	18 390	
Voluntary response rate	Not applicable	
Participation rate	= PA/EP	98.4%
Eligible/source population	= EP/SP	98.5%
Participants/source population	= PA/SP	96.9%

*Subjects lost to follow-up contribute to the analysis until their follow-up ends

Distribution of participants by exposure category	
Exposed	13 482
Probably exposed	416
Unknown exposure	541
Non-exposed	3951

Source: data from Rodolfo Saracci et al., 'Cancer mortality in workers exposed to chlorophenoxy herbicides and chlorophenols,' *The Lancet*, Volume 338, Issue 8774, p. 1027–32, © 1991 Published by Elsevier Ltd [1].

employed in the parts of the factories which produced the chemicals, and had never sprayed them; these workers are regarded as being non-exposed to the chemicals in question, although they were exposed to other chemicals. Therefore the study has an *external* control group, shown by the comparison of observed mortality with the mortality expected on the basis of national data, and also an *internal* comparison, comparing different categories of exposure.

Results for total mortality, major causes of mortality, and cancer mortality are presented. For this review, we will concentrate on the result that is emphasized by the authors, which is *mortality from soft-tissue sarcoma*. This is emphasized because previous studies had demonstrated excesses of incidence or mortality of soft-tissue sarcoma in relationship to exposure to these chemicals, so that the hypothesis of an increased mortality rate was established a priori, and the study is testing that hypothesis. For many of the other results, the study is a hypothesis generation study, as the findings are unanticipated.

The mortality of the identified cohorts is compared with the expected mortality based on national mortality statistics by sex, age, and calendar period for the country relating to the individual cohort. For each cause of mortality the observed number of deaths is compared with the expected number, the ratio being the standardized mortality ratio (SMR). This is expressed in percentage terms, the null value being 100 and higher values showing an excess mortality (see Chapter 7, 'Indirect standardization').

The main result for soft-tissue sarcoma (Table 15.1) is that for exposed and probably exposed workers combined; four deaths were observed compared with 2.04 expected, giving an SMR of 196, with 95 per cent confidence limits of 53–502. The confidence intervals are calculated from tables of the Poisson distribution [1]; the 95 per cent limits for the observed number of four deaths are 1.09 and 10.24, so the 95 per cent limits of the SMR are 1.09/2.04 ×100 and 10.24/2.04 × 100. For the non-exposed workers, there were no observed deaths, compared with 0.42 expected; the SMR of zero has confidence limits of 0–878. Therefore the main result is an excess mortality rate from soft-tissue sarcoma in workers exposed to chlorophenoxy herbicides or chlorinated phenols. We need to assess whether this association is likely to be due to a causal relationship.

B. Internal validity: consideration of non-causal explanations

6. Are the results likely to be affected by observation bias?

As the key result with regard to soft-tissue sarcomas is dependent on the observation of four deaths, observation bias and observation error are both relevant. If even one or two true occurrences of death from this disease have been missed, or if some of the deaths recorded are erroneous, the results could be greatly affected.

Table 15.1 Main results for deaths from soft-tissue sarcoma: from the retrospective cohort study of Saracci et al. [1]. Results taken from Table III of the paper, SMR = standardized mortality ratio (100 = null result); TCCD = 2,3,7,8-tetra chlorodibenzo-*p*-dioxin.

	Observed number of cases	Expected number of cases	SMR	95% confidence limits
Subgroups				
Exposure				
Exposed or probably exposed	4	2.04	196	53–502
Non-exposed	0	0.42	0	0–878
Type of work				
Production workers	1	1.03	97	3–541
Sprayers	3	1.01	297	61–868
Chemicals used				
Both	1	0.48	208	5–1161
Phenoxy	3	1.50	200	41–585
Chlorophenols	0	0.06	0	0–6148
Exposure to TCDD				
Probable	2	1.00	200	24–723
Unlikely	2	1.04	193	23–695
Years since first exposure				
30+	0	0.24	0	0–1537
20–29	0	0.52	0	0–709
10–19	4	0.66	606	165–1552
0–9	0	0.50	0	0–738
Duration of exposure				
20+	0	0.15	0	0–2459
10–19	2	0.29	690	84–2491
1–9	0	0.89	0	0–415
<1	2	0.59	339	41–1125

Source: data from Rodolfo Saracci et al., 'Cancer mortality in workers exposed to chlorophenoxy herbicides and chlorophenols,' *The Lancet*, Volume 338, Issue 8774, p. 1027–32, © 1991 Published by Elsevier Ltd [1].

In terms of *bias*, the essential issue is whether the recognition and recording, which includes the classification of the cause of death, was done in an identical manner in these workers as in the general population (with reference to the external control comparison), and whether it was done in an identical fashion in groups defined with different levels of exposure (for the internal comparison). Bias compared with the general population could arise if this disease or others like it were thought to be more common in such workers: if so, there could be greater clinical awareness for this condition, specific diagnostic procedures might be more likely to be done, if it did occur it could be more likely to be recorded on the clinical record or on a death certificate, and an ambiguous record might be more likely to be coded to sarcoma. A study of this issue done now would need to take account of such potential biases, as the possible association between herbicide exposure and soft-tissue sarcomas is now widely recognized. However, the observation period for mortality in this study largely preceded such interest. The period of observation varies with the different cohorts: the starting dates range from 1955 to 1975, and the cut-off dates range from 1982 to 1988. The earliest suspicion of a link, which can be judged from the extensive list of references given in this paper, appears to be from a case–control study published in 1979. It seems unlikely that this suspicion would have affected clinical practice or death certification until some years after that. The potential bias could be addressed by seeing if the excess mortality was confined to deaths occurring in the later years, when knowledge of the potential hypothesis would be more widespread. An analysis by calendar year of death would of course have to be appropriately adjusted for the associations between year of death, duration of exposure, and year since first exposure; no such analysis is presented here. Therefore while observation bias remains a theoretical possibility, it is unlikely to be a major issue.

The question of the *error* in the reported mortality from soft-tissue sarcomas is of greater significance. These cancers are not particularly easy to diagnose, and they are not very clearly defined in clinical or pathological terms; therefore some deaths from soft-tissue sarcomas could have been inadequately described on a death certificate and coded to some other category. It is less likely that any of the deaths recorded as being from soft-tissue sarcomas were in fact from something else. This type of inaccuracy, occurring without bias, would produce some misclassification of the outcome, and would weaken the power of the study to detect a real effect; this could mean that the observed result is an underestimate of the true relationship.

7. Are the results likely to be affected by confounding?

In assessing potential confounders, we need to ask the two general questions. First, apart from these herbicides, what factors are known to increase or decrease the risk of death from soft-tissue sarcoma? Second, what other exposures are likely to be associated with exposure to these chemicals? The first question is not addressed in the paper, and so further review of the literature is necessary. At the time of the study, this was rather unproductive. Apart from the general confounders of age, sex, and country (which are controlled in this study because the expected numbers of deaths are based on analyses specific to those factors), little is known about causal factors for soft-tissue sarcoma. The disease is not known to be related to smoking, which is often a confounding factor in occupational studies. In terms of factors associated with the exposure, the most obvious are other chemical exposures. The study participants have worked in jobs which involve using or manufacturing chemicals, and are very likely to have been exposed to many chemicals. This is discussed in the paper, and the authors indeed conclude that their attempt to relate risks to specific agents was 'only partially successful' (discussion, paragraph 1). They argue that the most specific exposure to chlorophenoxy herbicides would be in sprayers, rather than production workers. The results show that the excess mortality was confined to sprayers, with an SMR of 297 based on three deaths, whereas the SMR in production workers was not increased, being 97 based on one death.

There is information, based on the job history, with regard to whether exposure was likely to have been to phenoxy compounds, chlorophenols, or both, and whether exposure to TCDD was likely. There were no deaths in those exposed only to chlorophenols, with the excess mortality being seen both in those exposed to phenoxy compounds (three deaths, SMR 200) and in those exposed to both (one death, SMR 208). There was no difference in the SMR by likely exposure to TCDD (Table 15.1).

The information with regard to spraying versus production work, and the information on likely individual chemical exposure, suggest that the association is primarily with phenoxy herbicides, rather than with chlorophenols or TCDD. Given the limitations of the classification of exposure and the very small numbers, this conclusion can only be tentative.

Potential confounding factors can also be identified by examining other mortality outcomes. For example, if the exposed workers had increased mortality from cancers related to smoking, it would suggest that they smoked more than the general population. If, in addition, soft-tissue sarcoma were related to smoking, smoking would be a confounder. In fact, neither of these relationships is supported. In this study, the SMR for lung cancer in exposed workers was not increased, being 102, and review of the literature shows that sarcomas are not known to be related to smoking. The pattern of other mortality is difficult to interpret because of the small numbers. Results are presented for 29 different cancer sites, of which 17 have SMRs above 100 and 12 below; there is nothing in the pattern which suggests any other causal agent which could be a confounder in the association with soft-tissue sarcomas.

8. Are the results likely to be affected by chance variation?

The increased SMR in exposed and probably exposed workers is not statistically significant, being 196, with a 95 per cent confidence interval of 53–502. In other words, the result is compatible with a mortality rate from soft-tissue sarcomas of approximately half that of the general population, up to a rate of five times. This demonstrates the weakness of cohort studies in dealing with rare outcomes; this study involved nearly 19 000 workers and was a major logistic effort, but for this particular outcome it is a very weak study. The effective sample size depends on the four observed deaths. Therefore chance variation is a quite likely explanation of the overall result.

The SMR is the ratio of the observed to expected numbers of deaths from a particular cause, as noted in Chapter 7. The statistical assessment is based on the Poisson distribution, which is appropriate for rare events. The variance of the number of events on this distribution is equal to the expected number, so a chi-squared statistic (one degree of freedom) testing the difference in an SMR from the null value of 1 or 100 is given by $(Obs - Exp)^2/Exp$; for the data on sarcoma $\chi^2 = (4 - 2.04)^2 / 2.04 = 1.88$; $P = 0.17$ from Table A2.15. The confidence intervals are calculated from tables of the Poisson distribution [1]; the 95 per cent limits for the observed number of 4 deaths are 1.09 and 10.24, so the 95 per cent limits of the SMR are $1.09/2.04 \times 100$ and $10.24/2.04 \times 100$, giving 53–502.

C. Internal validity: consideration of positive features of causation

9. Is there a correct time relationship?

The first criterion for the time relationship is that exposure to these chemicals must have occurred before the onset of the sarcoma. Workers were included in the register and classified as exposed from the first year of the study or from the time they began a job falling into that exposure classification; in three of the cohorts, minimum employment periods of 1 month, 6 months, and 1 year were specified. Once enrolled, their time experience contributed to the person-years at risk denominator, continuing until death or the end of the follow-up period. The relevant biological effect, causing the sarcoma, could predate death from the sarcoma by several years. Therefore, in those workers who develop a sarcoma, exposure after causation has been added erroneously to the denominator, and this gives an error. However, the number of workers to whom this applies is so small that it would make no difference to the results. Some of the sarcomas may indeed have originated prior to first chemical exposure, or prior to the date of entry into the cohort. These issues are addressed in analyses which look at the time dimensions of the study. If the association is causal, we would not expect death to occur within a few years of first exposure; it would happen after a time interval representing the induction time of the cancer plus the interval from cancer development to death. We might expect risk to rise steadily with time since first exposure or, as an alternative, postulate that risk would peak at a certain time after exposure and then subsequently decrease. In fact, there were no deaths within 0–9 years after first exposure, and all four deaths occurred between 10–19 years, with no deaths in the categories of 20–29 years and over 30 years since first exposure. The expected numbers show that there were substantial person-years of follow-up in these categories. The 10–19-year time-frame is compatible with a causal relationship, although the very small number of observed deaths prevents any firm conclusion about the time-specificity of the risk relationship.

10. Is the relationship strong?

This relationship is not particularly strong; the overall effect is a doubling of risk, four observed deaths compared with two expected. Of course, it is likely that the observed SMR, if there is a true causal effect, is an underestimate, because the categorization of exposure must have a great deal of error. The exposure is based on a job history, and for some of the groups of workers is simply employment as no specific job history was available. Within those categorized as exposed there are probably many workers with minimal exposure, and perhaps only a small group with very high levels of exposure. The SMR relates to the average exposure of this overall group. The fact that it is not particularly large means that such a result could occur through a modest amount of error or bias in the observation of death from soft-tissue sarcoma, the effect on an unidentified confounding factor, or, of course, chance variation. As all four deaths occurred in one particular category of year since first exposure, 10–19 years, for this interval there were four observed deaths and 0.66 expected, giving an SMR of 606. This is statistically significant, with a lower 95 per cent confidence interval of 165, but as this is a post hoc choice of category, undue emphasis should not be put on this result.

11. Is there a dose–response relationship?

Dose–response relationships have been assessed in a number of ways in this study. First, results are presented for workers regarded as exposed or probably exposed (combined), and also for those regarded as non-exposed, with the relevant SMRs being 196 and zero. All four deaths in the combined exposure group were in exposed workers. Although this difference could be due to chance, it is consistent with causality. Similarly, those classified as sprayers have an increased SMR, with no increase being seen in production workers. This is consistent with causality if the level of exposure to these chemicals was higher in sprayers than in production workers. It is not clear whether this is true. The authors argue that the sprayers were more likely to be exposed *specifically* to these chemicals rather than to other chemicals, but they do not comment on the relative *intensity* of exposure of sprayers and production workers.

The other measure of dose–response is duration of exposure, and we would expect that the risk would increase with duration of exposure. In particular, those workers who had a very modest time of exposure might show little increase in risk. Duration of exposure was categorized into four groups, from less than 1 year up to 20 or more years. Two of the deaths occurred in workers with 10–19 years of exposure, giving an SMR of 690, and the other two deaths occurred in workers with less than 1 year of exposure, giving an SMR of 339. Thus these data do not show a dose–response relationship; indeed, the occurrence of two of the four deaths in workers with less than 1 year of exposure tends to argue against these chemicals being the cause of all four deaths.

12. Are the results consistent within the study?

Consistency in this study is assessed by the factors regarded as indicating high levels of exposure; these have been discussed. The number of outcome events is too small to assess other relevant aspects of consistency, for example, by country, or in men and women.

13. Is there any specificity within the study?

A particular association with soft-tissue sarcomas would be more convincing if it were strong, and if there were no other excesses from other causes of death. In the workers categorized as exposed, there are several causes of death with SMRs higher than 200, and they are a mixed group. They include cancers of unspecified digestive organs, nose or nasal cavities, the male breast, the testes, the thyroid gland, and other endocrine glands, and there is a high SMR for benign and unspecified neoplasms. There are high SMRs for several other cancer sites in workers classified as probably exposed. Therefore the association with sarcoma is not specific in terms of the outcome. Specificity in terms of the exposure has been discussed; it appears to be specific to phenoxy herbicides.

Conclusions with regard to internal validity

So what can we conclude about the internal validity of this study with regard to the association with sarcoma? The study seems unlikely to be open to systematic observation bias, but unsystematic error in the outcome could influence the study results. The classification of exposure is open to considerable error, reducing the power of the study to show a real association. Confounding by exposures to other chemicals seems a possible explanation of the results, and so little is known about the causation of this disease that unrecognized confounding factors cannot be ruled out. Chance variation is a quite likely alternative explanation of the results seen, as the overall result is not significant at conventional levels. Certain subcategorizations of the results are significant, and the authors put considerable stress on the SMR of 606 obtained by only assessing 10–19 years from first exposure, and the SMR of 882 by using the same criterion plus restricting to sprayers rather than production workers. While both of these examples of specificity can be justified, these justifications are essentially after the fact. Specific associations at this time period and in this particular group of workers were not clearly specified as a priori hypotheses to be tested, and so the statistical significance of these selected results has to be viewed with caution. In general, therefore, this study on its own cannot be regarded as pointing unequivocally towards a causal explanation, as the possibilities of observation bias, confounding, and chance variation all remain.

D. External validity: generalization of the results

14. Can the study results be applied to the eligible population?

Generalization of the results from the participant population, those who were followed up so that mortality could be determined, to the eligible population, those employees in workplaces cooperating with the international registry, seems without problems; the participation rate was 98.4 per cent (Box 15.1). The main issue is whether large numbers of workers within these cohorts were lost to follow-up, and so did not contribute to the results for the whole time period. In the methods section, the loss to follow-up overall is given as about 5 per cent of the total cohort, and did not exceed 10 per cent in any particular constituent cohort. This is a very high follow-up rate.

15. Can the study results be applied to the source population?

In this study the source and eligible populations are basically the same, if we can accept that all eligible male workers in the work forces in the study were enrolled in the documented cohorts. Problems would have arisen if workers for whom exposure could not be categorized were excluded, but this was not done; such workers were maintained in the study, and results for this 'unknown exposure category' are also shown.

16. Can the study results be applied to other relevant populations?

The generalization of the results to other target populations is more difficult. We need to review the objective of the study, and we can consider it as either pragmatic or explanatory. A pragmatic objective is to assess if occupational exposure to these chemicals is associated with an increase in the mortality from soft-tissue sarcoma, which clearly has implications for management, control, and industrial compensation. The relevant issue is whether these exposed workers are representative of a wider population of exposed workers. If the workplaces contributing to this international register had particularly high levels of exposure, the association seen, even if true, might not apply to workers in other workplaces with considerably lower levels of exposure. If the workplaces studied had particularly low exposures, perhaps by having particularly good industrial hygiene standards and practices, the results could underestimate the problem. As production of these compounds has been restricted or banned in recent years (as stated in the introduction), current industrial exposures may be more stringently controlled and exposure levels may be lower than they were in the workplaces studied here.

We could argue that the purpose of the study is explanatory—to assess whether there is a causal relationship between these chemicals and soft-tissue sarcoma in general scientific terms. In this argument, we view these occupational groups not as representing occupationally exposed subjects in general, but as a natural experiment to observe the results of in human subjects. Whereas the pragmatic objective would be best fulfilled if the exposures of these workers were typical of a wider workforce, this is not relevant to an explanatory objective; indeed, selection of workplaces with the highest exposure levels would maximize the power of the study.

The other limitations, applying to both interpretations, are in gender and geography. The participants were mainly men, and so the association, if valid, might not apply to women. The workforces represented are predominantly of European ethnic backgrounds; the results might not apply to other ethnic groups. These issues would need to be explored if the results from this study were much more striking.

E. Comparison of the results with other evidence

On its own, this study is rather unconvincing. Its generalizability, at least to adult males and with regard to the levels of exposure experienced in workplaces, are probably quite reasonable. The great weakness is the internal validity of the study. The association found is of modest size and could well occur through observational bias or error, confounding, or chance variation; none of these non-causal explanations can be ruled out confidently. Therefore the consistency with other evidence is critical.

17. Are the results consistent with other evidence, particularly evidence from studies of similar or more powerful study design?

We would expect any individual study of this question to be weak, because of the difficulties of studying a rare disease and a particular chemical exposure which is usually accompanied by other chemical exposures. Therefore the consistency of a large number of studies of different designs and different situations is crucial. Indeed, a meta-analysis of all available studies would give the best guidance on the topic. In the introduction to this paper it is stated that several studies had shown excesses of soft-tissue sarcoma linked to these or closely related chemicals. Given the rarity of soft-tissue sarcoma, a major problem with all studies will be small numbers, and because of this there could be a major problem of publication bias. A small study showing an excess may be published, but a small study showing no excess might not be published or even submitted for publication.

18. Does the total evidence suggest any specificity?

This total evidence does suggest a specific relationship between exposure to these chemicals and soft-tissue sarcoma, although associations with other diseases such as non-Hodgkin's lymphoma, which is also a tumour of non-epithelial tissue, have been suggested. Of course, a small increase in other more common diseases, such as lung cancer, would be even more difficult to detect.

19. Are the results plausible in terms of a biological mechanism?

Plausibility is quite important. It is relevant to know if these chemicals have carcinogenic actions, as tested on cell systems or animal models. The authors state that this evidence has been considered by the International Agency for Research in Cancer (IARC), which has a system of assessing evidence for carcinogenicity noted in Chapter 10, which concluded that there was 'limited' evidence of human carcinogenicity [2]. The IARC considers human studies (epidemiology) and also animal studies and other data. Here, there were several epidemiological studies, giving 'limited' evidence, but evidence of carcinogenicity in animals was 'inadequate', and the other studies, including tests of mutagenicity, were inconsistent. So the plausibility question is still unresolved.

20. If a major effect is shown, is it coherent with the distribution of the exposure and the outcome?

The argument of coherence is relevant only if the exposure in question is a major cause of the outcome, so that the occurrence of exposure and outcome would be linked, and this link would be detectable. A relative risk of the order of 2, as suggested here, means that this is not likely, although of course if real, this risk is likely to be an underestimate. A coherence argument predicts that the mortality from this disease would have increased since the 1950s when these herbicides were introduced. However, a time trend analysis of a rare condition which is difficult to classify is open to changes in diagnostic classification patterns, as well as to the influences of unidentified causal factors. It could also be argued that these sarcomas should be more common in populations with heavier exposures, which might include rural or agricultural populations, or specific workforces, and these issues could be explored in descriptive data sets looking at mortality by occupation or place of residence. It is unlikely that any of these types of analyses would add greatly to the arguments for and against causality, and they are much weaker methods than the cohort study presented here.

Conclusions

Assessed on its own, this study has produced results which are consistent with causality, but are not convincing, as other explanations cannot be excluded (Table 15.2). Taken with the background of several other studies cited in the paper, which also suggest an increase in this rare condition with this particular exposure, the overall evidence is stronger, but still not definitive. It appears from the literature reviewed in this paper that there are a considerable number of studies supporting this association. The balance of these reports may be influenced by publication bias. The association is plausible on the grounds of the potential carcinogenicity of these chemicals in non-human systems. Further consideration would have to assess the other published studies with a similar critical appraisal approach. The best method to assess the human evidence would be

Table 15.2 Summary of assessment of the retrospective cohort study of workers exposed to chlorophenoxy herbicides and chlorophenols [1].

A. Description of the evidence

1.	Exposure	Occupational exposure to chlorophenoxy herbicides or chlorophenols
2.	Outcome	Cancer mortality, by site
3.	Design	Retrospective cohort study, average follow-up 17 years
4.	Study population	20 employee groups in 10 countries since 1955, Europe, Australia, Canada, New Zealand; over 90% male
5.	Main result	Increased mortality from soft tissue sarcoma

B. Non-causal explanations

6.	Observation bias	Cancer deaths ascertained through routine methods; unlikely to be biased; may be incomplete ascertainment
7.	Confounding	Confounding by other chemical exposures, smoking, other factors possible, but few other causal agents known for these cancers
8.	Chance	Overall result non-significant, based on 4 observed deaths, SMR 196, 95% limits 53–502. For sprayers, also non-significant. Significant excesses at 10–19 years from first exposure; but this is a post hoc category

C. Features consistent with causation

9.	Time relationship	All 4 deaths occurred 10–19 years from first exposure; time relationship reasonable
10.	Strength	Not strong: relative risk about 2; in sprayers 3
11.	Dose–response	Not clear: 2 cases with duration of exposure less than 1 year
12.	Consistency	Numbers too small to assess usefully
13.	Specificity	Disease excess may be specific; no overall cancer excess; non-significant excesses of some other cancers

D. External validity

14.	Eligible population	Participants represent eligible employees
15.	Source population	May represent major exposed workers internationally; no data on how exposure levels compare with workplaces not included in the source population
16.	Target populations	Past exposures from 1955; current industrial exposures may be lower. Data may not apply to women

E. Comparison with other evidence

17.	Consistency	Consistent with some earlier small studies, which created the hypothesis in relation to soft-tissue sarcomas
18.	Specificity	Association with this type of cancer may be specific
19.	Plausibility	These chemicals are accepted as carcinogens; unclear why this cancer type should be affected particularly
20.	Coherence	Too little known about this disease to assess coherence

Source: data from Rodolfo Saracci et al., 'Cancer mortality in workers exposed to chlorophenoxy herbicides and chlorophenols,' *The Lancet*, Volume 338, Issue 8774, p. 1027–32, © 1991 Published by Elsevier Ltd [1].

a systematic meta-analysis, in which considerable efforts would have to be made to identify relevant sets of data which might not have been published in easily accessible sources.

Subsequent development

When published in 1991 [3], this study was the most powerful human study of exposure to these chemicals. Even before this study, in 1986, the IARC had classified chlorophenoxy herbicides as having 'limited evidence of carcinogenicity in humans', group 2B in their classification, on the basis of case–control studies and limited cohort studies [2,4]. The topic is complex because there are many related chemicals, and results can depend on whether specific compounds or groups such as chlorophenoxy herbicides are considered.

In terms of epidemiology, the cohort study has been expanded and continued, and a further report shows an SMR of 2.0 for soft-tissue sarcoma, based on six deaths, and of 1.12 for all cancers, both significantly increased, and also shows increases, although not significant, in mortality from non-Hodgkin's lymphoma and lung cancer [5]. These increased risks appeared to be restricted to workers who were exposed to TCDD or similar contaminants; those exposed to phenoxy herbicides with minimal or no contamination showed only a small excess of soft-tissue sarcoma (SMR 1.35) and no excess of other cancers. However, these results are based on small numbers, with only two deaths from soft-tissue sarcomas. Nested case–control studies of 11 incident cases of soft tissue sarcoma and of 32 cases of non-Hodgkin lymphoma within this cohort showed increased risks of sarcoma, but not restricted to TCDD exposed workers, and a small excess of lymphoma [6]. A study of the 701 female workers in this international cohort population [7] showed no overall excess cancer risk, but there was a significantly increased incidence (standardized incidence ratio 222) for total cancer in those exposed to TCDD. There were no cases of soft-tissue sarcoma or non-Hodgkin's lymphoma in the female workers. Non-cancer mortality has also been studied in this cohort, finding an increased rate of ischaemic heart disease in workers exposed to TCDD and similar contaminants [8]. A more recent cohort study of chlorophenoxy herbicide manufacturing workers in the Netherlands showed no excess in cancer in total or in non-Hodgkin lymphoma, but an excess in urinary cancers [9].

The IARC classification of chlorophenoxy herbicides as group 2B was based on 'limited' human evidence, with animal evidence for carcinogenicity in animals being 'inadequate' [4]. A detailed review in 2013 of some chlorophenoxy compounds challenges this classification, concluding that toxicology and experimental carcinogenesis studies have not shown a carcinogenic action, and that the epidemiological results are inconsistent, and suggesting that if there is an increased cancer risk, gene–environmental interactions involving polymorphisms, family history, or other exposures would need to be involved [10].

References

1. **Altman DG, Machin D, Bryant T, Gardner M (Eds.).** *Statistics with Confidence: Confidence Intervals and Statistical Guidelines*, 2nd edn. London: British Medical Journal; 2000.

2. **International Agency for Research on Cancer.** Occupational exposures to chlorophenoxy herbicides. *IARC Monogr Eval Carcinog Risk Chem Hum* 1986; **41**:357–406.

3. **Saracci R, Kogevinas M, Bertazzi P-A, de Mesquita BHB, Coggon D, Green LM, et al.** Cancer mortality in workers exposed to chlorophenoxy herbicides and chlorophenols. *Lancet* 1991; **338**:1027–1032.

4. **International Agency for Research on Cancer.** *IARC Monographs on the Evaluation of Carcinogenic Risks to Humans. Overall Evaluations of Carcinogenicity: An Updating of IARC Monographs 1 to 42. Supplement 7. Chlorophenoxy Herbicides (Group 2B)*. Lyon: International Agency for Research on Cancer; 1987:156–160.

5. **Kogevinas M, Becher H, Benn T, Bertazzi PA, Boffetta P, Bueno-de-Mesquita HB, et al.** Cancer mortality in workers exposed to phenoxy herbicides, chlorophenols, and dioxins. An expanded and updated international cohort study. *Am J Epidemiol* 1997; **145**:1061–1075.

6. **Kogevinas M, Kauppinen T, Winkelmann R, Becher H, Bertazzi PA, Bueno-de-Mesquita HB, et al.** Soft tissue sarcoma and non-Hodgkin's lymphoma in workers exposed to phenoxy herbicides, chlorophenols, and dioxins: two nested case-control studies. *Epidemiology* 1995; **6**:396–402.

7. **Kogevinas M, Saracci R, Winkelmann R, Johnson ES, Bertazzi PA, Bueno de Mesquita BH, et al.** Cancer incidence and mortality in women occupationally exposed to chlorophenoxy herbicides, chlorophenols, and dioxins. *Cancer Causes Control* 1993; **4**:547–553.

8. **Vena J, Boffetta P, Becher H, Benn T, Bueno-de-Mesquita HB, Coggon D, et al.** Exposure to dioxin and nonneoplastic mortality in the expanded IARC international cohort study of phenoxy herbicide and chlorophenol production workers and sprayers. *Environ Health Perspect* 1998; **106**(Suppl 2):645–653.

9. **Boers D, Portengen L, Bueno-de-Mesquita HB, Heederik D, Vermeulen R**. Cause-specific mortality of Dutch chlorophenoxy herbicide manufacturing workers. *Occup Environ Med* 2010; **67**:24–31.

10. **von Stackelberg K**. A systematic review of carcinogenic outcomes and potential mechanisms from exposure to 2,4-D and MCPA in the environment. *J Toxicol* 2013; **2013**:371610.

Chapter 16

Critical appraisal of a matched case–control study

Introduction

In this chapter, we review a small matched case–control study that was the first publication showing an important relationship between a disease and a widely used drug. It has been chosen because it is of historical importance, and is a good example of an individually matched study with several issues of interpretation. It also shows an interesting way of assessing confounding, which is valid although not usually used in current studies.

Increased risk of endometrial carcinoma among users of conjugated estrogens

Harry K Ziel, William D Finkle

Abstract

The possibility that the use of conjugated estrogens increases the risk of endometrial carcinoma was investigated in patients and a twofold age-matched control series from the same population. Conjugated estrogens (principally sodium oestrone sulfate) use was recorded for 57 per cent of 94 patients with endometrial carcinoma, and for 15 per cent of controls. The corresponding point estimate of the (instantaneous) risk ratio was 7.6 with a one-sided 95 per cent lower confidence limit of 4.7. The risk-ratio estimate increased with duration of exposure: from 5.6 for 1 to 4.9 years' exposure to 13.9 for seven or more years. The estimated proportion of cases related to conjugated estrogens, the etiologic fraction, was 50 per cent with cone-sided 95 per cent lower confidence limit of 41 per cent. These data suggest that conjugated estrogens have an etiologic role in endometrial carcinoma.

Reproduced with permission from the Harry K. Ziel, 'Increased Risk of Endometrial Carcinoma among Users of Conjugated Estrogens', *New England Journal of Medicine*, Volume 293, Number 23, pp. 1167–1170, © 1975, Massachusetts Medical Society, available from http://www.nejm.org/doi/full/10.1056/NEJM197512042932303 [1].

A. Description of the evidence

1. What was the exposure or intervention?
2. What was the outcome?
3. What was the study design?
4. What was the study population?
5. What was the main result?

Box 16.1 History of conjugated oestrogen use among 94 patients with endometrial cancer and 188 matched control subjects: the matching criteria were age, area of residence, duration of Health Plan membership, and intact uterus

ESTROGENS AND ENDOMETRIAL CANCER—RESULTS

Distribution of triples by use of conjugated oestrogens

Patients' use of conjugated oestrogens	Controls' use of conjugated oestrogens			
	Both	One	Neither	Totals
Used	1	16	37	54
Did not use	0	11	29	40
Totals	1	27	66	94

Exposure rates	Used conjugated oestrogens		Did not use conjugated oestrogens		Totals
	No.	%	No.	%	
Patients	54	(57)	40	(43)	94
Controls	29	(15)	159	(85)	188

Source: data from Harry K. Ziel, 'Increased Risk of Endometrial Carcinoma among Users of Conjugated Estrogens', *New England Journal of Medicine*, Volume 293, Number 23, pp. 1167–1170, © 1975, Massachusetts Medical Society [1].

The exposure is the use of conjugated oestrogenic drugs, as recorded in medical records up to 1 year before the date of diagnosis of the cases, or the equivalent time for the controls (using American spelling). The outcome is the pathologically confirmed diagnosis of endometrial adenocarcinoma or adenoacanthoma. The design is an individually matched retrospective case–control study. The case subjects were diagnosed at the Kaiser Permanente Medical Centre between 1970 and 1974, and were reported to its tumour registry. For each case, two controls were chosen from the membership files of the health plan that operates this hospital, matched for birth date within 1 year, area of residence by postal code, duration of health plan membership, and possession of an intact uterus. The main result of the study was that oestrogen use was recorded in 57 per cent of cases and in 15 per cent of controls, giving an odds ratio of 7.6 for 'ever use' (Box 16.1). The note at the end of this chapter explains how this is calculated.

B. Internal validity: consideration of non-causal explanations

6. Are the results likely to be affected by observation bias?

Since this is a case–control study, the major problems relate to the assessment of exposure. Assessment of disease status is straightforward. For the cases, this was a pathologically confirmed diagnosis, with little chance of inaccuracy. It is possible that some of the control subjects had undiagnosed endometrial adenocarcinoma, but this would result only in a reduction of the observed risk ratio.

The information on oestrogen use is based on a 'blind' medical record review. One clerk obtained the records for each set of cases and controls, and concealed all information recorded after a reference date 1 year before the date of diagnosis for the case and a corresponding date for the controls. A different clerk abstracted the information from each record, without knowing whether the record belonged to a case or a control. Further information on the quality of the medical records would be helpful, in particular any independent assessment of the completeness and accuracy of drug recording. There could be substantial under-reporting of drug usage, as drugs might have been used that were not prescribed within this particular health plan, or were not recorded; also, some drugs prescribed may not have been used. Such errors, if randomly distributed amongst all subjects, would serve only to reduce the observed association. The crucial question is whether oestrogen use was more completely recorded in subjects later diagnosed with endometrial cancer than in the control subjects. The blind procedure and the exclusion of any material relating to the period 1 year before diagnosis provide some protection. Could other factors affect this? Endometrial cancer is more common in the higher socioeconomic groups. Might such patients have more completely recorded drug histories? This seems unlikely as all the study participants used the same health care system. Could patients later diagnosed with endometrial cancer have had a more frequent history of other gynaecological or related problems, resulting not only in a greater prescribing of these drugs but also a greater recording of such prescribing? For parity, obesity, and age at menopause, the data were more complete for the cases than for the controls. Could the information on oestrogens also be more complete? Counter-arguments are that no excess was seen for several other drugs, an indication for the use of oestrogens was recorded more frequently in the controls, and that the association was very strong (please see '10. Is the association strong?'). It seems unwise to accept totally results based on review of one medical record, without independent verification, and the issue of observation bias cannot be dismissed.

7. Are the results likely to be affected by confounding?

The subjects were matched by age, area of residence (which probably gives some measure of socioeconomic matching), and duration of health plan membership; a matched analysis has been performed. Potential confounding factors are those related both to the incidence of endometrial cancer and to the use of oestrogenic drugs. The literature on endometrial cancer is reviewed in the paper; at that time there were several recognized risk factors such as high parity, obesity, and late age at menopause. For each of these, the authors used data from the medical records in a stratified analysis; but there was substantial missing data. Rather than giving unconfounded odds ratio estimates from the stratified analysis, the authors used a less common technique in calculating the 'confounding risk ratio', which is a measure of the extent to which the association is produced by confounding. An explanation of this method is given at the end of this chapter. The confounding effect for each of the three factors of parity, obesity, and age at menopause is very minor, but the analysis is limited by the missing data. No other confounding factors had been shown to have major associations. Some protection against the observed association being due to confounding is given by the strength of the association; the odds ratio is high compared with the odds ratio of 1.5–3 usually quoted for factors such as parity or obesity.

At the time this paper was published there was little written on the factors related to oestrogen use. Of prime importance is the indication for oestrogen usage, as the observed association with the drug could be disguising a true association with the indication for the drug. The most frequently recorded indication was hot flashes. If the case patients used more oestrogenic drugs, and if the indications for use of oestrogens were the same in cases and controls, this implies that the case subjects suffered from hot flashes more frequently than did the controls, suffered from them more severely, sought treatment more readily, or for some other reason were given these drugs as treatment more readily. Thus there is a competing hypothesis that endometrial cancer could be related to hot flashes, being caused by them or by the factors causing them. A further possibility is that cases might have a high usage of drugs in general; this can be dismissed as the cases were recorded as using diazepam, reserpine, and thyroid drugs less commonly than were the controls. Thus there is protection against confounding by most of the major known risk factors for endometrial carcinoma. However, there is a viable alternative hypothesis to causation—that the disease is related not to the use of oestrogens but to the indications for their use.

8. Are the results likely to be affected by chance variation?

The estimated odds ratio is 7.6, and the associated P-value is less than 10^{-8}, giving 95 per cent two-sided confidence limits of 4.3 and 13.4. Thus chance variation can be excluded. The methods used in the statistical analysis are a little different from those presented in this book; a note on them is given at the end of this chapter. Publications may use methods other than those described in this book, which may have particular advantages for that study. However, the results should not differ greatly from those obtained by the methods described here. Applying the methods for analysis of a matched case–control study presented in Table A2.6 gives similar results: an odds ratio of 8.2, and an associated χ^2 statistic of 48.8 giving $P < 10^{-8}$.

Summary: non-causal explanations

Thus of the three non-causal explanations, we can effectively exclude chance, but must keep in mind the possibilities of observation bias and of confounding, particularly by the indication for drug usage.

C. Internal validity: consideration of positive features of causation

9. Is there a correct time relationship?

This study, as is common with case–control studies, is fairly weak with regard to time relationships. By excluding information recorded in the year before clinical diagnosis, we can conclude that the drugs assessed were prescribed before the endometrial cancer was diagnosed. But could the disease or its precursor have been present even earlier, and have produced symptoms which led to the prescription for the drugs? We do not know if any of the case subjects had previous tests (e.g. a curettage) that would have detected the disease or a related state such as hyperplasia. The time relationship is not clear; no data for risk by time since first use of oestrogens are given. As it is unlikely that the records go back many years, we assume that the risk is seen only a few years from first exposure. If the risk is causal, it shows a short-term action, which is more consistent with a cancer promotor effect than a cancer initiator.

10. Is the association strong?

The relationship is strong, with a high odds ratio of 7.6. This odds ratio is greater than those associated with even extremes of parity, obesity, late menopause, and other recognized risk factors for endometrial carcinoma, making it unlikely that this association could be produced by confounding by such factors. However, it is no protection against the association being due to the indication for the drug rather than the usage of the drug, as the association between these two may be very close. To assess its relevance for observation bias, it is useful to go to the raw data, which show that oestrogen use was recorded for 57 per cent of the case subjects compared with 15 per cent of the controls. Thus for the association to be totally due to observation bias would require, for example, that oestrogen use was always recorded for the case subjects, but recorded on only about 25 per cent of occasions for the controls; this seems implausible. Thus the strength of the association protects against some aspects of confounding and against observation bias, but not against what is emerging as the chief competing hypothesis—an association with the indication rather than with the drug prescribed.

11. Is there a dose–response relationship?

Table 2 of the paper shows the odds ratio increasing from shorter to longer exposures, the odds ratios, with non-exposed as the referent, being 5.6 for up to 5 years' exposure, 7.2 for 5 up to 7 years, and 13.9 for 7 years' exposure or more; all are significantly different from the unexposed. This dose–response is not very helpful in interpretation; it could occur if the relationship were produced by confounding by the indication for the drug, or even from observation bias. It is important if causality is accepted, showing a substantial increased risk even with short durations of exposure. Information on the relationship between risk and time since first use or since last use might be of more help, but is not given.

12. Are the results consistent within the study?
And 13. Is there any specificity within the study?

The association shows some specificity, as no increased risks were seen with diazepam, reserpine, and thyroid drugs. This protects mainly against observation bias, that is, the possibility that all drugs would be recorded more frequently for the cases. Beyond that, a separation of patients with different indications for the use of the oestrogen drugs would be helpful, but this would probably need a further special study. Separation of different oestrogenic preparations would also help, but there is no information on the precise preparations used. An association with a particular drug is more convincing if no association is seen with other drugs used for the same indications.

Conclusions with regard to internal validity

The second part of our assessment of internal validity has not been particularly helpful, and this is often the situation in assessing a relatively small study. Larger studies give more opportunity to assess consistency between subgroups, dose–response relationships, and so on. Therefore the assessment of internal validity depends on the comparison of the causal hypothesis with the alternatives of bias and confounding. The main alternative hypothesis is that the association is not due to the drug itself, but to the symptoms for which the drug has been prescribed, which might be caused by the developing carcinoma, or be indications of an altered physiological state produced by mechanisms akin to those producing the tumour. To assess this alternative we need information from other studies, as will be seen.

D. External validity: generalization of the results

14. Can the study results be applied to the eligible population?

The eligible population comprises the members of the Kaiser Foundation Health Plan, and there is little problem applying the results to them. If we accept that they would all attend this medical centre and that the tumour registry is efficient, all patients with a histological diagnosis during the stated time period were included, and medical records on all of them were obtained. The control subjects, apart from the appropriate matching criteria, should be representative of unaffected members of the plan, with the limitation that they include only women with an intact uterus. This is an appropriate criterion, both on the argument that women without a uterus are not at risk of developing endometrial cancer and therefore are not eligible as cases, and also because women who have had their uterus removed may be different in terms of oestrogen usage.

15. Can the study results be applied to the source population?

The source and eligible populations in this study are essentially the same.

16. Can the study results be applied to other relevant populations?

The participants were members of the Kaiser Foundation Health Plan diagnosed between 1970 and 1974 in Los Angeles. Are members of this health plan different from women in Los Angeles in general? Further information would be required, but we might assume that plan members are likely to be fairly affluent stable subjects, who can afford a comprehensive prepaid health plan. No information is given on racial origin. However, the representativeness of the subjects in the study is not the most important issue. The main question is: is the *association* seen likely to apply to other women? If the true relationship is between the drug and the disease, the finding is likely to be widely applicable. In other populations, the value of the odds ratio maybe considerably different, depending on the usual dosage and length of time the drugs are used. If the true association is with a specific type of drug, the association may not be seen in societies where other types are used. Even if the association is consistent, its importance will depend on the type, frequency, and dosage of the drugs used, and on the level of background incidence of endometrial cancer, produced by other factors. In this study population, a strong association is seen with a drug used frequently—in 15 per cent of controls. The attributable proportion is 87 per cent in those exposed and 50 per cent in the study population—if causal, oestrogens are the main cause of the disease. (These calculations are shown at the end of this chapter.)

E. Comparison of the results with other evidence

17. Are the results consistent with other evidence, particularly evidence from studies of similar or more powerful study design?

This study was one of the first to suggest this association. In the same issue of the same journal another case–control study, from Seattle, was published, showing a similar association, and this strengthens the credibility of these results [2]. However, if this other study is assessed, bearing in mind the conclusion we have reached on the present study, that is, that the association is likely to be either causal or due to an association between the indication for the drug and endometrial cancer, we find that the same limitation applies to its interpretation. Because of the importance of the association suggested, these two papers were followed reasonably rapidly by several other case–control studies and some cohort studies. There have been randomized trials of oestrogen use, but these have often been too small to assess the outcome of endometrial cancer.

18. Does the total evidence suggest any specificity?

At the time this paper was published there was no relevant information. However, several later studies confirmed the association in the USA, where conjugated oestrogens were used widely, whereas studies in some other countries showed no risk because the use of conjugated oestrogens was much less. It appears that patients who would be treated with conjugated oestrogens in the United States would be treated with a mixture of oestrogens and progestogens in Europe, and this combination did not confer a marked increased risk of endometrial cancer.

19. Are the results plausible in terms of a biological mechanism?

The authors review epidemiological and experimental evidence that oestrogens may produce endometrial cancer, and the association seems biologically acceptable. The time issue is relevant. Cancer-initiating factors produce tumours only many years after exposure, but this association does not fit this pattern. Hormones in general are not initiators of cancer, but act as cancer promoters, and this action would be consistent with a short-term effect.

20. If a major effect is shown, is it coherent with the distribution of the exposure and the outcome?

This study does show a major effect, and the authors calculated that in this population approximately 50 per cent of endometrial cancer was caused by these drugs, if the association they have shown is causal. They also noted that the usage of these drugs quadrupled between 1962 and 1973, and therefore a noticeable increase in the incidence of endometrial carcinoma in the United States would be expected. They reviewed the literature available at that time, which did not show any such increase, but pointed out that an increase might be disguised by an increase in the prevalence of hysterectomy for non-cancer reasons. Subsequent work published some months later, using better information, did show a substantial rise in the incidence of endometrial cancer in the USA. Strong evidence of causality is given by the trends in the years after the publication of this and other studies; there was a reduction in the prescribing of these drugs, and a fairly rapid reduction in the incidence of this tumour [3]. As well as the time relationship, we would expect the excess incidence to occur in geographical areas, and in social groups, in which the usage of these oestrogenic drugs was maximum, and the difference between American and European experience in this regard has already been mentioned.

Coherence is the item on which the two major hypotheses can be separated. If the association with the drug is merely indicating a true association with symptoms, the rapid rise in use of the drugs will not affect the incidence rate, while a direct effect of the magnitude given will have doubled the previous incidence in this population. Thus, given the size of the effect, there should be a close association between the use of these drugs and the incidence of endometrial cancer in terms of time, place, and person. If the real relationship is with the indication, no such associations will be found. Therefore the concordance of drug usage and disease subsequently shown between countries, social groups, and over time is crucial.

Conclusions

The study shows a large and important association, which is most likely to be due to one of two mechanisms: either a causal relationship between the use of these particular drugs and the development of endometrial cancer, or an association between the indications for those drugs and an increased risk of endometrial cancer (Table 16.1). There are other possibilities, that the result reflects other confounding factors, or that it is produced by observation bias with regard to the medical records on which the data on oestrogen exposure were based, but these seem less likely. If the association is real, it is likely to apply to other women who are exposed to these same agents, and therefore is of substantial practical importance.

Thus, in assessing priorities for further investigation and for critical reading of subsequent results, we should look particularly for studies that can differentiate between a direct effect of the drug and an effect of the indications for the drug. One relevant issue is the time trends in the incidence of the disease. Studies in other countries, where women presumably have the same symptoms but may be treated differently, are helpful. Other than that, we look for studies using more reliable methods of assessing drug

Table 16.1 Summary of assessment of the case–control study of endometrial cancer by Ziel and Finkle [1].

A. Description of evidence

1. Exposure	Conjugated oestrogens; use in period up to 1 year before diagnosis; assessed from medical records
2. Outcome	Endometrial cancer; adenocarcinoma, adenoacanthoma
3. Design	Case–control study
4. Study population	Cases—all those diagnosed at Kaiser Permanente Medical Center, Los Angeles, July 1970–Dec. 1974; $n = 94$
	Controls—from LA members of Kaiser plan, matched for age, residence, length of membership; two per case
5. Main result	Odds ratio = 7.6; 95 per cent confidence limits = 4.3–13.4; strong positive association of oestrogen use with endometrial cancer

B. Non-causal explanations

6. Observation bias	Possible—recording of drug use might be more complete on cases, despite protection of blind abstraction and avoiding period immediately before diagnosis
7. Confounding	Major risk factors for endometrial cancer controlled by matching or stratification. Most likely non-causal hypothesis is an association with the indications for drug usage
8. Chance	Can be excluded

C. Features consistent with causation

9. Time relationship	Drug usage at least 1 year before clinical diagnosis, but it is possible that preclinical or precursor state might have existed prior to then
10. Strength	Strong association—protects against many alternative hypotheses but not helpful if the true association is with the indication for the drug
11. Dose–response	Seen with total duration of exposure
12. Consistency	Information not available
13. Specificity	Information not available

D. External validity

14. Eligible population	No difficulties in applying results
15. Source population	Same as eligible
16. Other populations	While frequency and mode of usage may vary, association, if causal, is likely to be widely applicable. Studies in other populations may help distinguish causal hypothesis from hypothesis of an association with the indication for the drug, and indicate which particular drugs are involved

E. Comparison with other evidence

17. Consistency	One other case–control study at time of publication. Further support later. No strong support for competing hypothesis of the association being with indications for the drug

18. Specificity	Evidence for specificity to unconjugated oestrogens used alone emerged later
19. Plausibility	Time relationship makes a long-term cancer initiator action unlikely. A short-term promoter action is plausible and supported by some experimental work
20. Coherence	Shown by later work. Evidence of incidence rate of endometrial cancer rising with use of oestrogenic drugs and later falling is strong evidence against the competing hypothesis of the association being with the indication

Source: data from Harry K. Ziel, 'Increased Risk of Endometrial Carcinoma among Users of Conjugated Estrogens', *New England Journal of Medicine*, Volume 293, Number 23, pp. 1167–1170, © 1975, Massachusetts Medical Society [1].

exposure, perhaps medical records supplemented by independent reviews or direct interviews, even though recall bias may then become an issue. Prospective studies of users of these drugs would be useful, and the ultimate would be a trial in which women regarded as eligible for treatment with conjugated oestrogens were randomized either to receive such treatment or to receive a non-oestrogen alternative. Such a study would be unethical in women with an intact uterus; such trials have been done with opposed oestrogen, that is, oestrogen and progestogen combinations [4].

Subsequent development

This paper [1], and the other case–control study published simultaneously [2], provided the first information on the important relationship between oestrogenic drugs and endometrial cancer. The studies raised much controversy and were vigorously criticized, primarily by gynaecologists who had used the drugs clinically for many years and were reluctant to accept epidemiological evidence of a major hazard. In arguments reminiscent of the debate about smoking and lung cancer in the 1950s, some of the criticisms were along the lines that case–control studies could not demonstrate causation. One anonymous editorialist in *The Lancet* criticized the studies because they were not prospective and randomized, without discussing the reality that a prospective randomized trial to answer this question would be logistically extremely difficult because of the numbers required, and of course ethically dubious [5]. In response to this, the authors of one of the observational studies commented that if such rules of evidence were applied generally, even the cause of pregnancy could not be regarded as established [6].

The main issue related to the difficulty of separating an association with a drug itself from an association with the indications for the drug. Studies comparing patients with endometrial cancer with other patients attending the same gynaecological services who had similar presenting symptoms, such as uterine bleeding, showed similar rates of oestrogen usage and therefore no association. However, subsequent studies demonstrated that the most reasonable explanation for these results was that oestrogenic drugs caused both benign hyperplasia leading to bleeding, and also endometrial cancer [7].

A meta-analysis of 30 observational studies showed an overall relative risk estimate of 2.3 comparing users with non-users, rising to 9.5 after 10 years of use [8]. The tumours produced tend to be diagnosed earlier because they bleed easily, and are usually of low grade and stage with an excellent prognosis [9]. This association between endometrial cancer and oestrogenic drugs is a good example of an important aetiological relationship being first demonstrated in a case–control study, and the Ziel and Finkle study is regarded as a classic [10].

The association of oestrogen drugs with endometrial cancer is now universally accepted, and use of oestrogenic drugs alone (unopposed by a progestogen) is contra-indicated in women with an intact uterus. However, if oestrogenic preparations are combined with progestogens, the risk of endometrial cancer is no longer increased. A Cochrane systematic review of 46 randomized trials of endometrial hyperplasia, which can precede cancer, showed increased risks with unopposed oestrogen, but no increase after the use of oestrogen combined with a progestogen [11]. The risks and benefits are complex; a recent review concludes that unopposed oestrogens in hysterectomized women are effective against menopausal vasomotor symptoms (hot flashes), do not increase risks of breast, colorectal, or lung cancers, but may reduce the risk of cardio-vascular events within 10 years of menopause [4]. However, in terms of the suggested longer-term benefits and risks, the US Preventive Services Task Force recommended, in 2013, against the use of either combined oestrogen and progestin, or oestrogen alone in hysterectomized women, as they are not convinced that the risks outweigh any bene-fits [12]. This is currently (2015) under further review.

The analysis used in the paper by Ziel and Finkle

Main analysis

The basic data for this matched case–control study with two controls per case are given in Box 16.1. The formula shown in Table A2.6 gives an odds ratio of 8.2. This is rather different from the maximum likelihood point estimate calculated by the authors by a more complicated iterative procedure, which is 7.6, and such disparity is to be expected with these relatively small numbers. The chi-squared statistic, cal-culated by the variant of the Mantel–Haenszel procedure given in Table A2.6 is 48.8, identical with that given in the paper. A chi statistic of 6.98 ($\sqrt{48.8}$) is out of the range of most conventional tables; but using the function shown in Table A2.16 gives the corresponding two-sided P-value as $<10^{-9}$.

The odds ratio calculated from an unmatched analysis can also be derived from Box 16.1, which gives a value of 7.4; the difference between this and the result of the matched paired analysis is small. In Table 2 of the paper, where results are subdivided by duration of exposure, unmatched analyses are used, and the appropriate chi-squared statistic can be derived by the usual formula for case–control studies given in Table A2.1; an exact test (Table A2.4) and a test for trend (Table A2.7) can also be applied.

Control of confounding

This study uses the concept of 'confounding risk ratio'. This is the odds ratio linking exposure to outcome, which is produced by the confounder; it can be thought of as the risk ratio which would be observed in the absence of any direct association [13]. If there is no confounding, it will be 1.0; if the crude association is totally due to confounding, the confounding risk ratio will equal the crude risk ratio. The crude risk ratio OR_c, the confounding risk ratio OR_f, and the unconfounded or standardized risk ratio OR_s are simply related as follows:

$$OR_c = OR_f \times OR_s.$$

Thus controlling for parity gives a crude odds ratio (OR_c) for oestrogens and endometrial cancer of 6.71 (different from the risk for the whole study because of the missing data), and a confounding odds ratio OR_f of 1.18 (showing very little confounding). The unconfounded odds ratio OR_s is given by 6.71/1.18 = 5.69. The authors also calculate a 'confounding effect' relating the extent of confounding to the size of the unconfounded risk ratio, giving $(1.18 - 1)/(5.69 - 1) = 4$ per cent.

Attributable proportion

Using the formulae shown in Chapter 4, the overall odds ratio is 7.6 and the proportion p of controls exposed is 15 per cent (Box 16.1). The attributable proportion (= 'aetiological fraction') in those exposed is

$$(OR-1)/OR = 87 \text{ per cent}$$

and the attributable proportion in the population is

$$p(OR-1)/(p(OR-1)+1) = 50 \text{ per cent}.$$

References

1. **Ziel HK, Finkle WD.** Increased risk of endometrial carcinoma among users of conjugated estrogens. *N Engl J Med* 1975; **293**:1167–1170.
2. **Smith DC, Prentice R, Thompson DJ, Herrmann WL.** Association of exogenous estrogen and endometrial carcinoma. *N Engl J Med* 1975; **293**:1164–1167.
3. **Austin DF, Roe KM.** The decreasing incidence of endometrial cancer: public health implications. *Am J Public Health* 1982; **72**:65–68.
4. **Mirkin S, Komm BS, Pickar JH.** Conjugated estrogens for the treatment of menopausal symptoms: a review of safety data. *Expert Opin Drug Saf* 2014; **13**:45–56.
5. **Anonymous.** Hormone replacement therapy and endometrial carcinoma. *Lancet* 1977; **1**:577–578.
6. **Mack TM, Pike MC.** Hormone replacement therapy and endometrial carcinoma. *Lancet* 1977; **309**:1358.
7. **Hulka BS, Grimson RC, Greenberg BG, Kaufman DG, Fowler WC, Jr.,** Hogue CJ, et al. 'Alternative' controls in a case-control study of endometrial cancer and exogenous estrogen. *Am J Epidemiol* 1980; **112**:376–387.
8. **Grady D, Gebretsadik T, Kerlikowske K, Ernster V, Petitti D.** Hormone replacement therapy and endometrial cancer risk: a meta-analysis. *Obstet Gynecol* 1995; **85**:304–313.
9. **Elwood JM, Boyes DA.** Clinical and pathological features and survival of endometrial cancer patients in relation to prior use of estrogens. *Gynecol Oncol* 1980; **10**:173–187.
10. **Anonymous.** Citation classic: Ziel and Finkle 1975. *CC Clin Practice* 1982; **26**:28.

11. **Furness S, Roberts H, Marjoribanks J, Lethaby A**. Hormone therapy in postmenopausal women and risk of endometrial hyperplasia. *Cochrane Database Syst Rev* 2012; **8**:CD000402.

12. **Moyer VA, US Preventive Services Task Force**. Menopausal Hormone Therapy for the Primary Prevention of Chronic Conditions: U.S. Preventive Services Task Force Recommendation Statement. *Ann Intern Med* 2013; **158**:47–54.

13. **Miettinen OS**. Components of the crude risk ratio. *Am J Epidemiol* 1972; **96**:168–172.

Chapter 17

Critical appraisal of a large population-based case–control study

Introduction

We will now discuss a large population-based case–control study [1], published in the *Journal of the National Cancer Institute*, June 21 1995, 87, 923–929, and available at http://jnci.oxfordjournals.org/content/87/12/923.abstract.

Risk of breast cancer in relation to lifetime alcohol consumption

Matthew P Longnecker, Polly A Newcomb, Robert Mittendorf, E Robert Greenberg, Richard W Clapp, Gregory F Bogdan, John Baron, Brian MacMahon, Walter C Willett

Abstract

Background. Although an association between alcohol consumption and risk of breast cancer has been observed in many studies, questions of major importance remain, including the nature of the dose–response relationship and the effects of drinking at various periods in life.

Purpose. Our goal was to address the issues listed above with a large case–control study.

Methods. We conducted a population-based case–control study in Maine, Massachusetts (excluding the four counties that include metropolitan Boston), New Hampshire, and Wisconsin. Case patients were eligible if their diagnosis of invasive breast cancer was first reported to one of the four statewide cancer registries during the period of 1988 through 1991. During the accrual period, 11 879 potentially eligible case patients and 16 217 control subjects were identified. After excluding ineligible women from the study, telephone interviews were obtained from 6888 case patients and 9424 control subjects. Complete data for recent alcohol consumption, and thus final eligibility for study participation, were determined for 6662 case patients and 9163 control subjects. The average age at time of interview was 58.7 years. The questions on alcohol use addressed average consumption during five periods of the subjects' lives: ages 16–19, 20–29, 30–39, 40–59, and 60–74 years. Similar responses from 211 control subjects upon reinterview 6–12 months later were taken to be indicative of the reliability of the questionnaire used in this study.

Results. Lifetime average alcohol consumption (measured as the average grams per day consumed from age 16 to the recent past) and recent alcohol consumption (average grams per day consumed in the previous age interval) were associated with risk of developing breast cancer. The multivariate relative risk of breast cancer, in those who drink compared with abstainers, associated with average lifetime consumption of 12–18 g/day of alcohol (about one drink) was 1.39 (95 per cent confidence interval [CI] = 1.16–1.67), of 19–32 g/day (about two drinks) was 1.69 (95 per cent CI = 1.36–2.10), of 33–45 g/day (about three drinks) was 2.30 (95 per cent CI = 1.51–3.51), and of greater than or equal to 46 g/day (four or more drinks) was 1.75 (95 per cent CI = 1.65–2.64) (*P* for trend <0.0001). The multivariate relative risk per 13 g/day (about one drink) of alcohol consumed before 30 years of age was 1.09 (95 per cent CI = 0.95–1.24), whereas the relative risk associated with recent consumption of 13 g/day was 1.21 (95 per cent CI = 1.09–1.34).

Conclusions. In these data, alcohol consumption was clearly related to breast cancer risk. Risk appeared to increase even at moderate levels of consumption. For women of all ages combined, consumption before 30 years of age was not an important determinant of risk.

Reproduced from Matthew P. Longnecker et al., 'Risk of Breast Cancer in Relation to Lifetime Alcohol Consumption,' *Journal of National Cancer Institute*, Volume 87, Issue 12, pp. 923–929, © 1995, Oxford University Press [1].

A. Description of the evidence

1. What was the exposure or intervention?
2. What was the outcome?
3. What was the study design?
4. What was the study population?
5. What was the main result?

The exposure in this study is previous alcohol consumption, and the outcome is breast cancer; this is a case–control study. The association between alcohol consumption and breast cancer was already established, as noted in the introduction, and this study was to measure the association more precisely, particularly with regard to the dose–response relationship and the effects of alcohol consumption at different ages. The study population comprised women resident in four defined areas of the United States with population-based cancer registries. Cases had breast cancer diagnosed at ages under 75 and reported by the registries between 1988 and 1991. Controls were selected from the general population within that age range from the same four areas. Finding a population list from which controls can be chosen is always a major issue; here the drivers' licence lists held at state level for subjects aged under 65, and the list of Medicare beneficiaries for subjects aged between 65 and 74 were used. Telephone interviews were used. As the controls aged under 65 had to have a driving licence and a listed telephone number, the same restrictions were made for the cases. For the age range 65–74, all subjects should be on Medicare files, and therefore the restriction was only in terms of telephone listings. The methods section as published is detailed and worth reading.

The main result was a positive association between increasing lifetime alcohol consumption and increasing risk of breast cancer. Table 17.1 shows numbers of cases and controls and crude odds ratios for seven categories of average daily alcohol consumption, each calculated with reference to the zero consumption category; calculated by the methods shown in Chapter 4 and Table A2.16. These crude odds ratios (relative risks) are not presented in the published paper as they do not take any confounding factors into account, but calculating the crude risks when appraising a paper is useful in understanding the data and may illustrate any major discrepancies. The published results show the odds ratios (described as relative risks) adjusted for age and state of residence by the Mantel–Haenszel method. The 'multivariate adjusted' relative risks are also shown; these will be discussed under 'confounding' later. These three sets of results are generally quite similar. The best results are the multivariate adjusted risk ratios, and these are given in the summary. There is a steadily increasing risk with increasing alcohol consumption except in the highest category, where the relative risk is lower than would be expected from a simple linear trend. The association can also be expressed as the relative risk per 13 g/day intake; this unit is equivalent to one drink of most types

Table 17.1 Format of the results of the large case–control study showing the ability to explore dose–response relationships and confounder control. The crude odds ratios (not in the published table) are calculated directly from the data given; the published data were the relative risks (odds ratios) after adjustment for age and state only, and after adjustment for several confounders using a logistic regression model (see text).

All subjects, by lifetime average alcohol consumption

Alcohol g/day	Numbers of cases	Numbers of controls	Crude odds ratio	RR: age and state adjusted	RR: multivariate adjusted risk ratio
0	698	1165	*1 (Ref)*	1 (Ref)	1 (Ref)
>0–5	4080	5864	*1.16*	1.11	1.13
6–11	900	1141	*1.32*	1.23	1.24
12–18	351	409	*1.43*	1.45	1.39
19–32	248	233	*1.78*	1.76	1.69
33–45	63	40	*2.63*	2.58	2.30
>=46	59	55	*1.79*	1.95	1.75

RR = relative risk (odds ratio)

Ref = referent group

Adapted from Matthew P. Longnecker et al., 'Risk of Breast Cancer in Relation to Lifetime Alcohol Consumption,' *Journal of National Cancer Institute*, Volume 87, Issue 12, pp. 923–929, © 1995, Oxford University Press [1].

of alcoholic beverage. This is a useful parameter for making comparisons between sub-groups, as will be shown. The statistical tests will be discussed in due course.

B. Internal validity: consideration of non-causal explanations

6. Are the results likely to be affected by observation bias?

The issue of observation bias concerns the relationship of the recorded information on alcohol intake to the biologically relevant level of alcohol intake. Non-differential error will reduce the observed relative risk towards the null value. Bias relates to a different relationship between recorded and true relevant alcohol intake in cases compared with controls, and could have any type of effect on the result. The information was collected by a standardized telephone interview taking on average less than 25 minutes. The questions were quite detailed, addressing five different time periods, and consumption of beer, wine, and liquor (spirits) separately. A typical question was 'On average, how often did you drink one bottle, glass, or can of beer when you were in your twenties?' There were also questions on lactation, hormone use, physical activity in adolescence and early adulthood, vitamin A intake, established breast cancer risk factors, and other characteristics. The data collected related to the time period prior to diagnosis or to the 'reference date' for control subjects, defined as the date of interview minus the median time between diagnosis and interview for case patients in that state. This is to produce the same time interval between interview and the last relevant time of alcohol consumption for the controls as for the cases.

The main protection against bias is the standardization of methods; the questions were identical and were presented in an identical fashion to both cases and controls. The interviewers were blind to the status of the interviewee at the start of the interview. Of course, many subjects would directly or indirectly make it clear to the interviewer whether they were breast cancer patients or not. The interview began with a request that participants not discuss their medical history until the end of the interview, and the interviewers were asked to record if they were still unaware of the case or control status of the interviewee by the end of the interview; this was so for 74 per cent of cases and 90 per cent of controls.

To assess the reproducibility of the questionnaire, 211 control subjects were re-interviewed after an interval of 6–12 months. Rank correlation coefficients between the average daily consumption of alcohol reported in the two interviews are given for four different time intervals; these range from 0.75 to 0.84. This re-test reliability is high compared with similar assessments of questionnaires or of clinical history items, although even a correlation of 0.8 suggests that an observed relative risk of 2.0 will relate to a true odds ratio of 2.4 (see Chapter 6).

The critical issue is whether there could be bias. If their actual consumption were the same, would women with breast cancer tend to report higher, or lower, alcohol consumption than comparison women from the general population? The authors cite two studies which looked at re-test consistency of alcohol consumption assessed for both breast cancer cases and controls; they showed similar results for the two groups, suggesting that bias is unlikely. A useful extension of the study would have been to assess re-test reliability on a sample of cases as well as on controls. The literature reviewed suggests that reporting is generally reasonable, but some under-reporting is more likely amongst those with a very high alcohol intake. Such bias could affect the results seen in Table 17.1; assuming there is a true relationship, if cases with the highest alcohol consumption tended to under-report this, the risks in the highest categories may be underestimated.

It could be argued that differential recall bias might be particularly strong either a considerable time after diagnosis, or (perhaps more likely) shortly after diagnosis. Results are given for cases interviewed within 14 months of diagnosis, and these were not substantially different from those based on all case patients. An analysis restricted to subjects where the interviewer was still blind to their status at the end of their interview would also be helpful, but is not reported. Thus some non-differential misclassification is inevitable, and so the reported relative risks are likely to underestimate the true relationship. Observation bias cannot be totally excluded, but it seems unlikely that the bias would be substantial enough to account for the main result, or to make a very large difference to it.

7. Are the results likely to be affected by confounding?

There are many potential confounding factors. Many factors affect the risk of breast cancer, including age, ethnic origin, social class, many aspects of reproductive history, diet, and obesity. Many factors would be expected to differ between women with different levels of alcohol consumption, including some of these risk factors. Individual matching for more than the general demographic factors would be difficult. Frequency matching was done by state and by age, to make the ratio of controls to case subjects at least one in each 5-year group. The main method of confounder control was to obtain information on potential confounding factors, and use this in a multivariate analysis. Therefore the results are expressed in two ways, showing the Mantel–Haenszel odds ratios adjusted only for age and state, and the multivariate adjusted odds ratio. These are from a logistic regression model (see Chapter 6) with 6390 case patients and 8794 control subjects, including as well as alcohol consumption, variables for age, state, age at first term pregnancy, parity, body mass index (an index of obesity), age at menarche, education, previous history of benign breast disease, and family history of breast cancer. The number of categories of each of these is given in the methods section; thus the model has many variables. The use of oral contraceptives and replacement oestrogens were also considered as potential confounding factors, but in these data they were not associated with alcohol consumption and therefore were not retained. As 98 per cent of the cases were white, race is not further considered. After all this analysis, the final multivariate adjusted results are not greatly different from the results adjusted only for age and state, or indeed from the crude results shown in Table 17.1.

There are two main issues in assessing if confounding has been adequately controlled. First, have the potential confounding factors that have been identified been adequately controlled? Good control depends on having accurate information on each factor, and using this in an appropriate analysis. If the data on confounders have a high degree of error, this compromises the ability to deal with confounding. While it is impossible to conclude that all confounding by these known factors has been totally removed, given that the approach used did not produce major differences in the association of alcohol intake and breast cancer, it seems unlikely that better control for these confounders would affect the results substantially.

The second issue is: are there other confounders that have not been included? Are there any established risk factors for breast cancer that could also be related to alcohol consumption, which have not been considered in this study? One possibility is diet. Obesity (body mass index) was included as a confounder, but no detailed dietary information was collected. Other dietary relationships with breast cancer were not very clear when this study was done; for example, a major meta-analysis of cohort studies showed no association with fat intake. The associations seen were not stronger than that seen here with alcohol consumption; it is possible that the relationship with diet is confounded by alcohol consumption, rather than the other way round. There could also be some further unrecognized factors, which would be important if they were true confounders, being a risk factor for breast cancer and also being independently association with alcohol consumption. This is always a possibility. There will also be factors which are intermediates in the association between alcohol consumption and breast cancer; alcohol consumption may produce some metabolic or hormonal change which in turn increases the breast cancer risk. Such a factor would not be a confounder, as it would be an intermediate on the causal pathway, as discussed in Chapter 7.

8. Are the results likely to be affected by chance variation?

Chance variation is appropriately assessed by looking at the results after multivariate adjustment, as in Table 17.1. For all women, the relative risk for lifetime average consumption rises from the referent value of 1 in those with no alcohol consumption up to 1.75 in the highest category, and the values in all six categories used are individually statistically significant, with the lower 95 per cent confidence limit being greater than 1 (Table 4 in the original paper). An appropriate overall statistical test is a test for trend; this is highly significant, with $P < 0.0001$. The statistical model used the square root of the alcohol consumption as this gave a better fit to the data, as described in the methods section. The overall association can also be expressed as the relative risk per 13 g/day, which is 1.31, with 95 per cent confidence limits of 1.20–1.43. The same format and statistical tests are applied to the results for more specific groups, as will be discussed. One of the objectives of this study was to compare the effects of alcohol consumption at different ages, as this should elucidate the mechanism of the association. We will discuss this further under the heading of specificity.

Summary: non-causal explanations

To summarize, observation bias has been as well controlled as is feasible in a retrospective study, but the possibility of biased responses from the subjects cannot be totally excluded. There will be some non-differential misclassification, although the re-test reliability of the methods used has been shown to be high. Confounding by most known potential confounding factors has been adequately controlled by multivariate methods, but there remains the possibility of confounding by other factors not included in the study. Chance variation can be confidently excluded because the size of the study gives narrow confidence limits for the estimates of effect, and there is a regular dose–response relationship.

C. Internal validity: consideration of positive features of causation

9. Is there a correct time relationship?

Alcohol consumption after the recognition of cancer is clearly irrelevant to the causal hypothesis. Case patients were interviewed at a median of 14 months after diagnosis, and the interviews were restricted to asking about intakes up to the time of diagnosis, or a corresponding date for the controls. The accuracy of this cut-off might be less good where the interval from diagnosis to interview was longer, and no detailed information (e.g. the maximum time interval) is given. However, as noted before, the results were similar in those interviewed within 14 months of diagnosis to those in all subjects. The relevant time of alcohol intake depends on whether the relevant process is the first initiation phase of cancer development, or a later stage such as promotion, and so could be from a few to many years before clinical diagnosis.

10. Is the association strong?

The relationship is moderately strong. For all women, the relative risks reach approximately 2.0 at the highest alcohol intake level measured. This is consistent with causality, but is not greater than some other breast cancer risk factors. Because of the high prevalence of alcohol consumption in the population, even this risk, if valid, is important in clinical and public health terms. However, it does raise the question of whether alcohol intake is merely a rather inaccurate estimator of a more fundamental causal factor which, if identified, might show a much stronger association.

11. Is there a dose–response relationship?

The dose–response relationship is one of the main features of this study. The dose–response relationship is shown for lifetime consumption in Table 17.1, and data are also given for recent consumption, for consumption before age 30, and for incidence in pre-menopausal and post-menopausal women separately. In each of these groups there is a regular positive dose–response relationship. The study was designed to be large enough to give reasonably precise relative risks at moderate levels of consumption; for example, for one alcoholic drink per day, the relative risk is 1.39 with a 95 per cent confidence level of 1.16–1.67, a quite precise measure of effect. The regular dose–response relationships give considerable protection against the association being due to observation bias, as observation bias would be unlikely to be consistently related to the amount of alcohol consumption; we might expect observation bias to apply particularly to those with very heavy consumption, giving a rather erratic dose–response relationship. It is less protection against confounding, as if a confounding factor were regularly and systematically related to alcohol consumption, it could be consistent with a regular dose–response relationship.

12. Are the results consistent within the study? And 13. Is there any specificity within the study?

In this study, specificity and consistency are assessed with respect to three factors: the consumption of alcohol at different ages, the occurrence of breast cancer at different ages, and the consumption of different types of alcohol.

For alcohol consumption at different ages, the comparison is made by taking subjects diagnosed at over age 40, further subdivided into pre-or post-menopausal at diagnosis, and comparing the effects of consumption before age 30 with consumption during a more recent time period. The full results have been condensed in Table 17.2 to show only the overall relative risk per 13 g/day alcohol consumption, derived from the multivariate model. These results are complex. For women diagnosed after the menopause, there was a significant positive association with consumption during the recent time period ($RR = 1.26$), but the association with consumption before age 30 was weak and not significant ($RR = 1.03$). However, for pre-menopausal women the association with consumption before age 30 is the stronger. Of course, these two time periods are close

Table 17.2 Relative risks per 13 g/day alcohol consumption, from logistic regression model, in various subgroups (table cross-references refer to original paper [1]).

Relative risk per 13 g/day alcohol intake, from multivariate model

	RR	95% confidence limits
All subjects		
All subjects, lifetime average consumption (Table 4)	1.31	1.20–1.43
All subjects, recent time interval (Table 1)	1.24	1.15–1.33
Subjects over age 40		
Recent time interval (all other results Table 2)	1.21	1.09–1.34
Consumption before age 30	1.09	0.95–1.24
Subjects over age 40, post-menopausal		
Recent time interval	1.26	1.12–1.42
Consumption before age 30	1.03	0.88–1.20
Subjects over age 40, pre-menopausal		
Recent time interval	1.05	0.85–1.31
Consumption before age 30	1.34	1.02–1.75

Source: data from Matthew P. Longnecker et al., 'Risk of Breast Cancer in Relation to Lifetime Alcohol Consumption,' *Journal of National Cancer Institute*, Volume 87, Issue 12, pp. 923–929, © 1995, Oxford University Press [1].

together for these younger women, and so the interpretation is not as clear as it is for post-menopausal women.

The other comparison made, for women aged over 40, was to assess the joint effect of consumption before age 30 and in a recent time period. The results are given in the paper for 16 subgroups representing four categories of consumption in each time period. These results are 'mutually adjusted'; that is, the relative risk for alcohol consumption before age 30 is adjusted for alcohol consumption in the recent time period, and vice versa. The results show that in women with no recent consumption, alcohol consumption before age 30 has a strong effect ($RR = 1.72$); and in women with no consumption before age 30, recent alcohol consumption has a strong effect ($RR = 1.90$). The authors suggest that this is consistent with a cumulative effect. These data do not support the prior hypothesis of a specific effect of alcohol consumption in early life.

Results are given for daily intake of alcohol for beer, wine, and liquor. Using data on alcohol consumption in the most recent age interval, a multivariate model was fitted with a continuous variable for each measure of alcohol consumption. As these factors are fitted simultaneously, the resulting odds ratios show of the change in risk associated with a unit change in alcohol consumption of 13 g/day, adjusting for the other sources of alcohol. The relative risk estimates for beer, liquor, and wine are 1.25, 1.18, and 0.93, respectively; the coefficients for beer and liquor are statistically significant, but that for wine is not significant. Thus the results show no association with wine, but positive associations with beer and liquor. We need to assess this result with regard to possible observational bias and confounding. The weaker association with the consumption of wine could arise if the degree of non-differential classification for this exposure were greater than that for the other types of alcohol, or if there were other confounding effects related to this exposure. If there is under-reporting of heavy consumption, this reduces the range of reported consumption, which thus reduces the ability to detect a real association; such an effect might have a greater influence where the range may be relatively small, as in wine consumption.

Conclusions with regard to internal validity

The internal validity of the result of this study is high. It is a large study. It has been carefully conducted with standardized and, to a large extent, interviewer-blind data collection, although of course the subjects providing the data are well aware of whether or not they have had breast cancer. The possibility of observation bias remains, but the methods used, the regularity of the dose–response relationships, and the high re-test reliability of the questionnaire together make observation bias an unlikely explanation of the results. Non-differential error will make the results underestimate the true association. Confounding by the accepted risk factors for breast cancer has been dealt with by multivariate analysis; this gave very little change in the risk ratios showing that confounding by these factors is minor, and also suggests that further control, for example, by having more comprehensive data on such factors, would be unlikely to greatly modify the result. However, the influence of unrecognized confounders cannot be dismissed. Diet has not been assessed and could be a confounder. Chance variation can be confidently excluded, as the study is large, and the probability of such results occurring by chance is extremely small. The time relationships are consistent with causality, the relationship is moderately strong, and there is a clear and regular dose–response relationship. There are many subgroup comparisons, for which the conclusions are less definitive. The results suggest generally similar effects for pre-menopausal and post-menopausal women. The relationship appears limited to beer or liquor consumption, with no association seen for wine. A causal explanation of the association seems more likely than any of the alternative non-causal explanations, and it is reasonable to proceed on this basis. The most plausible non-causal explanation would be confounding by factors not included in this study.

D. External validity: generalization of the results

14. Can the study results be applied to the eligible population?

Box 17.1 shows the typical complexity of a large population-based case–control study. The 6862 cases participating fully in the trial are derived from an eligible population of 8579. Of these, 14.9 per cent were not approached for interview for the reasons shown, 5.6 per cent of those approached refused the interview, and a further 3.3 per cent had missing data on some of the key variables. Therefore the voluntary response rate is extremely high at 91 per cent, and the participation rate (the participant group divided by the eligible population) is also substantial at 78 per cent.

For the control group, the 9163 controls are derived from 11 238 eligible control subjects. The proportion not approached (2.5 per cent) is much lower than that of the cases, because fewer died before interview and there was no requirement for a doctor to give permission. On the other hand, the 14 per cent refusal rate for interviews is much higher than that of the cases, although it is still very reasonable; a similar proportion of the interviews (2.8 per cent) were incomplete. The voluntary response rate for controls was 83.6 per cent, which is very high for a study of this nature in the United States, and the participation rate at 81.5 per cent is also high and very similar to that of the case series.

These results are impressive. The cases will tend to exclude women with very advanced disease who died before interview, and those whose doctor refused permission may also have had more advanced disease. This is relevant if the association between alcohol and breast cancer also relates to the extent of disease at diagnosis, for example, by affecting the growth speed of the tumour or the speed of diagnosis. Apart from that, the exclusion and voluntary refusals are minor. We might well expect that they could be related to alcohol consumption, and that the higher refusal rate amongst those approached for interview in the control group compared with the cases could lead to the exclusion of more controls with particularly high alcohol intakes. If this bias did occur, it would tend to exaggerate the observed relative risks; the recorded level of alcohol consumption in participating controls would underestimate the consumption in all eligible controls, with this bias occurring to a lesser extent among the cases.

Box 17.1 Derivation of the case and control groups contributing to the analysis of alcohol consumption and breast cancer in Longnecker et al. [1]

PROGRESS OF A CASE–CONTROL STUDY

	Cases		Controls	
	In study	Excluded	In study	Excluded
Source population (SP)	11 879	% of source	16 217	% of source
No phone number		2641 22.2		4442 27.4
Previous breast cancer		273 2.3		296 1.8
No driver's licence		297 2.5		47 0.3
Inadequate English		51 0.4		87 0.5
Missing data		38 0.3		107 0.7
Total excluded		3300 27.8		4979 30.7
Eligible population (EP)	8579	% of eligible	11 238	% of eligible
Died before interview		463 5.4		126 1.1
Doctor refused permission		761 8.9		0 0.0
Not located		55 0.6		153 1.4
Total not approached		1279 14.9		279 2.5
Approached for interview (AI)	7300	%	10 959	%
Refused interview		412 5.6		1535 14.0
Participants in study (PS)	6888	%	9424	%
Missing data		226 3.3		261 2.8
Participants in analysis (PA)	6662		9163	
Voluntary response rate (overall)		= PS/AI 94.4%		86.0%
Voluntary response rate (full data)		= PA/AI 91.3%		83.6%
Participation rate		= PA/EP 77.7%		81.5%
Eligible/source population		= EP/SP 72.2%		69.3%
Participants/source population		= PA/SP 56.1%		56.5%

Source: data from Matthew P. Longnecker et al., 'Risk of Breast Cancer in Relation to Lifetime Alcohol Consumption,' *Journal of National Cancer Institute*, Volume 87, Issue 12, pp. 923–929, © 1995, Oxford University Press [1].

15. Can the study results be applied to the source population?

The source population is women resident in the four geographical areas in 1988–91. Both cases and controls had to have a listed telephone number (excluding 22 per cent of cases and 27 per cent of controls) and possess a driver's licence (excluding 3 per cent of cases and 1 per cent of controls) (Box. 17.1). There is no discussion of the effects of these exclusions. There should be little effect on internal validity, as the restrictions apply to both cases and controls. Women in unfavourable socioeconomic circumstances maybe underrepresented; this restriction might exclude some women with high alcohol intake. However, it seems unlikely that these exclusions would greatly affect the relationship between alcohol consumption and breast cancer occurrence examined in this study.

16. Can the study results be applied to other relevant populations?

These results apply to women in the United States, almost all white, diagnosed in 1988–91. Breast cancer is more common in populations of European origin than in, for example, Asian or African populations. Alcohol consumption in women is a culturally specific exposure, and its associations with other social, economic, and cultural factors vary considerably in different societies; so, confounding relationships could be different in different societies and time periods. On the other hand, despite the considerable range of incidence rates, risk factors such as reproductive factors have reasonably consistent associations with the disease in a wide range of cultures. A fundamental biological association between alcohol consumption and breast cancer would be expected to be universal. Therefore, in general, the reasonably high internal validity suggests a biological causal relationship between alcohol consumption and breast cancer, which can be applied widely. The details of the relationship, such as the specificity to consumption of beer or liquor rather than wine, might suggest possible differences in confounding relationships, in that the social factors linked to these different drinks may vary. It would be reasonable to consider these results as applicable to generally similar societies, that is, affluent Western societies with women of predominantly European origin, but there would be more caution in applying the results to other social, ethnic, or racial groups.

E. Comparison of the results with other evidence

17. Are the results consistent with other evidence, particularly evidence from studies of similar or more powerful study design?

When published, this study, primarily because of its size, was one of the best individual case–control studies of this topic. Other case–control and cohort studies are reviewed in the discussion. Many studies have found a positive association between alcohol consumption and breast cancer; the inconsistencies are in terms of whether drinking at different ages has different effects, and in terms of specific relationships to the type of alcohol.

18. Does the total evidence suggest any specificity?

The results on variation by age at diagnosis, alcohol consumption at different ages, and specificity to different types of alcohol, have to be considered as less definitive than the overall association, so other studies are also needed. In the introduction and discussion, several papers giving inconsistent results on the age relationships are noted, and also papers giving different results in terms of types of alcohol.

19. Are the results plausible in terms of a biological mechanism?

Possible biological mechanisms of this association are discussed in some detail in this paper. Animal experiments have shown that alcohol intake increases the risk of breast tumours and the proliferation rate of breast tissue cells, although these results are inconsistent. Alcohol is not generally accepted as an initiator of the cancer transformation process in cells. However, it is recognized as a promoter, that is, it promotes the development of cells which have been transformed. The association is therefore plausible, although the mechanism is unclear. The authors cite studies showing that alcohol appears to increase serum oestradiol levels, which is relevant as other work links high oestradiol levels to breast cancer risk.

20. If a major effect is shown, is it coherent with the distribution of the exposure and the outcome?

The overall association is not strong enough to make an assessment of coherence useful. Breast cancer is a common disease, and several other factors have associations as strong as or stronger than that produced here. Therefore we would not anticipate a clear relationship between alcohol consumption and breast cancer incidence, for example, on a geographical or secular trend basis. However, the high incidence rate in Western countries, and perhaps the increasing trend in breast cancer incidence over recent decades, is consistent with differences in alcohol consumption. A positive association between breast cancer mortality and estimated alcohol intake per capita, comparing countries, has been shown [2], although the association with fat intake was greater. The limitation is that this type of evidence is open to so many other interpretations that it adds little to the argument for causality; the current study uses a much more powerful method of inquiry.

Conclusions

In conclusion, this large case–control study has shown a regular positive association between recorded alcohol intake and breast cancer risk (Table 17.3). The most convincing aspect of this is the clear and regular dose–response relationship. The least convincing aspect is the complex relationship with consumption at different ages, with curious results when age at diagnosis is also taken into consideration, which do not lead to a clear conclusion. The overall association is unlikely to be due to observation bias. Confounding by most well-established risk factors for breast cancer has been dealt with. Confounding by diet has not been addressed, and the disease is sufficiently complex that the possibility of unrecognized confounding factors remains. The associations

Table 17.3 Summary of assessment of the case–control study of breast cancer and alcohol consumption.

A. Description of the evidence	
1. Exposure	Alcohol consumption at different ages, dosages, and types
2. Outcome	Breast cancer incidence
3. Design	Retrospective case–control study, population based; telephone interviews
4. Study population	Breast cancer cases in four states in the United States, 1988–91; controls from community sources
5. Main result	Increased risk with increasing alcohol consumption, even at moderate levels; consumption before age 30 not specifically hazardous
B. Non-causal explanations	
6. Observation bias	Systematic methods and single-blind design may protect; evidence of acceptably high re-test consistency; cannot exclude some bias
7. Confounding	Controlled for most known confounders by multivariate methods. Confounding by diet still possible
8. Chance	Large study gives precise estimates; chance can be confidently excluded
C. Features consistent with causation	
9. Time relationship	Positive association seen with lifetime, recent, and before age 30 consumption, varying in different age groups of cases; consistent with a cumulative effect rather than specific to one age range at consumption
10. Strength	Overall effect not very strong: relative risk up to 2 at maximum consumption
11. Dose–response	Clearly seen over finely divided range; consistent with linear increase, no evidence of threshold effect
12. Consistency	Not consistent between pre- and post-menopausal women; generally positive but differences in detail
13. Specificity	Specific to beer or liquor consumption; no effect seen with wine consumption
D. External validity	
14. Eligible population	High participation rates; little difficulty in generalizing to eligible population
15. Source population	Eligible subjects had to have a listed phone and a driver's licence; may exclude some social groups
16. Target populations	Applicable to women in most developed countries; predominantly white ethnic groups

E. Comparison with other evidence

17. Consistency	Consistent with earlier studies; adds precision in dose response
18. Specificity	Specificity to beer or liquor not supported by other studies. Relationships in different age groups still unclear for all evidence
19. Plausibility	Plausible, although mechanism of action unknown
20. Coherence	Relationship too weak, and may be other aetiological factors for breast cancer, to expect clear coherence

Source: data from Matthew P. Longnecker et al., 'Risk of Breast Cancer in Relation to Lifetime Alcohol Consumption,' *Journal of National Cancer Institute*, Volume 87, Issue 12, pp. 923–929, © 1995, Oxford University Press [1].

seen are highly statistically significant. The results are generally consistent with the results of other observational studies, most of which, however, would be open to the same limitations. A reasonable conclusion is that a causal explanation is the most likely explanation of the results seen, but that confounding cannot be excluded. The aspect of the results suggesting that the association is specific to beer or liquor consumption, rather than wine consumption, is not consistent with the totality of other evidence, and can be regarded only as tentative.

Subsequent development

This study was a substantial contribution to knowledge about alcohol consumption and breast cancer. Its most important result was to show that risk increased even at moderate levels of consumption, of even one standard drink per day. The study also suggested that consumption before the age of 30 was less important than average lifetime consumption or alcohol consumption in recent years.

The association with modest levels of consumption has been confirmed. A meta-analysis including 110 studies of breast cancer shows that light drinking (up to one drink per day) has a small but significant increase in risk ($RR = 1.05$, 95 per cent limits 1.02–1.08), seen in both case–control and cohort studies; this small risk would lead to 5000 extra cases per year worldwide [3]. For heavy alcohol consumption, the overall risk ratio estimate was 1.61 (95 per cent limits 1.33–1.94) [4]. The association is greater in, but not restricted to, oestrogen receptor-positive tumours [5]. Whether risk of breast cancer varies by the type of alcohol consumed has not been confirmed, with some other studies showing no such variation [6].

The risk may be conferred through increased oestrogen levels, but many mechanisms including oxidative stress, epigenetic changes, folate metabolism, and decreased retinoic acid have been explored [5,6]. Alcohol intake is associated with several cancers in addition to breast cancer, and is categorized as a definitive type 1 carcinogen by the International Agency for Research on Cancer [7], and alcohol reduction is a key cancer prevention strategy [8].

References

1. **Longnecker MP, Newcomb PA, Mittendorf R, Greenberg ER, Clapp RW, Bogdan GF, et al.** Risk of breast cancer in relation to lifetime alcohol consumption. *J Natl Cancer Inst* 1995; 87:923–929.

2. **Schatzkin A, Piantadosi S, Miccozzi M, Bartee D.** Alcohol consumption and breast cancer: a cross-national correlation study. *Int J Epidemiol* 1989; **18**:28–31.

3. **Bagnardi V, Rota M, Botteri E, Tramacere I, Islami F, Fedirko V, et al.** Light alcohol drinking and cancer: a meta-analysis. *Ann Oncol* 2013; 24:301–308.

4. **Bagnardi V, Rota M, Botteri E, Tramacere I, Islami F, Fedirko V, et al.** Alcohol consumption and site-specific cancer risk: a comprehensive dose-response meta-analysis. *Br J Cancer* 2015; **112**:580–593.

5. **Seitz HK, Pelucchi C, Bagnardi V, La VC.** Epidemiology and pathophysiology of alcohol and breast cancer: Update 2012. *Alcohol Alcohol* 2012; **47**:204–212.

6. **Scoccianti C, Lauby-Secretan B, Bello PY, Chajes V, Romieu I.** Female breast cancer and alcohol consumption: a review of the literature. *Am J Prev Med* 2014; **46**:S16–S25.

7. **International Agency for Research on Cancer (IARC).** Alcohol consumption and ethyl carbamate. *IARC Monogr Eval Carcinog Risks Hum* 2010; **96**:3–1383.

8. **Scoccianti C, Cecchini M, Anderson AS, Berrino F, Boutron-Ruault MC, Espina C, et al.** European Code against Cancer 4th Edition: Alcohol drinking and cancer. *Cancer Epidemiol* 2015; **39**(Suppl 1):S67–74.

Appendix 1

Answers to self-test questions

Chapter 2

Q2.1

A factor is a cause of an event if its operation increases the frequency of the event.

Q2.2

(a) Sufficient causation for this person (with common-sense assumptions about the general circumstances).
(b) Necessary causation (but note that clinical polio is defined as involving infection with the virus).
(c) Common causation, that is, neither necessary (the lung cancer could be due to other factors) nor sufficient (lung cancer does not always occur even after heavy smoking).
(d) Sufficient and necessary causation. Most examples of sufficient and necessary causation are situations where there is enough knowledge to relate a specific genetic or biochemical abnormality to a clearly defined disease state.
(e) Common causation (if the evidence supports that interpretation), neither necessary nor sufficient.

Q2.3

(a) The prevalence of wearing glasses is 8 in 40, or 20 per cent.
(b) The incidence rate of road accidents was 1 per 1000 per year.
(c) The in-hospital mortality rate is 14 per cent (this is a cumulative incidence rate of death, but it would be better if the time period was known).
(d) The prevalence of breast malignancy is 25 per cent.

Q2.4

(a) The initial prevalence of hypertension is 16 per cent; the final prevalence is 28 per cent.
(b) The cumulative incidence of hypertension over 3 years is 120/840 = 14.3 per cent (as the number at risk at the beginning of the observation time is 840).

(c) In the 3 years recorded, the incidence is 120 new cases and the average population at risk is 780 (840 at risk at the start, 720 at risk after 3 years), so that the incidence rate is 120/780 over 3 years = 5.1 per cent per year.

Q2.5

(a) Population at risk at 1 January 2001 = 1000 − 180 = 820.

(b) Prevalence rate at 1 January 2002 = 200/1000 = 20 per cent.

(c) Number of new cases over 2 years = 250 − 180 = 70. Initial population at risk = 820. Cumulative incidence over 2 years = 70/820 = 8.5 per cent.

(d) Number of new cases in 2002 = 250 − 200 = 50. Population at risk at start of 2002 = 800; at end of 2002 = 750. Therefore average population at risk in 2002 = 775; hence average incidence rate in 2002 = 50/775 = 6.5 per cent per year.

Chapter 3

Q3.1

(a) Cohort study, as the subjects are selected on their exposure, air travel; cross-sectional.

(b) Case–control study, retrospective. The subjects are selected on their outcome, which is hypertension.

(c) Cohort study, retrospective. The comparison is based on the exposure, which is occupation.

(d) Case–control study, retrospective. The comparison is based on the outcome, which is infarction.

(e) Cohort study, prospective. The comparison is based on the exposure, which is smoking.

(f) Case–control study nested in a cohort study.

(g) Non-randomized intervention study (clinical trial): equally can be regarded as a cohort study.

Q3.2

(a) Perhaps, but as the time direction is unspecified, diabetes may lead to unemployment, or both may be consequences of other causal factors.

(b) Perhaps, but may be those who smoke at age 85 are less likely to survive to age 95.

(c) Perhaps, but in this retrospective case–control study the accuracy of the information on stressful events is questionable. A prospective study, where data on stressful events were collected before the breast cancer diagnosis, would be stronger.

(d) Perhaps, but this cross-sectional study will exclude any workers who developed repetitive strain injury and then stopped work. A prospective study of workers from their first employment would be better.

Q3.3

A cohort study addresses the question of the effects of a particular exposure, and will allow multiple end points to be assessed. The major disadvantages for an outcome such as cancer occurrence will be the large size of study (both exposed and unexposed comparison groups) which will be needed, and the long time period of follow-up necessary. The potential of the outcome ascertainment being biased by knowledge of the exposure is also a potential problem.

Q3.4

A case–control study can assess a large number of potential exposure factors, and is feasible even with a fairly small number of cases of the newly recognized disease. Questions can be asked about exposures at various times in the past, avoiding the time delay of prospective studies. The main difficulties are that the retrospective assessment of exposures will be open to inaccuracy, and perhaps bias. Defining an appropriate control group may be difficult.

Q3.5

Randomized trials are a direct method of testing a causal hypothesis by observing whether subjects offered the intervention under test have a different frequency of outcome to an appropriate comparison group. Randomization on an adequately large sample should mean that the two groups being compared are similar in all relevant factors, so that, without the intervention, they would have the same frequency of outcome. Randomization demands a precise protocol and concurrent controls, so that methods to avoid bias in the outcome assessment, such as double-blind techniques, can be used.

Chapter 4

Q4.1

(a) The mortality rates are 7.3 per cent in the treated group and 26.9 per cent in the controls. These are cumulative mortality rates over the follow-up period (which was 6 months).

(b) The relative risk of death is 0.27, or the relative risk of survival is 3.7.

(c) The odds ratio for death is 0.21, or the odds ratio of survival is 4.7. It is larger than the relative risk (greater difference from 1) as the risk of death is high.

(d) The attributable risk is −19.6 per cent.

(e) The attributable benefit is 19.6 per cent (i.e. 19.6 per cent of treated subjects benefit from the treatment in regard to this outcome).

(f) The number needed to treat for one death prevented is 100/19.6 = 5. There were 10 less deaths than expected in the 55 subjects treated.

Q4.2

(a) The mortality rates are 3.84 deaths per 1000 man-years in the high-fat group, and 2.91 per 1000 man-years in the lower-fat group

(b) The relative risk (high fat compared with lower fat) is 1.32.

(c) The attributable risk of the high-fat diet in this population is 0.93 deaths per 1000 man-years, if causality is accepted.

(d) The preventable proportion in the high-fat diet group is 0.93/3.84 = 24.2 per cent, again if causality is accepted.

(e) The preventable proportion in this whole population, in which the death rate is 3.25 per 1000 man-years, is (3.25 − 2.91)/3.25 = 10.5 per cent, again if causality is accepted, and if the study is representative in terms of the exposure distribution.

Q4.3

(a) Assuming an additive model, the expected incidence rate for joint exposure is 50 + 50 + 350 = 450 per 10 000 person-years.

(b) Assuming a multiplicative model, the relative risk for smoking is 8, and for air pollution is 2; therefore the joint relative risk is 8 × 2 = 16, and the expected incidence rate for joint exposure is 50 × 16 = 800 per 10 000 person-years.

Q4.4

(a) The relative risk cannot be directly assessed. The best estimate will be the odds ratio; it will be somewhat different from the relative risk as this disease is quite common.

(b) The odds ratio is (180 × 680)/(320 × 120) = 3.19, showing an increased risk in those with a prior knee injury.

(c) The attributable proportion in the exposed group = (3.19 − 1)/3.19 = 68.7 per cent, if the association is causal.

Q4.5

This describes incidence-based sampling, so that now the cross-products ratio of 3.19 is a valid estimate of relative risk. The odds ratio is not directly obtained.

Q4.6

(a) Assuming causality, and using the relative risk of 5.1, the preventable proportion is (5.1 − 1.0)/5.1 = 80 per cent. (Using 4.8 yields 79 per cent; the difference is a rounding error.)

(b) This is another application of the number needed to treat; as the risk difference is 3.8 per 100 000 population, the number affected is about 26 000 to reduce firearm-based murders by one per year.

(c) Here we use the total results; the preventable proportion is calculated as either (1.6 − 1)/1.6 = 38 per cent or (11.3 − 6.9)/11.3 = 39 per cent. This assumes that the results show causality, and that a change in the laws would produce the same effect as is seen in these observational data based on past experience.

Chapter 5

Q5.1

The participants are the children whose data are analysed even though their parents or other informants provide the data. The eligible population comprises all children with leukaemia seen in the particular hospital, in some specified time period, excluding those in a terminal stage. The age range and the definition of 'terminal stage' need to be clarified. The source population is all children seen in that hospital. The target population is probably all children with leukaemia in the country concerned, or internationally, but may be restricted to certain types of leukaemia or in other ways.

Q5.2

The internal validity concept addresses whether this association is due to a causal relationship between measles and leukaemia in the children participating in this study, or is produced by observation bias, confounding, or chance. The issue of external validity is whether the association, if internally valid, can be applied to 'measles' and 'childhood leukaemia' on a wider basis, for example, in all children, in those in certain age groups, in those with different types of measles or leukaemia, or in different geographical areas and times.

Q5.3

Selection bias can affect the external validity if the participants are not representative of a wider population, it can affect the internal validity if selection effects are different in the groups being compared, or it may modify the hypothesis being tested.

Q5.4

The source population is 1000, and the eligible population is 900. Of these, a total of 160 are not approached for administrative reasons, and so 740 are approached, of whom 500 agree to be interviewed, but only 450 give the information that is used in the analysis.

The participation rate (full participants divided by eligible subjects) is 450 out of 900, 50 per cent; the voluntary response rate for full participation is 450 out of 740, 61 per cent, and for any cooperation is 500 out of 740, 68 per cent. Thus the full participants represent 50 per cent of the eligible subjects and 45 per cent of the source population. The study results depend on the full participants, and the 50 per cent figure is the best indicator of their relationship to the ideal, which would be to have information on all eligible subjects.

Q5.5

Fifty per cent of those randomized to the intervention accepted the intervention, and of those 50 per cent quit smoking (total 25 per cent quit); 50 per cent did not accept, and of those 10 per cent quit (total 5 per cent). Therefore the success rate in the whole group randomized to intervention is 30 per cent. This can be compared with the success rate in the whole group randomized to no intervention (20 per cent), giving a relative risk of cessation of 1.5 (30/20), an odds ratio of 1.7, or a difference in rate of quitting of 10 per cent. All these are valid results. This comparison assesses the effect of *offering* the programme, and as it is based on the randomization, should have protection against confounding. Any comparison based on the 50 per cent success rate in those who accept the programme is no longer a randomized comparison, and must be interpreted as very likely to be influenced by confounding factors which relate to acceptance of the programme.

Q5.6

The exposed group should truly be exposed, they should be studied from the beginning of exposure or from some defined period after it, they should be representative of a defined eligible population of exposed subjects, and they should be chosen so that the further investigations and follow-up can be carried out in a similar manner as in the comparison group.

Q5.7

The controls will be chosen either to be representative of unaffected subjects, or to be representative of the entire study base; in this case, the former is more likely. They should be chosen so that the information can be gained in the same way as in the cases, that is, by telephone interviews. They should be representative of the same eligible population which provides the cases. Therefore it would be wise to select controls who are also patients in the same general practices.

Q5.8

In a single-blind trial, participating subjects are unaware of which intervention they are receiving; in a double-blind trial, neither the subjects nor those making the observations of outcome are aware of the intervention being received. This is frequently accomplished in drug trials by using an identical placebo to the active drug.

Q5.9

An internal control group would consist (for example) of other employees who were not exposed to that particular chemical; an external comparison group might consist of members of a different workforce or industry, or the general population of the geographical area or country. An internal control group will in general give better comparability, if an adequately large group can be found, and if there is little danger of contamination (in both chemical and epidemiological terms) by that control group also being exposed to the chemicals under study.

Chapter 6

Q6.1

Observation bias; because confounding and chance variation can only be assessed by using the data, which if biased will be misleading.

Q6.2

Bias refers to inaccuracy that is different in the different groups of subjects being compared; error refers to inaccuracy that is similar in the different groups.

Q6.3

Non-differential error will nearly always make the observed association closer to the null value than is the true association.

Q6.4

Observation bias, having different effects on the different groups being compared, can affect the results of a study in either direction, increasing or decreasing the measure of association compared with the true value.

Q6.5

In a single-blind assessment, the observer is unaware of the exposure or disease status of the subject; in a double-blind comparison, the subject is also usually unaware of their exposure or treatment classification; in a triple-blind design, the analysis is done without knowledge of the allocation of subjects.

Q6.6

Having a clear definition of the factors being assessed, and appropriate choices of instruments, standardization of methods, and good quality control, applied in identical fashions to all groups of subjects being assessed.

Q6.7

(a) The proportion showing agreement = $0.6 + 0.2 = 0.8 = 80$ per cent.
(b) The expected agreement by chance = $0.7 \times 0.7 + 0.3 \times 0.3 = 0.58 = 58$ per cent.
(c) Kappa = $(0.80 - 0.58)/(1 - 0.58) = 0.52 = 52$ per cent.

Q6.8

If kappa = 0.52 and observed odds ratio = 1.8, the estimated true odds ratio = $(0.52 + 1.8 - 1)/0.52 = 2.5$.

Q6.9

A kappa value of 0.9 shows very good agreement, 0.7 reasonable agreement, 0.5 moderate agreement, and 0.2 poor agreement, but this categorization is very approximate. Kappa values may be misleading, particularly when the prevalence of the factor assessed is very low or very high.

Q6.10

Sensitivity = $50/60 = 83$ per cent.
Specificity = $890/940 = 95$ per cent.
Predictive value positive = $50/100 = 50$ per cent.

Q6.11

As the validity coefficient is 0.9, the true odds ratio is exp $(\ln 1.2/0.9^2) = 1.25$.

Q6.12

The observed odds ratio is $(0.5 \times 0.75)/(0.5 \times 0.25) = 3.0$.

Using the formula shown in Table 6.7, the estimated 'true' proportion exposed is 60 per cent for the cases and 27 per cent for the controls; the true odds ratio is $(0.6 \times 0.73)/(0.4 \times 0.27) = 4.1$.

Chapter 7

Q7.1

Because D is associated with X, the results will show a negative association, that is, an apparent protective effect, of high intakes of D on cancer incidence rates.

Q7.2

As D itself has no effect, the randomized trial will show no effect on cancer incidence.

Q7.3

It is quite likely that the teachers who volunteer will be the more enthusiastic teachers and they will put extra effort into the programme because it is innovative. For that reason, children in the new curriculum will show better results. Any true effect of the new curriculum, positive or negative, will be supplemented (confounded) by this effect due to selection of teachers.

Q7.4

In assessing confounding, whether the difference in a characteristic between two groups being compared is statistically significant is not relevant; the size of the confounding effect produced depends on the size of the difference between the two groups, and also on the strength of the association between that factor and the outcome. Assessing the change in relative risk with or without control for the confounding factor is the appropriate way to assess if there is substantial confounding.

Q7.5

The ratio of success rates, comparing hospital B with hospital A, is 1.5 for early disease and 1.6 for late disease. However, the overall success rate is 37.5 per cent in hospital A, and 46.7 per cent in hospital B, giving a crude ratio of only 1.24. This is lower than the true effect, because hospital B, although it has superior results, has a higher proportion of patients with late disease.

Q7.6

The Mantel–Haenszel relative risk is 1.53, which is intermediate between the relative risks for each category of patients. See Box 7.2 (p.156).

Q7.7

This rate, which we could call the stage-standardized rate, is 28.8 per cent for hospital A and 45.0 per cent for hospital B. The stage-standardized risk ratio is the ratio of these two results, which is 1.56. It differs from the Mantel–Haenszel estimate because although both are weighted averages, the weighting factors are different.

Q7.8

The crude odds ratio is 2.22; the sex-specific odds ratios are 1.5 in men and 0.80 in women. The fact that the overall odds ratio is higher than either of the sex-specific odds ratios demonstrates confounding; here because exposure to injury is more common in men (in the controls) and arthritis is more common in men (in this study, in the unexposed). The Mantel–Haenszel odds ratio is 1.44, being predominantly influenced by the results for men, as these are based on larger numbers. However, the effects appear to be different in the two genders, and so there is effect modification and the summary estimate is less useful; it is better to report the results for men and women separately.

Q7.9

The matched odds ratio is 200/50 = 4. The (incorrect) unmatched odds ratio is 3.2. See Box 7.4 (p.169).

Q7.10

The odds ratio for ever use of oral contraceptives on the crude analysis is exp (0.45) = 1.57. However, controlling for weight changes this to an odds ratio of 0.92. Thus the positive association disappears. This would occur either if oral contraceptive use is more common in women of greater weight and greater weight is positively associated with cardiovascular risk; or if oral contraception was less common in heavier women and such women had a lower risk of cardiovascular events. Of course, the odds ratios and the change in them may also be due to chance variation, which would need to be assessed.

Chapter 8

Q8.1

First you should consider whether the studies have been appropriately performed and whether observation bias and confounding have been dealt with. Assuming that they have, the first study shows a relative risk of 2.2, and the probability of this or a larger difference occurring by chance is less than 0.01, from the chi-square statistic (the Excel routine gives the P-value as 0.002). Therefore, for practical purposes, we can exclude chance variation as a possible explanation, and so if the other issues have been dealt with, we can conclude that the treatment increases recovery. The second study shows a greater benefit with a relative risk of 4.6, but the chi-square statistic gives a probability value of 0.18; that is, about 18 per cent of trials similar to this study would produce a relative risk of 4.6 or greater, or an equivalently large effect in the opposite direction, if there were no true effect. The implication is that this study must be small, and we cannot be confident about the result. These results of the second trial could occur if the treatment were effective, had no effect, or even was detrimental.

Q8.2

Calculation by the methods shown in Box 8.3 gives $a = 16$, $E = 5.09$, $V = 4.60$, and $\chi^2 = 25.8$, giving a P-value of less than 0.000 001 (Box A2.15 and Table A2.1). The relative risk is 4.0, with 95 per cent limits of 2.25 to 7.12, using the formula for the standard deviation of In RR in Box A2.2, part 4A.

Q8.3

The odds ratio is 3.45; for the Mantel–Haenszel calculation $a = 34$, $E = 17.2$, $V = 11.42$, and the χ^2 statistic is 24.7. This corresponds to a P-value of less than 0.001. The 95 per cent limits are 2.08–5.72, using the formula for the standard deviation of In RR in Box A2.1, part 4A. A positive association is seen, and is very unlikely to be due to chance variation. The other non-causal explanations (observation bias and confounding) need to be assessed.

Q8.4

The best estimate of the true relative risk is 2.25. There is a range of true relative risks compatible with this result; 95 per cent of this range is from 0.88 to 5.75 and thus there is a 5 per cent probability that the true RR is below 0.88 or above 5.75. As this range includes the null hypothesis value of 1.0, the result is not 'statistically significant' at the 5 per cent two-sided level.

Q8.5

Assuming equal-sized groups, $p_1 = 0.1$ and $p_2 = 0.2$. The K constant for 90 per cent power, using cone-sided test at 0.05 level, is 8.6. This yields $n = 215$ which is the minimum number required in *each* of two equal groups.

Q8.6

A smaller number would be possible if the background rate of cessation were higher and the effect the same on a ratio basis, that is, a doubling of cessation rate, or if a larger absolute difference would be accepted as the quantity measurable, for example, a difference between 10 per cent and 30 per cent. This might be achievable by studying a different group, or using a longer follow-up time (or in this situation perhaps a shorter follow-up time, if the effect decreases over time, but the relevance of the outcome variable must not be compromised). If the power criterion is weakened, accepting a study with, say, only 80 per cent chance of detecting a true result, the numbers required are smaller, but the risk of missing a true effect is larger. A one-sided test has already been chosen. Thus if $p_1 = 0.2$ and $p_2 = 0.4$, and power = 80 per cent, $n = 62$.

Q8.7

From the formula in Box 8.9, $p_2 = 0.1$ and $OR = 2$, and hence $p_1 = 0.18$; $K = 7.9$ and hence $n = 282$. This is the minimum number of cases and controls assuming equal-sized groups.

Q8.8

If four controls per case are used, with other parameters being the same, a study with 179 cases and four times this number of controls will provide equivalent power (Box 8.9).

Q8.9

The odds ratio is 4 and the chi-square statistic is 90, giving $P < 0.000\,001$. For 99 per cent limits, we use $Z = 2.58$ in the approximate calculation shown in Box 8.5, giving limits of 2.74 and 5.83.

Q8.10

The odds ratios are 4.0 for men and 13.5 for women. The heterogeneity chi-square is 5.81 (using Box A2.1, part 5E) on 1 d.f., which is significant. Therefore the summary odds ratio is less useful; the results are best given as odds ratios of 4.0 (95 per cent limits 2.1–7.5) for men and 13.5 (95 per cent limits 6.3–29.0) for women.

Q8.11

The curves show better survival for group B, especially in the first 12 months. The survival at 18 months is 75.0 per cent in group B compared with 28.6 per cent in group A. This is consistent with the significant difference shown by the log-rank statistic, but this comparison at only one time point is a less useful than the overall difference shown by the log-rank analysis. However, as an artificial example, the trial is much too small, and the confidence limits are very wide: 0 to 60 per cent in group A, and 45 to 100 per cent in group B.

Chapter 9

Q9.1

Publication bias exists if the results of a study influence whether it is published or presented, or whether it is easily retrieved. The most likely effect is that small studies which show strong, significant, or unusual results are more likely to be published than small studies which show null results, or results in the expected direction. Publication bias can also mean that research in different countries, reported in different languages and from different disciplines, may differ in accessibility.

Q9.2

The prime argument for including all studies is to avoid publication bias. The main argument against is that some studies may have clear methodological weaknesses, and including them may bias the overall result. Some reviews use explicit quality criteria to select studies for inclusion, or else use quality criteria to rank studies and assess the influence on the overall result of including studies cumulatively in regard to the quality score.

Q9.3

Using the Peto method gives an odds ratio of 2.78, with a normal deviate of 3.66 ($P < 0.001$); the 95 per cent confidence limits for the odds ratio are 1.61–4.80. Using the Mantel–Haenszel method, the odds ratio is 2.79, with the same statistical test. The heterogeneity statistic is small (χ^2 is 0.11 by the Peto method, and 0.04 by the Mantel–Haenszel method).

Q9.4

Using the method shown in Table 9.2, the summary odds ratio is 3.21, with 95 per cent limits of 2.81–3.65. The heterogeneity statistic is 3.66, on three degrees of freedom, giving $P = 0.3$ (Table A2.1), which is non-significant. The analysis is heavily weighted by the third study; its narrow confidence limits show that it must be much larger than the rest.

Appendix 2

Methods of statistical analysis: formulae and worked examples

This appendix presents tables showing the calculations of measures of association and of statistical tests, for the main study designs discussed showing for each the formulae and worked examples. There are also reference tables for statistical issues.

Introduction

These tables will enable the reader to analyse most studies where the factors involved are discrete rather than continuous variables. Of course, major analyses should not be done without consideration of alternative methods and discussion with colleagues, including those more skilled in statistical and epidemiological methods.

The formulae are primarily those derived from the work of Mantel and Haenszel. These involve approximations which are appropriate if the numbers of observations available are adequate: in a 2 × 2 table each expected value should be greater than 5. For the formulae used to produce summary risk estimates and test statistics after confounder control by stratification, it is the total number of observations which is relevant; the formulae can be applied even if some strata have few observations. The statistics used to test whether an odds ratio or attributable risk estimate is constant over several strata do depend upon having reasonable numbers of observations within each stratum.

The one exception in this appendix to the limitation of small numbers is the 'exact' test for a 2 × 2 table presented in Table A2.4. This can be applied to simple tables with small numbers. For all the other designs considered, more precise formulae ('exact' tests) are also available, but these will usually give similar results except where the numbers of observations are small.

The sources of the formulae are given with each table. There are many texts which review these and related methods in detail, and discuss the situations in which more complex formulae may be appropriate, and provide information on them

TABLE A2.1: Case–control studies, unmatched

FORMULAE

1. *Format of table*

Exposed	a	b	N_1
Unexposed	c	d	N_0
Total	M_1	M_0	T

2. *Risks*

Odds ratio, $OR = \dfrac{a}{b} / \dfrac{c}{d} = \dfrac{ad}{bc}$.

3. *Statistical tests*

Observed exposed cases	=	a
Expected value of a	=	$E = N_1 M_1 / T$
Variance of a	=	$V = N_1 N_0 M_1 M_0 / T^2 (T-1)$

3A. Chi–squared statistic, χ^2, with 1 degree of freedom

$$= \frac{(a-E)^2}{V} = \frac{(a-N_1 M_1 / T)^2}{\dfrac{N_1 N_0 M_1 M_0}{\{T^2 (T-1)\}}}$$

3B. χ statistic, or normal deviate $= \chi = \sqrt{\chi^2}$.

3C. Continuity correction: reduce absolute value of numerator by $\dfrac{1}{2}$ before squaring; i.e. replace numerator by $\left(|a-E| - \dfrac{1}{2}\right)^2$, where $|a-E|$ means the absolute value of $(a - E)$, irrespective of being positive or negative.

WORKED EXAMPLE

Data from the case–control study shown in Table 7.13 (p. 165) and in Box 8.5 (p. 204): association between cervical carcinoma and smoking.

1.   Crude table:

	Cases	Controls	Total
Smokers	130	45	175
Non-smokers	87	198	285
Total	217	243	460

2.   Odds ratio = $(130 \times 198)/(45 \times 87) = 6.57$

3A, B.   Statistical test:

$$a = 130 \ E = 175 \times 217 / 460 = 82.55$$
$$V = (175 \times 285 \times 243 \times 217)/(460 \times 460 \times 459) = 27.08$$
$$\chi^2 = (130 - 82.55)^2 / 27.08 = 83.14 \ \chi = \sqrt{83.14} = 9.12$$
$$\text{d.f.} = 1 \ P < 0.000001 \text{(Tables A2.15 and A2.16)}$$

3C.   With continuity correction $\chi^2 = 81.4$

TABLE A2.1: FORMULAE (*continued*)

4. *Confidence limits (C.L.)*
   $y\%$ limits for logarithm of odds ratio $= \ln OR \pm Zy(\text{dev} \ln OR)$, where
   $Zy =$ appropriate normal deviate (see Table A2.15) and dev $\ln OR =$ standard
   deviation of $\ln OR$

4A. $$\text{dev} \ln OR = \sqrt{\frac{1}{a} + \frac{1}{b} + \frac{1}{c} + \frac{1}{d}}.$$

5. *Stratified analysis over I subtables of above format, values a_i etc.*

5A. $$\text{Summary odds ratio} = OR_s = \frac{\sum_i a_i d_i / T_i}{\sum_i b_i c_i / T_i}$$

5B.
$$\text{Summary } \chi^2 \text{ statistic, 1 d.f.} = \frac{\left(\sum_i a_i - \sum_i E_i\right)^2}{\sum_i V_i}$$

Each term analogous to 3 above.

TABLE A2.1: WORKED EXAMPLE (*continued*)

4A.
$$\text{dev ln } OR = \sqrt{(1/130+1/45+1/87+1/198)}$$
$$= 0.216$$

$$\text{and } 95\% \text{ c.l.} = \exp\left[\ln 6.57 \pm (1.96 \times 0.216)\right]$$
$$= 4.3, 10.0$$

---

5. Stratified analysis:
Data are shown in Box 8.5. Totals in the three subtables are 113, 211, 136 (p. 204).

5A.
$$\text{Summary } OR = \frac{(41 \times 53/113)+(66 \times 83/211)+(23 \times 62/136)}{(6 \times 13/113)+(25 \times 37/211)+(14 \times 37/136)}$$
$$= 6.27$$

5B. Summary χ^2: calculate for each subtable a_i, E_i, V_i; and sum each of these.

		a_i	E_i	V_i
Subtable	1	41	22.46	6.91
	2	66	44.42	12.99
	3	23	16.32	6.69
Sum		130	83.20	26.59

$$\chi^2 = (130-83.2)^2 / 26.59 = 82.4 \quad \chi = \sqrt{82.4} = 9.08$$

TABLE A2.1: FORMULAE (*continued*)

5C. Continuity correction: reduce absolute value of numerator by $\frac{1}{2}$ before squaring.

5D. A formula for the variance of the logarithm of the summary odds ratio is given by Robins et al.[1]

For each stratum, these quantities are calculated. The subscripts have been omitted.

$$F=ad(a+d)/T^2 \quad G=\left[ad(b+c)+bc(a+d)\right]/T^2 \quad H=bc(b+c)/T^2$$
$$R=ad/T \qquad\qquad S=bc/T$$

Then the variance of ln Mantel–Haenszel summary odds ratio is:

$$\text{variance} = \frac{\sum F}{2\left(\sum R\right)^2} + \frac{\sum G}{2\sum R \sum S} + \frac{\sum H}{2\left(\sum S\right)^2}$$

and $y\%$ confidence limits for ln OR_s

$$= \ln OR_s \pm Z_y \sqrt{\text{variance}}$$

5E. Test of homogeneity $= \sum\limits_i \frac{\left(\ln OR_i - \ln OR_s\right)^2}{\text{var} \ln OR_i}$ where variance of ln OR_i =square of standard deviations given in 4A above. Gives a χ^2 on I – 1 degrees of freedom.

TABLE A2.1: WORKED EXAMPLE (*continued*)

5C. χ^2 with continuity correction = 80.6

d.f. = 1 P <0.000001 (Table A2.15)

. . . .

5D. Using Robins formula, var ln OR_{MH} = 0.0456, and 95 per cent confidence limits of OR_{MH} = 4.12, 9.53.

. . . .

5E. Test of homogeneity: calculate for each table OR_i and use formula 4A to obtain dev ln OR_i

		OR_i	dev ln OR_i (formula 4A)
Subtable	1	27.86	0.536
	2	5.92	0.307
	3	2.75	0.398

Hence test of homogeneity =sum of {(ln OR_i – ln OR_s)^2/var ln OR_i} where var ln OR_i =dev ln OR_i^2 and OR_s = 6.27 or, equivalently, test = sum of {(ln OR_i/ln OR_s)/dev ln OR_i}^{2}

$$\chi^2 = (7.74+0.04+4.29)=12.1$$
$$P=0.002$$

d.f. = 2, P-values from Table A2.16. The odds ratios vary significantly.

TABLE A2.1: FORMULAE (*continued*)

Sources

3A, 5A, and 5B: Mantel N and Haenszel W, 'Statistical aspects of the analysis of data from retrospective studies of disease', *Journal of the National Cancer Institute*, Volume 22, Issue 4, pp. 719–748, Copyright © 1959 Oxford University Press [2].

4A: Wolff B, 'On estimating the relationship between blood group and disease', *Annals of Human Genetics*, Volume 19, Issue 4, pp. 251–253, Copyright © May 1955 John Wiley and Sons [3].

5D: Robins JM et al., 'Estimation of the Mantel–Haenszel variance consistent with both sparse-data and large-strata limiting models', *Biometrics*, Volume 42, Number 2, pp. 311–323, Copyright © 1986 [1].

5E: Rothman KJ and Greenland S, *Modern Epidemiology, Third Edition*, Wolters Kluwer Lippincott, Philadelphia, USA, Copyright © 2008 [4].

TABLE A2.1: WORKED EXAMPLE (*continued*)

Data Sources

Table A2.1: Lyon JL et al., 'Smoking and carcinoma in situ of the uterine cervix,' *American Journal Public Health*, Volume 73, Issue 4, pp. 558–562, Copyright © 1983. All rights reserved.

TABLE A2.2: Cohort studies, count data

COHORT STUDIES COUNT DATA: FORMULAE

1.   *Format of table*

	Affected	Unaffected	Total	Risk
Exposed	a	b	N_1	$a/N_1 = r_e$
Unexposed	c	d	N_0	$c/N_0 = r_0$
Total	M_1	M_0	T	

2.   *Risks*

Relative risk $= r_e / r_0$ Odds ratio $= \dfrac{ad}{bc}$ Attributable risk $= r_e - r_0$

3.   *Statistical tests*

Observed exposed cases $= a$

Expected value of $a = E = N_1 M_1 / T$

Variance of $a = V = N_1 N_0 M_1 M_0 / T^2 (T-1)$

3A.   Chi–squared statistic, χ^2, with 1 degree of freedom $= (a - E)^2 / V$

$$= \frac{\left(a - N_1 M_1 / T\right)^2}{\dfrac{\left(N_1 N_0 M_1 M_0\right)}{\left\{T^2 (T-1)\right\}}}$$

3B. χ statistic, or normal deviate $= \chi = \sqrt{\chi^2}$.

3C.   Continuity correction: reduce absolute value of numerator by $\dfrac{1}{2}$ before squaring, i.e. replace numerator by $\left(|a - E| - \dfrac{1}{2}\right)^2$, $|a - E|$ means the absolute value of $(a - E)$, irrespective of being positive or negative.

COHORT STUDIES COUNT DATA: WORKED EXAMPLE

Data from a prospective cohort study; association between maternal epilepsy in pregnancy and malformation in infants; Shapiro et al. [5]

(Box 4.1 (p. 46) showed another study in the same format).

1. Crude table:

	Malformed	Not malformed	Total	Prevalence of malformation (%)
Exposed—epilepsy	32	273	305	10.49
Unexposed—no epilepsy	3216	46 761	49 977	6.43
Total	3248	47 034	50 282	

2. Relative risk = 1.63 Odds ratio = 1.70 Attributable risk = 4.06 per cent

3A. Statistical test:

$$a = 32 \ E = 305 \times 3248 / 50282 = 19.70$$
$$V = (305 \times 49977 \times 47034 \times 3248) / (50282 \times 50282 \times 50281)$$
$$= 18.32$$

3B $$\chi^2 = (a - E^2) / V = 8.26 \quad \chi = \sqrt{\chi^2} = 2.87$$

d.f. = 1 $\quad$ P < 0.01 (Table A2.15 and Table A2.16)

3C. With continuity correction $\chi^2 = 7.60$.

TABLE A2.2: FORMULAE (*continued*)

4.	*Confidence limits (C.L.)*
	(i) for logarithm of *RR*
	$= \ln RR + Zy \operatorname{dev} \ln RR$
	(ii) for logarithm of *OR*; analogous to *RR*, hence
	$= \ln OR \pm Zy \operatorname{dev} \ln OR$
	(iii) for attributable risk
	$= AR \pm Zy \operatorname{dev} AR$
	where Zy = appropriate normal deviate (see Table A2.15) and dev = standard deviation

4A.	Formulae for standard deviation

$$\text{(i)} \quad \operatorname{dev} \ln RR = \sqrt{\frac{b}{aN_1} + \frac{d}{cN_0}} \qquad \text{equivalently,} \quad = \sqrt{\frac{1}{a} - \frac{1}{N_1} + \frac{1}{c} - \frac{1}{N_0}}$$

$$\text{(ii)} \quad \operatorname{dev} \ln RR = \sqrt{\frac{1}{a} + \frac{1}{b} + \frac{1}{c} + \frac{1}{d}}$$

$$\text{(iii)} \quad \operatorname{dev} AR = \sqrt{\frac{ab}{N_1^3} + \frac{cd}{N_0^3}}$$

5.	*Stratified analysis*

5A.	Risks

(i) Summary RR_S	(ii) Summary OR_S	(iii) Summary AR_S
$\dfrac{\sum\limits_i a_i N_{0i} / T_i}{\sum\limits_i c_i N_{1i} / T_i}$	$\dfrac{\sum\limits_i a_i d_i / T_i}{\sum\limits_i b_i c_i / T_i}$	$\dfrac{\sum\limits_i w_i AR_i}{\sum\limits_i w_i}$

$$\text{where } w_i = 1/\left(\operatorname{dev} AR_i\right)^2$$

TABLE A2.2: WORKED EXAMPLE (*continued*)

4A.   Confidence limits:

for RR, dev ln $RR = 0.168$; limits $=$ exp(ln $RR \pm 1.96 \times$ dev ln RR)

$=$ 1.17, 2.27

for OR, dev ln $OR = 0.188$; limits $=$ exp(ln $OR \pm 1.96 \times$ dev ln OR)

$=$ 1.18, 2.46

for AR, dev $AR = 1.758\%$; limits $=$ $AR \pm 1.96 \times$ dev AR

$=$ 0.61, 7.51%

5.   Stratified analysis:

Analogous to Table A2.1. If the above data were one stratum of a stratified table, the weight w_i for use in formula 5A(iii) would be $1/(\text{dev } AR_i)^2 = 1/(0.0176)^2$.

TABLE A2.2: FORMULAE (*continued*)

5B. Summary χ^2 statistic on 1 d.f. $= \dfrac{\left(\sum_i a_i - \sum_i E_i\right)^2}{\sum_i V_i}$

Each term analogous to 3 above.

5C. Continuity correction: reduce absolute value of numerator by $\dfrac{1}{2}$ before squaring.

5D. Tests of homogeneity; χ^2 on I-1 degrees of freedom; variances are squares of standard deviations given in 4.

Relative risk

$$\sum_i \frac{\left(\ln RR_i - \ln RR_s\right)^2}{\text{var} \ln RR_i}$$

Attributable risk

$$\sum_i \frac{\left(AR_i - AR_s\right)^2}{\text{var } AR_i}$$

Sources

3A, 5A, and 5B Mantel N and Haenszel W, 'Statistical aspects of the analysis of data from retrospective studies of disease,' *Journal of the National Cancer Institute*, Volume 22, Issue 4, pp. 719–748, Copyright © 1959 Oxford University Press [2].

4A: Wolff B, 'On estimating the relationship between blood group and disease,' *Annals of Human Genetics*, Volume 19, Issue 4, pp. 251–253, Copyright © May 1955 John Wiley and Sons [3] and Rothman KJ and Greenland S, *Modern Epidemiology, Third Edition*, Wolters Kluwer Lippincott, Philadelphia, USA, Copyright © 2008 [4].

5D: Rothman KJ and Greenland S, *Modern Epidemiology, Third Edition*, Wolters Kluwer Lippincott, Philadelphia, USA, Copyright © 2008 [4].

TABLE A2.2: WORKED EXAMPLE (*continued*)

Data Sources

Table A2.2: Shapiro S, Slone D, Hartz SC, et al. Anticonvulsants and parental epilepsy in the development of birth defects. *Lancet* 1976; **i**:272–275.

TABLE A2.3: Cohort studies, person-time data

FORMULAE

1. *Format of table*

	Affected	Person-time	Risk
Exposed	a	N_1	$a/N_1 = r_e$
Unexposed	c	N_0	$c/N_0 = r_0$
Total	M_1	T	

2. *Risks*

Relative risk $= r_e/r_0$ Attributable risk $= r_e - r_0$

3. *Statistical tests*

Observed exposed cases $= a$

Expected value of $a = E = N_1 M_1 / T$

Variance of $a = V = N_1 N_0 M_1 / T^2$

3A. Chi-squared statistic, χ^2 with 1 degree of freedom $= (a - E)^2 / V$

$$= \frac{(a - N_1 M_1 / T)^2}{(N_1 N_0 M_1)/T^2}$$

3B. χ statistic, or normal deviate $= \chi = \sqrt{\chi^2}$

3C. Continuity correction: reduce absolute value of numerator by $\frac{1}{2}$ before squaring; i.e. replace numerator by $\left(|a - E| - \frac{1}{2} \right)^2$, $|a - E|$ means the absolute value of $(a - E)$, irrespective of being positive or negative.

WORKED EXAMPLE

Data from the prospective cohort study shown in Table 7.3 (p. 139); association between exercise and coronary heart disease mortality.

1.   Crude table:

	Deaths	Man-years	Rate/10 000
Light or moderate exercise	532	65 000	81.85
Heavy exercise	66	27 700	23.83
Total	598	92 700	

2.   Relative risk = 81.85/23.83 = 3.43

Attributable risk = 81.85 – 23.83 = 58.02/10 000 man-years

3A.   Statistical test:

$a = 532$ $E = 65\,000 \times 598/92\,700 = 419.31$

$V = 65\,000 \times 27\,700 \times 598/92\,700^2 = 125.30$

3B. $\chi^2 = (a - E)^2 / V = 101.35$ $\chi = \sqrt{101.35} = 10.07$

d.f. $= 1$ $P < 0.000001$ (Tables A2.15 and A2.16)

3C.   With continuity correction $\chi^2 = 100.45$.

TABLE A2.3: FORMULAE (*continued*)

4.	*Confidence limits (C.L.)*

(i) for logarithm of RR (ii) for attributable risk

$\quad = \ln RR + Zy \text{ dev } \ln RR \qquad\qquad = AR \pm Zy \text{ dev } AR$

where Zy = appropriate normal deviate (Table A2.15) and dev = standard deviation

---

4A.   Formulae for standard deviation

$$\text{dev} \ln RR = \sqrt{\frac{1}{a} + \frac{1}{c}} \qquad \text{dev } AR = \sqrt{\frac{a}{N_1^2} + \frac{c}{N_0^2}}$$

---

5.   *Stratified analysis over I subtables of above format, values, a_i etc.*

5A.   Summary relative risk, RR_s Summary attributable risk, AR_s

$$= \frac{\sum_i a_i N_{0i} / T_i}{\sum_i c_i N_{1i} / T_1} \qquad\qquad = \frac{\sum_i w_i AR_i}{\sum_i w_i}$$

$$w_i = 1 / (\text{dev } AR_i)^2$$

5B.   Summary χ^2 statistic $= \dfrac{\left(\sum_i a_i - \sum_i E_i \right)^2}{\sum_i V_i}$

Each term analogous to 3 above.

5C.   Continuity correction: reduce absolute value of numerator by $\dfrac{1}{2}$ before squaring.

TABLE A2.3: WORKED EXAMPLE (*continued*)

4A. $\text{dev} \ln RR \;=\; 0.131 \qquad 95\% \text{limits} = \exp\{\ln 3.43 \,\pm\, (1.96 \times 0.131)\}$

$\qquad\qquad\quad =\; 2.66, 4.44$

$\qquad \text{dev } AR \;=\; 4.60 / 10\,000 \quad 95\% \text{limits} = 58.8 \pm (1.96 \times 4.60)$

$\qquad\qquad\quad =\; 49.0, 67.0$

5. Stratified analysis. Analogous to Table A2.1.

TABLE A2.3: FORMULAE (*continued*)

5D. Tests of homogeneity; χ^2 on $I - 1$ degrees of freedom; variances are squares of standard deviations given in 4.

Relative risk   Attributable risk

$$= \sum_i \frac{\left(\ln RR_i - \ln RR_s\right)^2}{\text{var } \ln RR_i} \qquad = \sum_i \frac{\left(AR_i - AR_s\right)^2}{\text{var } AR_i}$$

Odds ratio: analogous to relative risk

Sources

3A: Mantel N and Haenszel W, 'Statistical aspects of the analysis of data from retrospective studies of disease,' *Journal of the National Cancer Institute*, Volume 22, Issue 4, pp. 719–748, Copyright © 1959 Oxford University Press [2].

5D: Rothman KJ and Greenland S, *Modern Epidemiology, Third Edition*, Wolters Kluwer Lippincott, Philadelphia, USA, Copyright © 2008 [4].

TABLE A2.3: WORKED EXAMPLE (*continued*)

Data Sources

Table A2.3: Paffenbarger RS and Hale WE, 'Work activity and coronary heart mortality,' *New England Journal of Medicine,* Volume 292, Number 11, pp. 545–550, Copyright © 1975 Massachusetts Medical Society. All rights reserved.

TABLE A2.4: Cohort (count data) or case–control, with small numbers; exact test for a fourfold table

FORMULAE

1.   *Format of table*

	Affected	Unaffected	Total
Exposed	a	b	N_1
Unexposed	c	d	N_0
Total	M_1	M_0	T

2.   *Risks*

As in Table A2.2; the small numbers make no difference.

3.   *Statistical test*

Probability of a particular table occurring $= \dfrac{N_1!N_0!M_1!M_0!}{T!a!b!c!d!}$.

To calculate one-sided probability of a or a more extreme value: if a is greater than expected, i.e. $a > N_1 M_1 / T$, calculate quantity above for each value of a from observed value to the maximum, given when $a = N_1$ or $a = M_1$; sum these values. If a is less than expected, calculate for values of a down to zero. For two-sided tests, the one-sided value is usually doubled.

! represents a factorial; e.g. 5! is $5 \times 4 \times 3 \times 2 \times 1$.

WORKED EXAMPLE

Saral et al. [8] performed a double-blind randomized trial of the drug acyclovir, compared with placebo, as prophylaxis against herpes simplex infection in 20 bone marrow transplant recipients who were seropositive for herpes simplex before randomization; the outcome was development of active herpes simplex infection.

1. Table of results:

	Infection	No infection	Total
Acyclovir	0	10	10
Placebo	7	3	10
Total	7	13	20

2. Risk: the relative risk and odds ratio are both zero.

3. Statistical test:

Probability of this set of data, given the null hypothesis

$$P = \frac{10!10!13!7!}{20!0!10!7!3!}$$

$$= \frac{10!13!}{20!3!} \quad (0!=1)$$

$$= \frac{10\times9\times8\times7\times6\times5\times4}{20\times19\times18\times17\times16\times15\times14}$$

$$= 0.0015$$

This is the one-sided P-value; the two-sided value of $P = 0.003$.

As the result obtained was an extreme one, only one calculation is necessary. Otherwise, further calculations are needed. For example, suppose there had been two infections in the acyclovir group compared with seven in the placebo. To assess significance, we add the probability of the observed table to the probability of more extreme results with the same marginal totals: the observed table is:

	Infection	No infection	Total	
Aciclovir	2	8	10	
Placebo	7	3	10	$P = \dfrac{10!10!11!9!}{20!2!8!7!3!}$
Total	9	11	20	$= 0.032$

TABLE A2.4: FORMULAE (*continued*)

Sources

This test was developed independently in the 1930s by R.A. Fisher, J.O. Irwin, and F. Yates. Exact confidence limits and stratified analysis will not be presented: see, for example, Breslow and Day [6] or Armitage et al. [7]

TABLE A2.4: WORKED EXAMPLE (*continued*)

More extreme results, given that a is less than its expected value, are $a = 1$ and $a = 0$ with the same marginal totals:

	Infection	No infection	Total	
Acyclovir	1	9	10	$P = 0.0027$
Placebo	8	2	10	
Total	9	11	20	

	Infection	No infection	Total	
Acyclovir	0	10	10	$P = 0.00006$
Placebo	9	1	10	
Total	9	11	20	

giving the final P-value (one-sided) of $0.032 + 0.0027 + 0.00006 = 0.035$ or (two-sided) $= 0.07$

Data Sources

TABLE A2.5: Case–control, 1:1 matching

FORMULAE

1. *Format of table: numbers of pairs*

		Controls	
		Exposed	Unexposed
Cases	Exposed	u	s
	Unexposed	t	v

2. *Risks*

Odds ratio = s/t

3A. *Statistical tests*

χ^3 statistic on 1 d.f. $= \dfrac{(s-t)^2}{s+t}$

3B. χ statistic, or normal deviate $= \sqrt{\chi^2}$.

3C. Continuity correction: reduce absolute value of numerator by 1 before squaring; it becomes $(|s-t|-1)^2$.

4. *Confidence limits*

The derivation of confidence limits is complex but online calculators are available.

Sources

Source: McNemar Q, 'Note on the sampling of the difference between corrected proportions or percentages,' *Psychometrika*, Volume 12, Issue 2, pp. 153–157, Copyright © 1947 [9]. Stratified analysis of matched data is not frequently performed; matched multivariate models are more useful.

WORKED EXAMPLE

Data from the case–control study shown in Box 7.4 (p. 169) and Box 8.7 (p. 208), association between nasal cancer and smoking.

1.   Table:

		Controls	
		Smokers	Non-smokers
Cases	Smokers	31	7
	Non-smokers	30	52

2.   Odds ratio = 30/7 = 4.29

3A,B. $\chi^2 \text{ statistic} = (30-7)^2 / (30+7) = 14.30$ $\chi = \sqrt{14.30} = 3.78$

3C.   With continuity correction, $\chi^2 = 13.1$.

4.   Using Open Epi (http://www.openepi.com) gives 95 per cent limits for OR of 1.88 to 9.76.

Data Sources

Table A2.5: Elwood JM, 'Wood exposure and smoking: association with cancer of the nasal cavity and paranasal sinuses in British Columbia,' *Canadian Medical Association Journal*, Volume 124, Issue 12, pp. 1573–1577, © 1981 [27].

TABLE A2.6: Case–control studies, fixed 1:m matching

FORMULAE

1. *Format of table: numbers of pairs*

    No. of controls exposed (maximum = m)

Cases	0	1	2	...	m	...
Exposed	a_0	a_1	a_2	...	a_m	...
Unexposed	c_0	c_1	c_2	...	c_m	...

    The pairs of sets (a_{m-1}, c_m) form the basis for the calculations. The values a_m (sets where all are exposed) and c_0 (sets where none is exposed) do not contribute.

2. *Risks*

    $$\text{Odds ratio} = \frac{\sum_{m-1}^{M}(M+1-m)a_{m-1}}{\sum_{m-1}^{M}mc_m}$$

    $$= \frac{Ma_0 + (M-1)a_1 + (M-2)a_2 + \cdots + a_{M-1}}{c_1 + 2c_2 + 3c_3 + \cdots + Mc_M}$$

3. *Statistical tests*

    $$\chi^2 \text{ statistic on 1 d.f.} = \frac{\left[\sum_{m=1}^{M}(M+1-m)a_{m-1} - \sum_{m=1}^{M}mc_m\right]^2}{\sum_{m=1}^{M}(a_{m-1}+c_m)m(M+1-m)}$$

    For the continuity correction, reduce the absolute value of the numerator by $\frac{1}{2}$ $(M+1)$ before squaring.

WORKED EXAMPLE

Data from Collette et al. [10]. A 1:3 matched case–control study assessing the value of screening for breast cancer by physical examination and xeromammography. The cases were women from the defined population who had died from breast cancer; the controls were age-matched women randomly selected from this population.

1. Table:

No. of matched controls screened (m)				
Cases:	0	1	2	3
Screened	1	4	3	1
Unscreened	11	10	12	4

Here $M = 3$; summations are from $m = 1$ to $m = 3$.

2.
$$\text{Odds ratio} = \frac{(3 \times 1) + (2 \times 4) + (1 \times 3)}{(1 \times 10) + (2 \times 12) + (3 \times 4)}$$
$$= 14 / 46 = 0.30$$

3.
$$\chi^2 \text{ statistic} = \frac{(14 - 46)^2}{(11 \times 1 \times 3) + (16 \times 2 \times 2) + (7 \times 3 \times 1)}$$
$$= 1024 / 118$$
$$= 8.68 \quad \chi = 2.95$$

With continuity correction, $\chi^2 = 7.63$

TABLE A2.6: FORMULAE (*continued*)

4.   *Confidence limits*

         The derivation of confidence limits is complex, see Breslow and Day [6].

Sources

2 and 3: Mantel N and Haenszel W, 'Statistical aspects of the analysis of data from retrospective studies of disease,' *Journal of the National Cancer Institute*, Volume 22, Issue 4, pp. 719–748, Copyright © 1959 Oxford University Press [2]. For more complex matched designs, see Breslow and Day [6], pp. 169–187.

TABLE A2.6: WORKED EXAMPLE (*continued*)

Data Sources

Table A2.6: Collette HJA et al., 'Evaluation of screening for breast cancer in a non-randomised study (the DOM project) by means of a case-control study,' *The Lancet*, Volume 1, Number 8388, pp. 1224–1226, Copyright © 1984 Published by Elsevier Ltd [10].

TABLE A2.7: Cohort (count data) or case–control studies: test for trend

FORMULAE

1.   *Format of table*

		Cases (affected)	Controls (unaffected)	Total	Score
Exposure level	0 (referent)	c	d	N_0	x_0
	1	a_1	b_1	N_1	x_1
	2	a_2	b_2	N_2	x_2
	3 … k	a_k	b_k	N_k	x_k
Total		M_1	M_0	T	

2.   *Risks*

Odds ratio for exposure level $k = \dfrac{a_k d}{b_k c} = \dfrac{a_k}{b_k} \Big/ \dfrac{c}{d}$

3.   *Statistical tests*

3A.   For each level k against the referent level: tests and confidence limits as in Table A2.1.

Heterogeneity χ^2 for the table above, on $k-1$ degrees of freedom

$$= (T-1)\left(\frac{1}{M_1} + \frac{1}{M_0}\right) \sum_k \frac{(a_k - E_k)^2}{N_k}$$

where E_k = expected value of $a_k = N_k M_1 / T$.

This test assesses whether the odd ratios, or more directly the proportions of cases, in the various exposure levels are consistent with the overall value—it does not take into account the order of the levels of exposure.

WORKED EXAMPLE

These are data from a case–control study relating the occurrence of twin births to maternal parity (the number of previous births the mother has had). The cases were mothers of twin births, the controls a sample of mothers of single births. From Elwood [11].

1.   Table and elements of calculations:

Category	Cases (twins)	Controls (single births)	Total	Score	Odds ratio	E	$a - E$
Parity 0	716	1833	2549	0	1.0(R)	848.07	– 132.07
1	582	1269	1851	1	1.17	615.84	– 33.84
2	454	853	1307	2	1.36	434.85	– 19.15
3+	720	1003	1723	3	1.84	573.25	146.75
Total	2472	4958	7430				

2.   Risks:

Given above: e.g. for parity 2 odds ratio = (454 × 1833)/ (853 × 716)

= 1.36

3A.   Global or heterogeneity, χ^2. For each level $E_k = N_K M_1/T$

e.g. for parity 2, $E_2 = 1307 \times 2472 / 7430 = 434.85$

$$\chi^2 = 7429 \left(\frac{1}{2472} + \frac{1}{4958} \right) \left(\frac{(716 - 848.07)^2}{2549} + \text{etc. for each level} \right)$$

= 91.16 d.f. = 3 $P < 0.001$ (Table A2.16).

TABLE A2.7: FORMULAE (*continued*)

3B. Test for trend from regression of the values $a_k - E_k$ on the score x_k; χ^2 on 1 d. f.

$$= \frac{T^2(T-1)\left\{\sum_k x_k(a_k - E_k)\right\}^2}{M_1 M_0 \left\{T\sum_k x_k^2 N_k - \left(\sum_k x_m N_k\right)^2\right\}}.$$

For a continuity correction, if x_k scores are one unit apart, replace

$$\left\{\sum_k x_k(a_k - E_k)\right\}^2 \text{ by } \left\{\left|\sum_k x_k(a_k - E_k)\right| - \frac{1}{2}\right\}^2.$$

3C. An approximate test of departure from the linear trend is given by the difference between the heterogeneity and the trend χ^2 statistics, on $k - 2$ degrees of freedom: this tests the adequacy of the linear trend in describing the data.

4. *Stratified analysis*

The trend statistic above can be generalized to a stratified analysis over I sub-tables of the format above, but the formula is tedious for hand calculation; see Breslow and Day [6] pp.148–150.

The stratified χ^2 statistic on 1 d.f. is

$$= \frac{\left\{\sum_k x_k \left(\sum_i a_{ki} - \sum_i E_{ki}\right)\right\}^2}{\sum_i \frac{M_{0i}}{T_i - 1}\left[\sum_k x_k^2 E_{ki} - \frac{1}{M_{1i}}\left(\sum_k x_k E_{ki}\right)^2\right]}.$$

where $E_{ki} = N_{ki} M_{1i}/T_i$.

Sources

3A: Armitage P., 'Test for linear trend in proportions and frequencies,' *Biometrics* 1955; Volume 11, Issue, pp. 375–386, Copyright © 1955 [12]; and Armitage P et al., *Statistical Methods in Medical Research, Fourth Edition*, Blackwell Scientific, Oxford, UK, Copyright © 2002 [7].

3B: Mantel N, 'Chi-square tests with one degree of freedom; extensions of the Mantel–Haenszel procedure,' *Journal of the American Statistical Association*, Volume 58, Number 303, pp. 690–700, Copyright © 1963 [13].

TABLE A2.7: WORKED EXAMPLE (*continued*)

3B. Test for trend

$$\chi^2 = \frac{7430^2 \times 7429(-33.84 + 2 \times 19.15 + 3 \times 146.7)^2}{2472 \times 4958 \left\{ 7430(1851 + 4 \times 1307 + 9 \times 1723) - (1851 + 2 \times 1307 + 3 \times 1723)^2 \right\}}$$

$$= \frac{7430^2 \times 7429 \times 444.71^2}{2472 \times 4958(7430 \times 22586 - 9634^2)}$$

$$= 88.24 \quad \text{with continuity correction}, \chi^2 = 88.04$$

d.f. = 1 $P < 0.000001$ (Table A2.15).

3C. Test for departure from linear trend:

$\chi^2 = 91.2 - 88.2 = 3.0$ d.f.=2 $\qquad P > 0.2$ (Table A2.16).

Data Sources

Table A2.7: data from Elwood JM., 'Maternal and environmental factors affecting twin births in Canadian cities,' *BJOG: An International Journal of Obstetrics and Gynaecology*, Volume 85, Issue 5, pp. 351–358, Copyright © 1978 John Wiley and Sons.

TABLE A2.8: Formulae for sample size determination

FORMULAE

1.   *Unmatched studies, equal groups*

Basic formula

$$n = \frac{(p_1 q_1 + p_2 q_2).K}{(p_1 - p_2)^2}$$

Approximately equivalent to

$$n = \frac{2\overline{pq}.K}{(p_1 - p_2)^2}$$

To calculate power

$$Z_\beta = \frac{(p_1 - p_2).\sqrt{n}}{\sqrt{(p_1 q_1 + p_2 q_2)}} - Z_\alpha$$

Case–control studies, given OR and p_2, then

$$p_1 = \frac{p_2.OR}{1 + p_2(OR - 1)}$$

2.   *Multiple controls per case*

Given c controls per case: n = no. of cases or exposed subjects,

$$cn = \text{no. of controls.}$$

$$n = \frac{(1 + 1/c).\overline{pq}.K}{(p_1 - p_2)^2}$$

$$Z_\beta = \frac{(p_1 - p_2).\sqrt{n}}{\sqrt{\{(1 + 1/c).\overline{pq}\}}} - Z_\alpha$$

3.   *1:1 matched studies*

$$M = \left[\frac{Z_\alpha/2 + Z_\beta \sqrt{\{H(1-H)\}}}{H - 0.5} \right]^2 \Big/ (p_2 q_1 + p_1 q_2)$$

where $H = OR/(1 + OR)$ OR =odds ratio and M =number of matched pairs.

Notation:

n = number of subjects in each group
p_1 = probability of outcome in group 1 $q_1 = 1 - p_2$
p_2 = probability of outcome in group 2 $q_2 = 1 - p_2$
$\overline{p}$ = probability of outcome in whole study group $\overline{q} = 1 - \overline{p}$
K= constant dependent on significance level and power = $(Z_\alpha + Z_\beta)^2$ (see Table A2.9)
Z_α = normal deviate corresponding to significance level (see Table A2.9)
Z_β = normal deviate corresponding to power (see Table A2.9)
c = number of controls per case
M = number of matched pairs

WORKED EXAMPLE

Please see Chapter 8 'Estimating the size of study which is needed', pp. 218.

TABLE A2.9: Constants for use in sample size

FORMULAE

A. *Table relating normal deviates to power and to significance level*

Power $(1 - \beta)$ (%)	Z-value (Normal deviate)	Significance level (α) One-sided	Two-sided
99.5	2.58	0.005	0.01
99	2.33	0.01	0.02
98	1.96	0.025	0.05
95	1.4	0.05	0.1
90	1.28	0.1	0.2
80	0.84	0.2	0.4
70	0.52	0.3	0.6
50	0.0	0.5	

B. *Values of $K = (Z_\alpha + Z_\beta)^2$, for commonly used values of α and β*

Power

		50%	80%	90%	95%		
Significance level:						Significance level:	
Two-sided	0.1	2.7	6.2	8.6	10.8	005	One-sided
value	0.05	3.8	7.9	10.5	13.0	0.025	Value
	0.02	5.4	10.0	13.0	15.8	0.01	
	0.01	6.6	11.7	14.9	17.8	0.005	

Normal deviates corresponding to frequently used values for significance levels (Z_α) and for power (Z_β); and table of K where $K = (Z_\alpha + Z_\beta)^2$. The value of Z_β is the normal deviate corresponding to the one-sided test for (1–power).

WORKED EXAMPLE

Please see Chapter 8 'Estimating the size of study which is needed', pp. 218.

TABLE A2.10: Calculation of kappa to compare two sets of observations

FORMULAE

1. *Format of table.* Shown for three categories.

p_{ij} = proportions of total subjects in cell i, j of the table

		Second survey			
		$j = 1$	2	3	Sum over j
First	$i = 1$	P_{11}	P_{12}	P_{13}	$P_{1\cdot}$
Survey	2	P_{21}	P_{22}	P_{23}	$P_{2\cdot}$
	3	P_{31}	P_{32}	P_{33}	$P_{3\cdot}$
	Sum over i	$P_{\cdot 1}$	$P_{\cdot 2}$	$P_{\cdot 3}$	$P_{\cdot\cdot} = 1.0$

Note: $p_{\cdot 1}$ means summation of p_{ij} over all i values where $j = 1$; $p_{1\cdot}$ means summation of p_{ij} over all j values where $i = 1$.

2. *Calculation of kappa, κ*

Observed agreement $= O = \sum_i p_{ii}$ i.e. summation of cells showing agreement (on the diagonal of the table).

Expected agreement
by chance $= E = \sum_{ij} p_{i\cdot} p_{\cdot i}$ i.e. summation of products of marginal totals.

Kappa, κ

$= (\text{observed agreement} - \text{expected agreement}) / (1 - \text{expected agreement})$

$= (O - E) / (1 - E)$

WORKED EXAMPLE

Data from Westerdahl et al.; [14].

1. Question: Have you ever been sunburned causing erythema and pain for a few days? If yes, how many times after the age of 19 years?

Data: numbers of subjects

		Second survey:			
		>5 times	1–5 times	Never	Total
First survey	>5 times	57	37	4	98
	1–5 times	30	312	36	378
	Never	3	40	74	117
	Total	90	389	114	593

Proportions of total subjects

		Second survey:			
		>5 times	1–5 times	Never	Total
First survey	>5 times	*0.096*	0.062	0.007	0.165
	1–5 times	0.051	*0.526*	0.061	0.637
	Never	0.005	0.067	*0.125*	0.197
	Total	0.152	0.656	0.192	1.000

2. *Calculation of kappa*

Observed agreement = (0.096 + 0.526 + 0.125) = 0.747
Expected agreement by chance

$$= (0.165 \times 0.152 + 0.637 \times 0.656 + 0.197 \times 0.192) = 0.481$$

Kappa, κ

$$= (\text{observed agreement} - \text{expected agreement})/ (1 - \text{expected agreement})$$
$$= (0.747 - 0.481)/(1 - 0.481) = 0.512$$

TABLE A2.10: FORMULAE (*continued*)

---

3.   *Standard error of kappa, SE(κ)*
          n =total number of subjects.
          Let $u_i = p_i. \, p._i(p_i. + p._i)$ u_i uses only the marginal totals.
          then

$$SE(k) = \frac{\sqrt{E + E^2 - \sum_i u_i}}{(1-E)\sqrt{n}}$$

Test of significance of kappa compared with null value of 0 is given by $z = \kappa/SE(\kappa)$, but this is not very useful.

---

4.   *Confidence limits for kappa*
          Using the Z-values given in Table A2.9
          two-sided limits $= K \pm Z_{\alpha}/_2.SE(\kappa)$
          Other formulae are available to test the significance of a difference in kappa from a pre-specified value, and for weighted kappa.

---

5.   *Relationship of kappa to odds ratio* (approximate)
          Let OR_0 =observed odds ratio and OR_T =true odds ratio
          then $OR_T = (\kappa + OR_0 - 1)/\kappa$
          and $OR_0 = \kappa \, (OR_T - 1) + 1$

Sources

2: Cohen J, 'A coefficient of agreement for nominal scales,' *Educational and Psychological Measurement*, Volume 20, Number 1, pp. 27–46, Copyright © 1960 SAGE Publications [15].

3 and 4: Fleiss JL et al., 'Large sample standard errors of kappa and weighted kappa,' *Psychological Bulletin*, Volume 72, Issue 5, pp. 323–327, Copyright © 1969 [16]; and Fleiss JL et al., Statistical methods for rates and proportions, Third Edition, John Wiley & Sons, New York, USA, Copyright © 2003 [17].

5: Thompson WD and Walter SD, 'Variance and dissent: A reappraisal of the kappa coefficient,' *Journal of Clinical Epidemiology*, Volume 41, Issue 10, pp. 949–958, Copyright © 1988 [18].

For weighted kappa and further development see Fleiss et al. [17]

For discussion of applications to study results see Armstrong et al. [19]

TABLE A2.10: WORKED EXAMPLE (*continued*)

---

3. *Standard error of kappa*

Number of subjects, $n = 593$

$u_1 = 0.00795$ from $0.165 \times 0.152 \times (0.165 + 0.152)$

$u_2 = 0.54084$ from $0.637 \times 0.656 \times (0.637 + 0.656)$

$u_3 = 0.01478$ from $0.197 \times 0.192 \times (0.197 + 0.192)$

hence $\sum_i u_i = 0.56357$

$$SE = \frac{\sqrt{0.481 + 0.481^2 - 0.564}}{(1 - 0.481)\sqrt{593}} = 0.031$$

Test of significance $Z = \dfrac{0.512}{0.031} = 16.8 \; p < 0.001$ (Table A2.15).

---

4. Confidence limits

95 per cent two-sided confidence limits = $0.512 \pm 1.96 \times 0.031 = 0.45, 0.57$

---

5. Relationship of kappa to odds ratio

Suppose a study using this measure yields an odds ratio (observed) of 1.80, then estimated true odds ratio = $(0.512 + 1.80 - 1)/0.512 = 2.56$

Data Sources

Table A2.10: Westerdahl J et al., 'Reproducibility of a self-administered questionnaire for assessment of melanoma risk,' *International Journal of Epidemiology*, Volume 25, Issue 2, pp. 245–251, Copyright © 1996 Oxford University Press.

TABLE A2.11: Adjustment of results of a case–control study using values of sensitivity and specificity

FORMULAE

1. *Observed results of case–control study: proportions of cases and controls exposed:*

	Cases	Controls
Exposed	e_1	e_0
Unexposed	$1 - e_1$	$1 - e_0$
Total	1	1

Observed odds ratio $= e_1(1 - e_0)/e_0(1 - e_1)$

2. *Sensitivity and specificity values for exposure, for cases and for controls:*

		Cases	Controls
Sensitivity =	$S =$	S_1	S_0
Specificity =	$F =$	F_1	F_0

WORKED EXAMPLE

1. *Observed results of case–control study (hypothetical data)*

	Cases	Controls
Exposed	200	100
Unexposed	300	400
Total	500	500

    Observed odds ratio = $(200 \times 400)/(300 \times 100) = 2.67$

    Results expressed as proportions exposed

	Cases	Controls
Exposed	0.40	0.20
Unexposed	0.60	0.80
Total	1	1

    Observed odds ratio = $(0.40 \times 0.80)/(0.20 \times 0.60) = 2.67$

2. *Sensitivity and specificity of exposure assessment, in cases and in controls, from other sources*

		Cases	Controls
Sensitivity =	$S =$	0.90	0.85
Specificity =	$F =$	0.80	0.83

TABLE A2.11: FORMULAE (*continued*)

3.　　*Hence estimated 'true' values:*

	Cases	Controls
Exposed	$e_1' = (e_1 - 1 + F_1) / (S_1 + F_1 - 1)$	$e_0' = (e_0 - 1 + F_0) / (S_0 + F_0 - 1)$
Unexposed	$1 - e_1'$	$1 - e_0'$
Total	1	1

Estimated true odds ratio $= e_1'(1 - e_0') / e_0'(1 - e_1')$

TABLE A2.11: WORKED EXAMPLE (*continued*)

3. For cases, 'true' proportion exposed = $(0.40 - 1 + 0.80)/(0.90 + 0.80 - 1) = 0.286$
and proportion unexposed = $1 - 0.286 = 0.714$
For controls, 'true' proportion exposed = $(0.20 - 1 + 0.83)/(0.85 + 0.83 - 1) = 0.044$
and proportion unexposed = $1 - 0.055 = 0.956$

Hence: estimated 'true' values for proportions exposed:

	Cases	Controls
Exposed	0.286	0.044
Unexposed	0.714	0.956
Total	1	1

Estimated true odds ratio = $(0.286 \times 0.956)/(0.044 \times 0.714) = 8.67$

TABLE A2.12: Meta-analysis: Mantel–Haenszel and Peto methods

FORMULAE

1. *Format for each study is the same as given in Table A2.2*

	Success	Failure	Total
Treated	a	b	N_1
Control	c	d	N_0
	M_1	M_0	T

For each study i,

observed number of successes on new treatment $= a_i$

expected number $E_i = N_{1i}M_{1i}/T_i$

variance of a_i

$$V_i = \frac{N_{1i}N_{0i}M_{1i}M_{0i}}{T_i^2(T_i-1)}$$

as in Table A2.2.

For meta-analysis of a number of studies, a format of one line per study is useful.

2. *Mantel–Haenszel method*

	Observed successes	Expected	Variance	ad/T	bc/T	Odds ratio
Each study	a_i	E_i	V_i	a_id_i/T_i	b_ic_i/T_i	a_id_i/b_ic_i
Summation overall studies	$\sum_i a_i$	$\sum_i E_i$	$\sum_i V_i$	$\sum_i a_id_i/T_i$	$\sum_i b_ic_i/T_i$	

2A. Summary results: summary odds ratio $= \dfrac{\sum_i a_id_i/T_i}{\sum_i b_ic_i/T_i}$

2B. χ statistic $= \dfrac{\sum a_i - \sum E_i}{\sqrt{\sum V_i}}$

WORKED EXAMPLE

1. *Format of table*

Data from three randomized trials assessing clomiphene in inducing ovulation [20]

Study	Treated group:		Control group:		Total
	Success	Fail	Success	Fail	
	a	*b*	*c*	*d*	*T*
1	20	4	8	14	46
2	16	6	5	14	41
3	35	30	7	58	130

2. *Mantel–Haenszel method*

Study	*a* = obs	E	V	ad/T	bc/T	ORi
1	20	14.6087	2.7947	6.0870	0.6957	8.75
2	16	11.2683	2.6109	5.4634	0.7317	7.47
3	35	21.0000	7.1628	15.6154	1.6154	9.67
Sum:	71	46.8770	12.5684	27.1658	3.0427	

2A. Summary odds ratio: $OR_S = sum(ad/T)/sum(bc/T) = 8.93$

2B. Chi statistic $Chi = (sum\ a - sum\ E)/sum\ \sqrt{V} = 6.80$

Chi sq $= \chi2 = 46.30$

TABLE A2.12: FORMULAE (*continued*)

2C. *Confidence limits for summary odds ratio*

Precise limits given using the Robins et al. [1] formula for the variance of the ln summary odds ratio, given in Table A2.1, 5D

$y\%$ limits for summary $OR = \exp\left[\ln OR_s \pm Z_y.\sqrt{\text{var}}\right]$

2D. *Test for heterogeneity*

For each study calculate $Q_i = w_i(\ln OR_i - \ln OR_s)^2$

where w_i = weight = 1/variance of ln OR_i, from Table A2.1.

ln OR_i = ln OR for study i

ln OR_s = ln summary OR

then $\sum_i Q_i$ is distributed as a χ^2 statistic on $n-1$ degrees of freedom, where n = number of studies.

3. *Peto method*

	Ob-served successes	Expected	Variance	obs-exp.	ln(odds ratio)	Odds ratio
Each study	a_i	E_i	V_i	$a_i - E_i$	$(a_i - E_i)/V_i$	$\exp(a_i - E_i)/V_i$
Summa-tion overall studies	$\sum_i a_i$	$\sum_i E_i$	$\sum_i V_i$	$\sum_i (a_i - E_i)$		

3A. Summary ln odds ratio $= \dfrac{\sum_i (a_i - E_i)}{\sum_i V_i}$

Summary odds ratio $= \exp\left[\dfrac{\sum_i (a_i - E_i)}{\sum_i V_i}\right]$

3B. Summary χ (normal deviate) $= \dfrac{\sum_i (a_i - E_i)}{\sqrt{\sum_i V_i}}$

3C. *Confidence limits for summary odds ratio* $= \exp\left[\ln OR_s \pm Z_\alpha \Big/ \sqrt{\sum_i V_i}\right]$

where Z_α is the normal deviate for the significance level α, from Table A2.9.

TABLE A2.12: WORKED EXAMPLE (*continued*)

2C. *Confidence limits for* OR_s $\ln OR_s = 2.1892$

variance of $\ln OR_S$ from Robins et al. [1] formula: 0.1173

95 per cent confidence limits using this variance 4.56, 17.47

2D. Test of heterogeneity

Study	ln OR	var ln OR	w_i	Q_i
1	2.1691	0.4964	2.0144	0.0008
2	2.0104	0.5006	1.9976	0.0638
3	2.2687	0.2220	4.5044	0.0285
Sum				0.0931

Sum Q_i is a χ^2 on two degrees of freedom: clearly non-significant

3. *Peto method*

Study	a = obs	E	V	a – E	ln OR_i	OR_i
1	20	14.6087	2.7947	5.3913	1.9291	6.88
2	16	11.2683	2.6109	4.7317	1.8123	6.12
3	35	21.0000	7.1628	14.0000	1.9545	7.06
Sum:	71	46.8770	12.5684	24.1230		

3A. Summary odds ratio

$\ln OR_s = \text{sum}(a - E)/\text{sum } V = 1.92$

$OR_s = \exp(\ln OR_s) = 6.82$

3B. Normal deviate

normal deviate $= \text{sum}(a - E)/\text{sum}\sqrt{V} = 6.80$

3C. *Confidence limits for summary odds ratio*

95 per cent limits for $OR = 3.92, 11.85$

TABLE A2.12: FORMULAE (*continued*)

3D. *Test of heterogeneity*

For each study V_i and $a_i - E_i$ have been defined as in 3 above, and $(a_i - E_i)^2$ is also calculated. The heterogeneity statistic Q is calculated as

$$Q = \sum_i \frac{(a_i - E_i)^2}{V_i} - \frac{\left[\sum_i (a_i - E_i)\right]^2}{\sum V_i}$$

Q is distributed as a χ^2 statistic on $n - 1$ degrees of freedom,

where n = number of studies.

As $\sum a_i - \sum E_i = \sum_i (a_i - E_i)$, the statistics produced by these two methods are the same. The odds ratio estimates are different.

Sources

Source: Mantel N and Haenszel W, 'Statistical aspects of the analysis of data from retrospective studies of disease,' *Journal of the National Cancer Institute*, Volume 22, Issue 4, pp. 719–748, Copyright © 1959 Oxford University Press [2]; Peto R et al., 'Design and analysis of randomized clinical trials requiring prolonged observation of each patient. II. Analysis and examples,' *British Journal of Cancer,* Volume 35, Issue 1, pp. 1–39, Copyright © 1977 Cancer Research UK [21]; and Petitti DB, *Meta-Analysis, Decision Analysis, and Cost-Effectiveness Analysis. Methods for Quantitative Synthesis in Medicine, Second Edition,* Oxford University Press, New York, USA, Copyright © 2000 [22].

TABLE A2.12: WORKED EXAMPLE (*continued*)

3D. *Test for heterogeneity*

Study	$(a - E)^2/V$
1	10.4004
2	8.5751
3	27.3636
Sum:	46.3391

Heterogeneity $\chi^2 = 46.339 - [(24.12)^2/12.57] = 0.04$

TABLE A2.13 Meta-analysis: confidence limits method

FORMULAE

1. *Data required*

   The information required from each study is an appropriate measure of odds ratio *, OR, and its variance, V, which can be calculated if the lower and upper confidence limits OR_L and OR_u are given, as

   $$V = \left(\frac{\ln (OR_u / OR)}{Z} \right)^2 = \left(\frac{\ln (OR / OR_L)}{Z} \right)^2$$

   where Z corresponds to the significance level: e.g. for 95 per cent two-sided confidence limits, $Z = 1.96$ (Table A2.9).

   Then, for each study, the weight w is $1/V$

	Odds ratio	Variance	Weight	wt. ln OR	Heterogeneity
Each study	OR_i	Vi	$w_i = 1/V_i$	$w_i \ln OR_i$	$Q_i = w_i(\ln OR_i - \ln OR_s)^2$
Summation over all studies			$\sum_i w_i$	$\sum_i (w_i \ln OR_i)$	$\sum_i Q_i$

2. *Calculation of summary odds ratio*

   $$\text{Summary } \ln OR_s = \frac{\sum_i (w_i \ln OR_i)}{\sum_i w_i}$$

   hence, $OR_s = \exp(\ln OR_s)$

3. *Confidence limits for the summary odds ratio*

   $$\text{variance of } \ln OR_s = V_s = \frac{1}{\sum_i w_i}$$

   95 per cent confidence limits for $\ln OR_s = \ln OR_s \pm 1.96\sqrt{V_s} = \ln OR_s \pm 1.96 / \sqrt{\sum_i w_i}$

   95 per cent confidence limits for $OR_s = \exp \left(\ln OR_s \pm 1.96 / \sqrt{\sum_i w_i} \right)$

WORKED EXAMPLE

1. Meta-analysis of seven case–control studies relating sunburn to melanoma.

Study i	Odds ratio OR_i	95% CL lower	95% CL upper	Variance v_i	Weight w_i w_i	ln OR_i	Hetero-geneity Q_i
1	1.30	0.90	1.80	0.03	31.86	8.36	4.39
2	1.20	0.60	2.30	0.12	8.50	1.55	1.73
3	3.70	2.30	6.10	0.06	16.14	21.12	7.35
4	2.40	0.80	7.30	0.32	3.14	2.75	0.18
5	6.50	3.40	12.30	0.11	9.29	17.40	14.25
6	1.49	0.97	2.32	0.05	20.20	8.06	1.11
7	1.60	1.00	2.60	0.06	16.83	7.91	0.45
Summation					105.97	67.14	29.47

2. Summary ln $OR_S = 67.14/105.97 = 0.63$
Summary $OR_S = \exp(0.63) = 1.88$

3. 95 per cent CL for summary $OR_s = \exp\left(0.63 \pm 1.96/\sqrt{105.97}\right) = \text{lower} \, 1.56$

upper 2.28

TABLE A2.13: FORMULAE (*continued*)

4.　　　*Heterogeneity test*

Heterogeneity statistic $= \sum_i Q_i = Q \quad I^2 = [Q-(n-1)]/Q$

which is a χ^2 statistic on $n-1$ degrees of freedom, where n = number of studies

---

*Note: This method is applicable to relative risk also, and (without the log transformation) to risk difference

Sources

Source: Prentice RL and Thomas DB., 'On the epidemiology of oral contraceptives and disease,' p. 285–401, in Klein G, and Weinhouse S (Eds.), *Advances in Cancer Research*, Volume 49, Academic Press, Orlando, Florida, USA, Copyright © 1987 [23]; and Greenland S, 'Quantitative methods in the review of epidemiologic literature', *Epidemiologic Reviews*, Volume 9, Issue 1, pp. 1–30, Copyright © 1987 by The Johns Hopkins University School of Hygiene and Public Health [24].

TABLE A2.13: WORKED EXAMPLE (*continued*)

4. Test for heterogeneity: sum $Q_i = 29.47$

Sum Q is a χ^2 statistic on $n - 1 =$ six degrees of freedom; from Table A2.1 $P < 0.0001$, so consideration has to be given to the results which are discordant, as shown by their Q_i results.

$I^2 = (29.47-6)/29.47 = 0.80$

$= 80$ per cent

TABLE A2.14: Random effects model (DerSimonian–Laird) applied to confidence limits data

FORMULAE

1.   The random effects model of DerSimonian and Laird uses the same data as the fixed effects model shown in Table A2.13. For each study, the odds ratios OR_i, and their variances v_i are as in Table A2.13.

Weights $w_i = 1/v_i$ are calculated. The fixed effects summary odds ratio OR_s is calculated as before, and the quantities $Q_i = w_i(\ln OR_i - \ln OR_s)^2$ and sum $Q_i = Q$

2, 3.   For the random effects model, revised weights dw_i are used where

$$dw_i = \frac{1}{(D + w_i)}$$

$$D = \frac{(Q - n - 1) \times \text{sum } w_i}{(\text{sum } w_i)^2 - \text{sum}(w_i^2)}$$

where n is the number of studies.

D cannot be negative. If $(n-1)$ is greater than Q, then $D = 0$.

If there is little heterogeneity, Q will be small, so D will be small, and the DerSimonian and Laird weights will be similar to the fixed effects weights.

WORKED EXAMPLE

1. Data as in Table A2.13: seven studies relating sunburn to melanoma

Fixed effects model (as in Table A2.13)						Random effects model			
Odds ratio and 95%limits			Variance	Weight		Heterog.		DL weight	
Study	OR	Lower Upper	v	w	w^2	$w \ln RR$	Q	DL w	DL $w \ln OR$
1	1.30	0.90 1.80	0.03	31.86	1015.34	8.36	4.39	3.55	0.93
2	1.20	0.60 2.30	0.12	8.50	72.28	1.55	1.73	2.72	0.50
3	3.70	2.30 6.10	0.06	16.14	260.56	21.12	7.35	3.20	4.19
4	2.40	0.80 7.30	0.32	3.14	9.88	2.75	0.18	1.76	1.54
5	6.50	3.40 12.30	0.11	9.29	86.37	17.40	14.25	2.80	5.23
6	1.49	0.97 2.32	0.05	20.20	408.15	8.06	1.11	3.34	1.33
7	1.60	1.00 2.60	0.06	16.83	283.12	7.91	0.45	3.23	1.52
Summations				105.97	2135.70	67.14	29.47	20.597	15.241

2. **Fixed effects model:**

As in Table A2.13:

Summary odds ratio	**1.88**	
$\ln OR_s$	0.634	
Variance of $\ln OR_s = 1/(\text{sum } w) =$	0.0094	
95 per cent C.I. For summary OR	1.56	2.28
Heterogeneity test $Q =$	29.47	
Degrees of freedom, P-value	6	0.00005
$I^2 = 79.60$ per cent		

3. **Random effects model:**

Number of studies (k)		7
$Q = 29.47$		
$D = ((29.47 - 6) \times 105.97) / (105.972 - 2135.70) =$		0.2502
DL summary odds ratio		**2.10**
$\ln OR_s$		0.740
Variance of $\ln OR_s = 1/(\text{sum } w) =$		0.0486
95 per cent C.I. for summary OR	1.36	3.23

TABLE A2.14: FORMULAE (*continued*)

4.	The percentage distribution of weights is shown, showing how the D–L method gives a more even weight distribution than the fixed effects method.

Sources

Source: DerSimonian R and Laird N, 'Meta-analysis in clinical trials,' *Control Clinical Trials*, Volume 7, Issue 3, pp. 177–188, Copyright © 1986Published by Elsevier Inc [25].

TABLE A2.14: WORKED EXAMPLE (*continued*)

4.   Weight distribution

	Weight%	
Study	**Fixed**	**Random**
1	30.1	17.2
2	19.1	16.2
3	15.9	15.74
4	15.2	15.6
5	8.8	13.6
6	8.0	13.2
7	3.0	8.5
Sum	100.0	100.0

TABLE A2.15: Table of probabilities (*P*-values) and corresponding values of χ^2 on 1 d.f., standardized normal deviate 2-sided, and 1-sided

P-values	χ^2 1 d.f.	Normal deviate 2-sided	Normal deviate 1-sided
0.000001	23.9	4.89	4.75
0.00001	19.51	4.42	4.27
0.0001	15.14	3.89	3.72
0.001	**10.83**	**3.29**	**3.09**
0.01	**6.63**	**2.58**	**2.33**
0.02	5.41	2.33	2.05
0.03	4.71	2.17	1.88
0.04	4.22	2.05	1.75
0.05	**3.84**	**1.96**	**1.64**
0.06	3.54	1.88	1.55
0.07	3.28	1.81	1.48
0.08	3.06	1.75	1.41
0.09	2.87	1.70	1.34
0.10	**2.71**	**1.64**	**1.28**
0.11	2.55	1.60	1.23
0.12	2.42	1.55	1.18
0.13	2.29	1.51	1.13
0.14	2.18	1.48	1.08
0.15	2.07	1.44	1.04
0.16	1.97	1.41	0.99
0.17	1.88	1.37	0.95
0.18	1.80	1.34	0.92
0.19	1.72	1.31	0.88
0.20	**1.64**	**1.28**	**0.84**
0.25	1.32	1.15	0.68
0.3	1.07	1.04	0.52
0.35	0.87	0.93	0.39
0.4	0.71	0.84	0.25
0.45	0.57	0.76	0.13
0.5	0.45	0.67	0.0
0.6	0.27	0.52	
0.7	0.15	0.39	
0.8	0.06	0.25	
0.9	0.02	0.13	

The values tabulated

1. *The chi-square χ^2 statistic on one degree of freedom. For any other number of degrees of freedom, use Table A2.16.*

The table gives the probability of the given χ^2 or a larger value under the null hypothesis.

Although this is a one-tail probability on a χ^2 distribution, because the χ^2 distribution is given by a normal deviate squared, this gives a two-sided test; assessing a variable x^2 using a χ^2 distribution is equivalent to assessing x using a normal distribution and a two-sided test.

2. *The standardized normal deviate (often called Z or chi) using a two-sided test.*

The probability given is that of the given value $\pm Z$ or a more extreme value of either sign, under the null hypothesis.

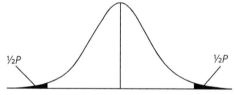

3. *The standardized normal deviate (often called Z or chi), using a one-sided test.*

The probability given is that of the given value Z or a more extreme value of the same sign.

Relationships between these

1. For a given value of P, the corresponding $\chi^2_{(1)}$ value is equal to the two-sided standardized normal deviate squared.

    e.g. for $P = 0.05$ $\chi^2 = 3.84$ $Z = 1.96 = \sqrt{3.84}$

2. For a given normal deviate, the two-sided probability is twice the one-sided.
    e.g. for $Z = 1.96$, two-sided probability $= 0.05$, one-sided $= 0.025$

TABLE A2.16: Functions in Microsoft Excel spreadsheets to convert between test statistics and probability (*P*) values

To get from	to:	Function	Example			
Z-statistic	P-value, 2-sided	=2*(1-normsdist(z))	Z-stat	1.96	P-value	0.049996
			Z-stat	3	P-value	0.002700
			Z-stat	4.89	P-value	0.000001
Z-statistic	P-value, 1-sided	=(1-normsdist(z))	Z-stat	1.96	P-value	0.024998
			Z-stat	1.64	P-value	0.050503
			Z-stat	4.75	P-value	0.000001
P-value, 2-sided	Z-statistic	=abs(normsinv(P/2))	P-value	0.05	Z-stat	1.96
			P-value	0.001	Z-stat	3.29
			P-value	0.1	Z-stat	1.64
P-value, 1-sided	Z-statistic	=abs(normsinv(P))	P-value	0.05	Z-stat	1.64
			P-value	0.1	Z-stat	1.28
			P-value	0.01	Z-stat	2.33
Chi-squared stat, df	P-value	=chidist(chi, df)	Chi stat, df	3.84	1	P-value	0.050044
			Chi stat, df	10.3	3	P-value	0.016181
			Chi stat, df	38.932	21	P-value	0.010000
P-value, df	Chi-sq	=chiinv(P,df)	P-value, df	0.01	1	Chi-sq	6.63
			P-value, df	0.2	1	Chi-sq	1.64
			P-value, df	0.05	30	Chi-sq	43.77
t-test result, df	P-value	=tdist(test, df, tails)	t-test, df, tails	4	1	P-value	0.077979
			t-test, df, tails	4	1	2	P-value	0.155958
			t-test, df, tails	1.96	160	2	P-value	0.051733

How to use Table A2.15

1.   Be sure you know which statistic you wish to use!

2.   To find the value of a statistic corresponding to a given P-value: look down the table to find the P-value or the nearest to it; read off the corresponding statistic.

Examples: What $\chi^2_{(1)}$ value corresponds to $P = 0.05$? Result: 3.84 What one-sided deviate corresponds to $P = 0.01$? Result: 2.33

3.   To find the P-value corresponding to a given statistic:
Find the correct column.
Look down the table to find the given value or the nearest to it; read off the corresponding P-value.
Examples: What P-value corresponds to $\chi^2_{(1)} = 7.4$? Result between 0.001 and 0.01; can be written $0.001 < P < 0.01$. What P-value corresponds to a one-sided test giving a deviate of 1.04? Result: 0.15.

References

1. **Robins JM, Breslow NE, Greenland S**. Estimation of the Mantel–Haenszel variance consistent with both sparse-data and large-strata limiting models. *Biometrics* 1986; **42**:311–323.
2. **Mantel N, Haenszel W**. Statistical aspects of the analysis of data from retrospective studies of disease. *J Natl Cancer Inst* 1959; **22**:719–748.
3. **Wolff B**. On estimating the relationship between blood group and disease. *Ann Hum Genet* 1955; **19**:251–253.
4. **Rothman KJ, Greenland S**. *Modern Epidemiology*, 3rd edn. Philadelphia, PA: Wolters Kluwer Lippincott; 2008.
5. **Shapiro S, Slone D, Hartz SC, et al**. Anticonvulsants and parental epilepsy in the development of birth defects. *Lancet* 1976; **i**:272–275
6. **Breslow NE, Day NE**. *Statistical Methods in Cancer Research. Volume 1: The Analysis of Case-Control Studies*. Lyon: IARC Scientific Publication No 32; 1980.
7. **Armitage P, Berry G, Matthews JNS**. *Statistical Methods in Medical Research*, 4th edn. Oxford: Blackwell Scientific; 2002.
8. **Saral R, Burns WH, Laskin OL, Santos GW, Lietman PS**. Acyclovir prophylaxis of herpes-simplex-virus infections: a randomized, double-blind, controlled trial in bone-marrow-transplant recipients. *N Engl J Med* 1981; **305**:63–67.
9. **McNemar Q**. Note on the sampling of the difference between corrected proportions or percentages. *Psychometrika* 1947; **12**:153–157.
10. **Collette HJA, Day NE, Rombach JJ, de Waard F**. Evaluation of screening for breast cancer in a non-randomised study (the DOM project) by means of a case-control study. *Lancet* 1984; **1**:1224–1226.
11. **Elwood JM**. Maternal and environmental factors affecting twin births in Canadian cities. *Br J Obstet Gynaecol* 1978; **85**:351–358.
12. **Armitage P**. Test for linear trend in proportions and frequencies. *Biometrics* 1955; **11**:375–386.
13. **Mantel N**. Chi-square tests with one degree of freedom; extensions of the Mantel–Haenszel procedure. *Am Stat Assoc J* 1963; **58**:690–700.
14. **Westerdahl J, Anderson H, Olsson H, Ingvar C**. Reproducibility of a self-administered questionnaire for assessment of melanoma risk. *Int J Epidemiol* 1996; **25**(2):245–251.

15. **Cohen J**. A coefficient of agreement for nominal scales. *Educ Psychol Meas* 1960; **20**:27–46.

16. **Fleiss JL, Cohen J, Everitt BS**. Large sample standard errors of kappa and weighted kappa. *Psychol Bull* 1969; **72**:323–327.

17. **Fleiss JL, Levin B, Paik MC**. *Statistical Methods for Rates and Proportions*, 3rd ed. New York: John Wiley & Sons; 2003.

18. **Thompson WD, Walter SD**. Variance and dissent. A reappraisal of the kappa coefficient. *J Clin Epidemiol* 1988; **41**:949–958.

19. **Armstrong BK, White E, Saracci R**. *Principles of Exposure Measurement in Epidemiology*. Oxford: Oxford University Press; 1992.

20. **Hughes E, Collins, J.**, Vandekerckhove, P. Clomiphene citrate vs. placebo for ovulation induction in oligo-amenorrhoeic women. *Cochrane Database Syst Rev* 1995; **2** (CD-ROM). [This review has since been updated.]

21. **Peto R, Pike MC, Armitage P, Breslow NE, Cox DR, Howard SV, et al**. Design and analysis of randomized clinical trials requiring prolonged observation of each patient. II. Analysis and examples. *Br J Cancer* 1977; **35**(1):1–39.

22. **Petitti DB**. *Meta-Analysis, Decision Analysis, and Cost-Effectiveness Analysis. Methods for Quantitative Synthesis in Medicine*, 2nd edn. New York: Oxford University Press; 2000.

23. **Prentice RL, Thomas DB**. On the epidemiology of oral contraceptives and disease. In: Klein G, Weinhouse S (Eds) *Advances in Cancer Research, Volume 49*. Orlando, FL: Academic Press; 1987:285–401.

24. **Greenland S**. Quantitative methods in the review of epidemiologic literature. *Epidemiol Rev* 1987; **9**:1–30.

25. **DerSimonian R, Laird N**. Meta-analysis in clinical trials. *Control Clin Trials* 1986; **7**:177–188.

Index